**Workbook
to
Accompany**

Diversified Health Occupations 5th EDITION

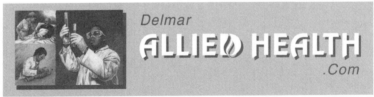

**Workbook
to
Accompany**

Diversified Health Occupations 5th EDITION

Louise Simmers, M.Ed., R.N.

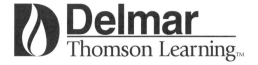

Africa • Australia • Canada • Denmark • Japan • Mexico • New Zealand • Philippines
Puerto Rico • Singapore • Spain • United Kingdom • United States

NOTICE TO THE READER

Delmar Staff

Business Unit Director: William Brottmiller
Acquisitions Editor: Doris Smith
Development Editor: Marah E. Bellegarde
Executive Marketing Manager: Dawn Gerrain

Project Editor: Stacey Prus
Production Coordinator: Barbara A. Bullock
Production Editor: Mary Colleen Liburdi
Cover Design: TDB Publishing Services

Asia:
Thomson Learning
60 Albert Street, #15-01
Albert Complex
Singapore 189969
Tel: 65 336 6411
Fax: 65 336 7411

Japan:
Thomson Learning
Palaceside Building 5F
I - I - I Hitotsubashi, Chiyoda-ku
Tokyo 100 0003 Japan
Tel: 813 5218 6544
Fax: 813 5218 6551

Australia/New Zealand:
Nelson/Thomson Learning
102 Dodds Street
South Melbourne, Victoria 3205
Australia
Tel: 61 39685 4111
Fax: 61 39 685 4199

UK/Europe/Middle East
Thomson Learning
Berkshire House
168-173 High Holborn
London
WC IV 7AA United Kingdom
Tel: 44 171497 1422
Fax: 44 171497 1426

Thomas Nelson & Sons LTD
Nelson House
Mayfield Road
Walton-on-Thames
KT 12 5PL United Kingdom
Tel: 44 1932 2522111
Fax: 44 1932 246574

Latin America:
Thomson Learning
Seneca, 53
Colonia Polanco
11560 Mexico D.F. Mexico
Tel: 525-281-2906
Fax: 525-281-2656

Canada:
Nelson/Thomson Learning
1120 Birchmount Road
Scarborough, Ontario
Canada MIK 5G4
Tel: 416-752-9100
Fax: 416-752-8102

Spain:
Thomson Learning
Calle Magallanes, 25
28015-Madrid
España
Tel: 34 91446 33 50
Fax: 34 91445 62 18

International Headquarters:
Thomson Learning
International Division
290 Harbor Drive, 2nd Floor
Stamford, CT 06902-7477
Tel: 203-969-8700
Fax: 203-969-8751

ISBN-13: 978-0-7668-1822–4
ISBN-10: 0-7668-1822–5
Library of Congress Cataloging-in-Publication Data 99–058899

CONTENTS

TO THE STUDENT

Two different types of worksheets are provided in this workbook: assignment sheets and evaluation sheets. These sheets are designed to correlate with specific information and procedures discussed in the textbook, *Diversified Health Occupations, 5th Edition.*

The assignment sheets are designed to allow you to review the main facts/information about a procedure. After you read the information about a specific procedure in the textbook, try to answer the questions on the corresponding assignment sheet. Refer to the information in the text to obtain the correct answers to the questions or statements. Then check the information to be sure your answers are correct. Let your instructor grade the completed assignment sheet. Note any points that are not correct. Be sure you understand these points before you perform the procedure. This will provide you with the basic knowledge or facts necessary before a procedure is done.

The evaluation sheets are designed to set criteria or standards that should be observed while a specific procedure is being performed. They follow the steps of the procedure as listed on the procedure sections in the textbook. As you practice each procedure, use the specific evaluation sheet to judge your performance. When you feel you have mastered a particular procedure, sign the evaluation sheet and give it to your instructor. The instructor will use this sheet to grade you on your performance.

The format of the evaluation sheet is designed to provide for both practice and the final evaluation of the procedure. The appearance of the evaluation sheet and the meaning of each of the abbreviations and parts is as follows:

DHO Evaluation Sheet

Name _____ Date _____

Evaluated by _____

DIRECTIONS:

		PROFICIENT				
Name of Procedure	Points Possible	Peer Check Yes No	Final Check* Yes No	Points Earned**	Comments	

Name: Sign your name in this area.

Date: The date you are given your final evaluation can be placed in this area.

Evaluated by: The person who is evaluating you (usually the instructor) on your final check of this procedure will sign his/her name in this area.

Directions: Basic directions for using the sheet are provided in this area.

Name of Procedure: The specific name of the procedure will be noted in this area.

Points Possible: A number will appear in this column—beside each step of the procedure. The number represents the points you will receive if you do this step of the procedure correctly.

Peer Check: These columns are used for practice when your peer (another student) watches as you perform the procedure. If you complete the step correctly, the peer (student) should check the "Yes" column. If you omit a step, or do not complete it correctly, the peer (student) should check the "No" column. After you complete the procedure, you can use this checklist as an indication of steps completed correctly and those needing additional practice.

Final Check: These columns will be used by the person (usually the instructor) doing your final check or evaluation on the procedure. Two columns are provided, one labeled "Yes" and one labeled "No." If you perform a step of the procedure correctly, the evaluator will place a check in the "Yes" column. If you do not perform a step of the procedure, or perform a step incorrectly, the evaluator will place a check in the "No" column.

Points Earned: In this column the evaluator will give you the correct number of points (as stated in the "Points Possible" column) for each step of the procedure on which you received a check in the "Yes" column. You will not receive the points for a particular step if you received a check in the "No" column. The number of points earned can then be totaled. A grade can be assigned by a scale determined by your instructor.

Comments: This column is for comments regarding your performance of the procedure. Any check in the "No" column should be explained by a brief explanation opposite the step in which the error occurred. In addition, positive comments on your performance of the procedure should be noted in this area.

As you can see, the evaluation sheet provides you with an opportunity to actually practice your performance test on a particular procedure before you have to take the final performance evaluation. By utilizing this sheet, you will achieve higher standards of performance and learn to master all steps of each procedure.

The sheets in this book follow the same order of procedures/skills found in the textbook. Each information section in the textbook refers you to a specific assignment sheet in the workbook. Each procedure section in the textbook refers you to a specific evaluation sheet in the workbook. By following the directions in the textbook and the directions on each of the sheets in this workbook, you can master the procedures/skills and become a competent health worker.

Matrix of Skills Used in Health Occupations
&
Correlation to National Health Care Skill Standards

x

Matrix of Skills Used in Health Occupations

SKILLS	CLINICAL LABORATORY SERVICES	DENTISTRY	DIETETICS AND NUTRITION	EDUCATION	HEALTH INFORMATION AND COMMUNICATION	HEALTH SERVICES ADMINISTRATION	MEDICINE	MENTAL, PHYSICAL, SOCIAL SPECIALTIES	NURSING	PHARMACY	PODIATRY	SCIENCE AND ENGINEERING	TECHNICAL INSTRUMENTATION	VETERINARY MEDICINE	VISION CARE
Unit 1: Health Care Systems															
Health care facilities	X	X	X	X	X	X	X	X	X	X	X	X	X	X	X
Government agencies	X	X	X	X	X	X	X	X	X	X	X	X	X	X	X
Nonprofit agencies	X	X	X	X	X	X	X	X	X	X	X	X	X	X	X
Health insurance plans	X	X	X	X	X	X	X	X	X	X	X	X	X	X	X
Organizational structure	X	X	X	X	X	X	X	X	X	X	X	X	X	X	X
History of health care	X	X	X	X	X	X	X	X	X	X	X	X	X	X	X
Trends in health care	X	X	X	X	X	X	X	X	X	X	X	X	X	X	X
Unit 2: Careers in Health Care															
Introduction to Health Careers	X	X	X	X	X	X	X	X	X	X	X	X	X	X	X
Dental careers		X		X	X										
Diagnostic services	X	X	X	X	X	X	X	X	X	X	X	X	X	X	X
Emergency medical services	X	X	X	X	X	X	X	X	X	X	X	X	X	X	X
Health information and communication services	X	X	X	X	X	X	X	X	X	X	X	X	X	X	X
Hospital/health care facility services	X		X	X	X	X	X	X	X	X	X				
Medical careers				X		X	X		X		X				X
Mental and social services				X	X	X	X	X	X						
Mortuary careers				X	X	X	X	X	X						
Nursing careers				X	X	X	X	X	X		X				
Nutrition and dietary services		X	X	X	X	X	X	X	X						
Therapeutic services	X	X	X	X	X	X	X	X	X	X	X	X	X	X	X
Veterinary careers				X	X									X	
Vision services				X	X	X	X	X	X	X			X		X
Unit 3: Personal Qualities of a Health Care Worker															
Personal characteristics	X	X	X	X	X	X	X	X	X	X	X	X	X	X	X
Personal appearance	X	X	X	X	X	X	X	X	X	X	X	X	X	X	X
Unit 4: Legal and Ethical Responsibilities															
Legal responsibilities	X	X	X	X	X	X	X	X	X	X	X	X	X	X	X
Ethics	X	X	X	X	X	X	X	X	X	X	X	X	X	X	X
Patient's rights	X	X	X	X	X	X	X	X	X	X	X	X	X	X	X
Advance directives for health care	X	X	X	X	X	X	X	X	X	X	X	X	X	X	X
Professional standards	X	X	X	X	X	X	X	X	X	X	X	X	X	X	X

Matrix of Skills Used in Health Occupations

SKILLS	CLINICAL LABORATORY SERVICES	DENTISTRY	DIETETICS AND NUTRITION	EDUCATION	HEALTH INFORMATION AND COMMUNICATION	HEALTH SERVICES ADMINISTRATION	MEDICINE	MENTAL, PHYSICAL, SOCIAL SPECIALTIES	NURSING	PHARMACY	PODIATRY	SCIENCE AND ENGINEERING	TECHNICAL INSTRUMENTATION	VETERINARY MEDICINE	VISION CARE
Unit 5: Medical Terminology															
Using medical abbreviations	X	X	X	X	X	X	X	X	X	X	X	X	X	X	X
Interpreting word parts	X	X	X	X	X	X	X	X	X	X	X	X	X	X	X
Unit 6: Anatomy and Physiology															
Basic structure of the human body	X	X	X	X	X	X	X	X	X	X	X	X	X	X	X
Body planes, directions, and cavities	X	X	X	X	X	X	X	X	X	X	X	X	X	X	X
Integumentary system	X	X	X	X	X	X	X	X	X	X	X	X	X	X	X
Skeletal system	X	X	X	X	X	X	X	X	X	X	X	X	X	X	X
Muscular system	X	X	X	X	X	X	X	X	X	X	X	X	X	X	X
Nervous system	X	X	X	X	X	X	X	X	X	X	X	X	X	X	X
Special senses	X	X	X	X	X	X	X	X	X	X	X	X	X	X	X
Circulatory system	X	X	X	X	X	X	X	X	X	X	X	X	X	X	X
Lymphatic system	X	X	X	X	X	X	X	X	X	X	X	X	X	X	X
Respiratory system	X	X	X	X	X	X	X	X	X	X	X	X	X	X	X
Digestive system	X	X	X	X	X	X	X	X	X	X	X	X	X	X	X
Urinary system	X	X	X	X	X	X	X	X	X	X	X	X	X	X	X
Endocrine system	X	X	X	X	X	X	X	X	X	X	X	X	X	X	X
Reproductive system	X	X	X	X	X	X	X	X	X	X	X	X	X	X	X
Unit 7: Human Growth and Development															
Life stages		X	X	X	X		X	X	X	X					X
Death and dying			X	X	X	X	X	X				X	X	X	
Human needs	X	X	X	X	X	X	X	X	X	X	X	X	X	X	X
Effective communication	X	X	X	X	X	X	X	X	X	X	X	X	X	X	X
Unit 8: Cultural Diversity															
Culture, ethnicity, and race	X	X	X	X	X	X	X	X	X	X	X	X	X	X	X
Bias, prejudice, and stereotyping	X	X	X	X	X	X	X	X	X	X	X	X	X	X	X
Understanding cultural diversity	X	X	X	X	X	X	X	X	X	X	X	X	X	X	X
Respecting cultural diversity	X	X	X	X	X	X	X	X	X	X	X	X	X	X	X
Unit 9: Geriatric Care															
Myths on aging	X	X	X	X	X	X	X	X	X	X	X		X	X	X
Physical changes of aging	X	X	X	X	X	X	X	X	X	X	X		X	X	X
Psychosocial changes of aging	X	X	X	X	X	X	X	X	X	X	X		X	X	X
Confusion and disorientation in the elderly	X	X	X	X	X	X	X	X	X	X	X		X	X	X
Meeting the needs of the elderly	X	X	X	X	X	X	X	X	X	X	X		X	X	X

Matrix of Skills Used in Health Occupations

SKILLS	CLINICAL LABORATORY SERVICES	DENTISTRY	DIETETICS AND NUTRITION	EDUCATION	HEALTH INFORMATION AND COMMUNICATION	HEALTH SERVICES ADMINISTRATION	MEDICINE	MENTAL, PHYSICAL, SOCIAL SPECIALTIES	NURSING	PHARMACY	PODIATRY	SCIENCE AND ENGINEERING	TECHNICAL INSTRUMENTATION	VETERINARY MEDICINE	VISION CARE
Unit 10: Nutrition and Diets															
Fundamentals of nutrition	X	X	X	X	X	X	X	X	X	X	X	X	X	X	X
Essential nutrients	X	X	X	X	X	X	X	X	X	X	X	X	X	X	X
Utilization of nutrients	X	X	X	X	X	X	X	X	X	X	X	X	X	X	X
Maintenance of good nutrition	X	X	X	X	X	X	X	X	X	X	X	X	X	X	X
Therapeutic diets		X	X	X			X	X	X					X	
Unit 11: Computers in Health Care															
Introduction to computers	X	X	X	X	X	X	X	X	X	X	X	X	X	X	X
What is a computer system?	X	X	X	X	X	X	X	X	X	X	X	X	X	X	X
Computer applications	X	X	X	X	X	X	X	X	X	X	X	X	X	X	X
Unit 12: Promotion of Safety															
Using body mechanics	X	X	X	X	X	X	X	X	X	X	X	X	X	X	X
Preventing accidents and injuries	X	X	X	X	X	X	X	X	X	X	X	X	X	X	X
Observing fire safety	X	X	X	X	X	X	X	X	X	X	X	X	X	X	X
Unit 13: Infection Control															
Understanding the principles of infection control	X	X	X	X	X	X	X	X	X	X	X	X	X	X	X
Washing hands	X	X	X	X	X	X	X	X	X	X	X	X	X	X	X
Observing standard precautions	X	X	X	X	X		X	X	X	X	X	X	X	X	X
Sterilizing with an autoclave	X	X	X	X		X	X	X	X	X	X	X	X	X	X
Using chemicals for disinfection	X	X	X	X		X	X	X	X	X	X	X	X	X	X
Cleaning with an ultrasonic unit	X	X	X	X		X	X	X	X	X	X	X	X	X	X
Using sterile techniques	X	X	X	X		X	X	X	X	X	X	X	X	X	X
Maintaining isolation	X	X	X	X		X	X	X	X	X	X	X	X	X	X
Unit 14: Vital Signs															
Measuring and recording vital signs	X	X		X			X	X	X	X	X	X	X	X	X
Measuring and recording temperature	X	X		X			X	X	X	X	X	X	X	X	X
Measuring and recording pulse	X	X		X			X	X	X	X	X	X	X	X	X
Measuring and recording respirations	X	X		X			X	X	X	X	X	X	X	X	X
Graphing temperature, pulse, and respiration (TPR)	X	X		X			X	X	X	X	X	X	X	X	X
Measuring and recording apical pulse	X	X		X			X	X	X	X	X	X	X	X	X
Measuring and recording blood pressure	X	X		X			X	X	X	X	X	X	X	X	X

Matrix of Skills Used in Health Occupations

SKILLS	CLINICAL LABORATORY SERVICES	DENTISTRY	DIETETICS AND NUTRITION	EDUCATION	HEALTH INFORMATION AND COMMUNICATION	HEALTH SERVICES ADMINISTRATION	MEDICINE	MENTAL, PHYSICAL, SOCIAL SPECIALTIES	NURSING	PHARMACY	PODIATRY	SCIENCE AND ENGINEERING	TECHNICAL INSTRUMENTATION	VETERINARY MEDICINE	VISION CARE
Unit 15: First Aid															
Providing first aid	X	X	X	X	X	X	X	X	X	X	X	X	X	X	X
Performing cardiopulmonary resuscitation (CPR)	X	X	X	X	X	X	X	X	X	X	X	X	X	X	X
Providing first aid for bleeding and wounds	X	X	X	X	X	X	X	X	X	X	X	X	X	X	X
Providing first aid for shock	X	X	X	X	X	X	X	X	X	X	X	X	X	X	X
Providing first aid for poisoning	X	X	X	X	X	X	X	X	X	X	X	X	X	X	X
Providing first aid for burns	X	X	X	X	X	X	X	X	X	X	X	X	X	X	X
Providing first aid for heat exposure	X	X	X	X	X	X	X	X	X	X	X	X	X	X	X
Providing first aid for cold exposure	X	X	X	X	X	X	X	X	X	X	X	X	X	X	X
Providing first aid for bone and joint injuries	X	X	X	X	X	X	X	X	X	X	X	X	X	X	X
Providing first aid for specific injuries	X	X	X	X	X	X	X	X	X	X	X	X	X	X	X
Providing first aid for sudden illness	X	X	X	X	X	X	X	X	X	X	X	X	X	X	X
Applying dressings and bandages	X	X	X	X	X	X	X	X	X	X	X	X	X	X	X
Unit 16: Preparing for the World of Work															
Developing job-keeping skills	X	X	X	X	X	X	X	X	X	X	X	X	X	X	X
Writing a letter of application and preparing a resumé	X	X	X	X	X	X	X	X	X	X	X	X	X	X	X
Completing job application forms	X	X	X	X	X	X	X	X	X	X	X	X	X	X	X
Participating in a job interview	X	X	X	X	X	X	X	X	X	X	X	X	X	X	X
Determining net income	X	X	X	X	X	X	X	X	X	X	X	X	X	X	X
Calculating a budget	X	X	X	X	X	X	X	X	X	X	X	X	X	X	X
Unit 17: Dental Assistant Skills															
Identifying the structures and tissues of a tooth		X	X	X			X	X	X					X	
Identifying the teeth		X	X	X			X	X	X				X	X	
Identifying teeth using the Universal Numbering System and the Federation Dentaire International System		X	X	X	X			X	X					X	X
Identifying the surfaces of the teeth		X	X	X			X	X	X				X	X	
Charting conditions of the teeth		X	X	X			X	X	X				X	X	
Operating and maintaining dental equipment		X		X				X				X	X	X	
Identifying dental instruments and preparing dental trays		X		X									X	X	
Positioning a patient in the dental chair		X		X				X					X	X	

Matrix of Skills Used in Health Occupations

SKILLS	CLINICAL LABORATORY SERVICES	DENTISTRY	DIETETICS AND NUTRITION	EDUCATION	HEALTH INFORMATION AND COMMUNICATION	HEALTH SERVICES ADMINISTRATION	MEDICINE	MENTAL, PHYSICAL, SOCIAL SPECIALTIES	NURSING	PHARMACY	PODIATRY	SCIENCE AND ENGINEERING	TECHNICAL INSTRUMENTATION	VETERINARY MEDICINE	VISION CARE
Unit 17: Dental Assistant Skills (cont.)															
Demonstrating brushing-flossing techniques		X	X	X	X		X	X	X					X	
Taking impressions and pouring models	X	X		X									X	X	
Making custom trays	X	X		X									X	X	
Maintaining and loading an anesthetic aspirating syringe		X		X					X	X	X		X	X	X
Mixing dental cements and bases		X		X						X			X	X	
Preparing restorative materials		X		X						X			X	X	
Developing and mounting dental X rays	X	X		X			X	X					X	X	
Unit 18: Laboratory Assistant Skills															
Operating the microscope	X	X	X	X			X	X	X	X	X	X	X	X	X
Obtaining/handling cultures	X	X	X	X			X	X	X	X	X	X	X	X	X
Puncturing the skin to obtain capillary blood	X	X		X			X	X	X		X	X	X	X	X
Performing a microhematocrit	X	X		X			X	X	X		X	X	X	X	X
Measuring hemoglobin	X	X		X			X	X	X		X	X	X	X	X
Counting blood cells	X	X		X			X	X	X		X	X	X	X	X
Preparing and staining a blood film or smear	X	X		X			X	X	X		X	X	X	X	X
Testing for blood types	X	X		X			X	X	X		X	X	X	X	X
Performing an erthrocyte sedimentation rate	X	X		X			X	X	X		X	X	X	X	X
Measuring blood sugar (glucose) level	X	X	X	X			X	X	X	X	X	X	X	X	X
Testing urine	X	X	X	X			X	X	X	X	X	X	X	X	X
Using reagent strips to test urine	X	X	X	X			X	X	X	X	X	X		X	
Measuring specific gravity	X			X			X	X	X		X	X		X	
Preparing urine for microscopic examination	X			X			X	X	X		X	X		X	
Unit 19: Medical Assistant Skills															
Measuring/recording height and weight	X	X	X	X			X	X	X	X	X	X	X	X	X
Positioning a patient	X	X	X	X	X		X	X	X	X	X	X	X	X	X
Screening for vision problems				X			X	X	X				X		X
Assisting with physical examinations				X			X	X	X		X		X	X	X
Assisting with minor surgery and suture removal		X		X			X	X	X		X	X	X	X	X
Recording and mounting an electrocardiogram	X			X			X					X	X	X	

Matrix of Skills Used in Health Occupations

SKILLS	CLINICAL LABORATORY SERVICES	DENTISTRY	DIETETICS AND NUTRITION	EDUCATION	HEALTH INFORMATION AND COMMUNICATION	HEALTH SERVICES ADMINISTRATION	MEDICINE	MENTAL, PHYSICAL, SOCIAL SPECIALTIES	NURSING	PHARMACY	PODIATRY	SCIENCE AND ENGINEERING	TECHNICAL INSTRUMENTATION	VETERINARY MEDICINE	VISION CARE
Unit 19: Medical Assistant Skills (cont.)															
Using the *Physicians' Desk Reference* (PDR)	X	X	X	X			X	X	X	X	X	X	X	X	X
Working with math and medications	X	X		X			X	X	X	X	X	X	X	X	X
Unit 20: Nurse Assistant Skills															
Admitting, transferring, and discharging patients				X		X	X	X	X		X			X	X
Positioning, turning, moving, and transferring patients	X	X	X	X			X	X	X		X	X	X	X	X
Bedmaking	X			X		X	X	X	X		X		X		
Administering personal hygiene				X			X	X	X		X		X	X	
Measuring and recording intake and output	X		X	X			X	X	X	X		X		X	
Feeding a patient			X	X				X	X					X	
Assisting with bedpan/urinal	X			X			X	X	X						
Providing catheter and urinary drainage unit care	X			X			X	X	X				X	X	
Providing ostomy care				X			X	X	X				X	X	
Collecting stool/urine specimens	X			X			X	X	X					X	
Giving enemas and rectal treatments				X			X	X	X				X	X	
Applying restraints	X	X		X			X	X	X		X			X	X
Administering pre- and postoperative care		X		X			X		X		X		X	X	X
Applying binders				X			X	X	X		X		X	X	
Administering oxygen	X			X			X	X	X		X		X	X	X
Providing postmortem care	X			X			X	X	X						
Unit 21: Physical Therapy Skills															
Performing range of motion (ROM) exercises	X			X			X	X	X		X			X	
Ambulating patients who use transfer (gait) belts, crutches, canes, or walkers	X	X		X			X	X	X		X		X	X	X
Administering heat/cold applications	X	X		X			X	X	X	X	X		X	X	X

Matrix of Skills Used in Health Occupations

SKILLS	CLINICAL LABORATORY SERVICES	DENTISTRY	DIETETICS AND NUTRITION	EDUCATION	HEALTH INFORMATION AND COMMUNICATION	HEALTH SERVICES ADMINISTRATION	MEDICINE	MENTAL, PHYSICAL, SOCIAL SPECIALTIES	NURSING	PHARMACY	PODIATRY	SCIENCE AND ENGINEERING	TECHNICAL INSTRUMENTATION	VETERINARY MEDICINE	VISION CARE
Unit 22: Business and Accounting Skills															
Filing records	X	X	X	X	X	X	X	X	X	X	X	X	X	X	X
Using the telephone	X	X	X	X	X	X	X	X	X	X	X	X	X	X	X
Scheduling appointments	X	X	X	X	X	X	X	X	X	X	X	X	X	X	X
Completing medical records and forms	X	X	X	X	X	X	X	X	X	X	X	X	X	X	X
Composing business letters	X	X	X	X	X	X	X	X	X	X	X	X	X	X	X
Completing insurance forms	X	X	X	X	X	X	X	X	X	X	X	X	X	X	X
Maintaining a bookkeeping system	X	X	X	X	X	X	X	X	X	X	X	X	X	X	X
Writing checks, deposit slips, and receipts	X	X	X	X	X	X	X	X	X	X	X	X	X	X	X

Correlation to National Health Care Skill Standards

UNIT	Academic Foundation	Communication	Systems	Employability Skills	Legal Responsibilities	Ethics	Safety Practices	Teamwork	Health Maintenance Practices	Client Interaction	Intrateam Communication	Monitoring Client Status	Client Movement	Data Collection	Treatment Planning	Implementing Procedures	Client Status Evaluation
	Health Care Core Standard								Therapeutic/ Diagnostic Core					Therapeutic Cluster			
Unit 1	X	X	X	X	X		X	X	X		X						
Unit 2	X		X	X	X			X			X			X			
Unit 3		X	X	X	X	X	X	X	X	X	X						
Unit 4		X	X	X	X	X				X	X	X		X	X	X	
Unit 5	X	X															
Unit 6	X								X		X	X					
Unit 7	X	X		X	X	X		X		X	X	X		X	X		X
Unit 8	X	X		X	X	X		X	X	X	X	X	X	X	X	X	X
Unit 9	X	X			X	X	X	X	X	X	X	X	X	X	X		X
Unit 10	X								X	X				X	X		X
Unit 11	X	X		X	X						X			X			X
Unit 12				X			X				X	X	X	X	X	X	X
Unit 13	X			X		X	X		X		X			X		X	X
Unit 14	X			X			X		X	X	X	X		X		X	X
Unit 15				X	X	X					X	X	X	X	X	X	X
Unit 16	X	X		X	X	X		X		X							
Unit 17				X	X	X			X	X	X	X	X	X	X	X	X
Unit 18				X	X	X			X	X	X	X					
Unit 19				X	X	X			X	X	X	X	X	X	X	X	X
Unit 20				X	X	X			X	X	X	X	X	X	X	X	X
Unit 21				X	X	X			X	X	X	X	X	X	X	X	X
Unit 22	X	X								X	X			X			

Correlation to National Health Care Skill Standards

UNIT	Diagnostic Cluster					Information Services Cluster					Environmental Services Cluster			
	Planning	Preparation	Procedure	Evaluation	Reporting	Analysis	Abstracting and Coding	Information Systems	Documentation	Operations	Environmental Operations	Aseptic Procedures	Resource Management	Aesthetics
Unit 1						X							X	
Unit 2	X									X	X			
Unit 3												X		
Unit 4	X				X	X		X	X		X	X		
Unit 5					X		X		X					
Unit 6												X		
Unit 7								X	X		X		X	
Unit 8	X	X	X	X	X	X		X	X				X	
Unit 9		X			X							X		X
Unit 10												X		X
Unit 11					X	X		X	X	X				
Unit 12	X	X	X	X	X						X		X	X
Unit 13		X	X								X	X	X	
Unit 14	X	X	X	X	X		X		X		X			
Unit 15	X	X	X	X	X									
Unit 16													X	
Unit 17	X	X	X	X	X		X							
Unit 18	X	X	X	X	X									
Unit 19	X	X	X	X	X									
Unit 20	X	X	X	X	X				X			X		
Unit 21														
Unit 22					X	X	X	X	X	X				

UNIT 1 HEALTH CARE SYSTEMS

ASSIGNMENT SHEET

Grade _____ Name _____

INTRODUCTION: An awareness of the many different kinds of health care systems is important for any health care worker. This assignment will help you review the main facts on health care systems.

INSTRUCTIONS: Read the information on Health Care Systems. Then follow the instructions by each section to complete this assignment.

A. Completion or Short Answer: In the space provided, print the word(s) that best completes the statement or answers the question.

  1. Unscramble the following words to identify some health care facilities.

    a. RAALOTBYRO

    b. TLEHHA NNCIAMTNAEE

    c. OLGN ETMR AREC

    d. UNLTISIDAR ETHLAH

    e. MNCEGEREY AECR

    f. LNTEMA LHTEHA

    g. LNCCII

    h. EAIINRIABHTLTO

    i. POTSAHIL

  2. Place the name of the type of health care facility by the brief description of the facility.

    a. _____ provide assistance and care for mainly elderly patients

    b. _____ provide special care for accidents or sudden illness

    c. _____ deal with mental disorders and disease

    d. _____ health centers located in large companies or industries

    e. _____ offices owned by one or more dentists

    f. _____ perform special diagnostic tests

    g. _____ provide care in a patient's home

    h. _____ provide physical, occupational, and other therapies

  3. Hospitals are classified into four types depending on the sources of income received. List the four (4) main types.

4. List three (3) services offered by medical offices.

5. Identify at least three (3) different types of clinics.

6. List three (3) examples of services that can be provided by home health care agencies.

7. What is the purpose or main goal for the care provided by rehabilitation facilities?

8. Identify three (3) services offered by school health services.

9. An international agency sponsored by the United Nations is the _____.
   A national agency that deals with health problems in America is the _____. Another
   national organization that is involved in the research of disease is the_____.
   A federal agency that establishes and enforces standards that protect workers from job-related injuries
   and illnesses is the _____.

10. List (4) services that can be offered by state and local health departments.

11. Nonprofit or voluntary agencies provide many services.

    a. How do these agencies receive their funding?

    b. List two (2) services provided by these facilities.

12. Define the following terms related to insurance plans.

    premium:

    deductible:

    75/25% co-insurance:

    HMOs:

    PPOs:

13. What is one advantage to HMOs? What is one disadvantage to HMOs?

14. Why has the concept of managed care developed? What is the principle behind managed care?

15. Identify the individuals who are usually covered under the following plans.

   Medicare:

   Medicaid:

   Workers' Compensation:

16. What is the purpose for an organizational structure in a health care facility?

17. What is holistic health care?

18. The Omnibus Budget Reconciliation Act (OBRA) of 1987 established standards for geriatric assistants in long-term care facilities. List four (4) requirements that all geriatric assistants must meet as a result of OBRA.

19. Describe what is meant by the following trends in health care. Include a brief explanation of why it is important to be aware of these trends.

   a. cost containment:

   b. diagnostic related groups (DRGs):

c. home health care:

d. geriatric care:

e. Omnibus Budget Reconciliation Act (OBRA):

f. wellness:

g. alternative methods of health care:

20. Do you think a national health care plan should be established to provide coverage for all individuals? Why or why not?

B. Matching: Place the letter of the person in Column B in the space provided by the person's contribution to the history of health care in Column A.

Column A   **Column B**

____ 1. Isolated radium in 1910   A. Clara Barton

____ 2. Established the patterns of heredity   B. Chinese

____ 3. Developed a vaccine for smallpox in 1796   C. Marie Curie

____ 4. Described the circulation of blood to and from the heart   D. Leonardo da Vinci

____ 5. Began public health and sanitation systems   E. Dark Ages

____ 6. Discovered X rays in 1895   F. Dorthea Dix

____ 7. The father of medicine   G. Egyptians

____ 8. Discovered penicillin in 1932   H. Gabrial Fahrenheit

____ 9. Artist who used dissection to draw the human body   I. Sir Alexander Flemming

____ 10. Pandemic of bubonic plague killed millions of people   J. Benjamin Franklin

____ 11. Founded the American Red Cross in 1881   K. Sigmund Freud

____ 12. Earliest people known to maintain accurate health records   L. William Harvey

____ 13. Began pasteurizing milk to kill bacteria   M. Hippocrates

____ 14. Used acupuncture to relieve pain and congestion   N. Edward Jenner

____ 15. Developed the culture plate method to identify pathogens   O. Robert Koch

____ 16. Founder of modern nursing   P. Joseph Lister

____ 17. Began using disinfectants and antiseptics during surgery   Q. Gregory Mendel

____ 18. Created the first mercury thermometer   R. Florence Nightengale

____ 19. Developed the polio vaccine in 1952   S. Louis Pasteur

____ 20. An Arab physician who began the use of animal gut   T. Rhazes

      for suture material   U. William Roentgen

                                                                   V. Romans

                                                                   W. Jonas Salk

     5

UNIT 2 CAREERS IN HEALTH CARE

ASSIGNMENT SHEET

Grade _____   Name _____

INTRODUCTION: An individual who wants to work in health care has a wide variety of career choices. This assignment will help you review some of the different careers.

INSTRUCTIONS: Read the information on Careers in Health Care. Then follow the instructions by each section to complete this assignment.

A. Health Career Search: All of the careers listed are hidden in the following word search puzzle. Locate and circle the careers.

admitting officer	home health care	pedodontics
animal technician	internist	perfusionist
athletic trainer	licensed practical nurse	pharmacist
biomedical equipment	medical laboratory	physical therapist
central supply	medicine	physician
chiropractic	music therapist	podiatric
dental hygienist	neurologist	psychologist
dentist	nurse	radiologic technologist
dialysis technician	occupational therapist	recreational therapist
dietitian	optician	respiratory therapy
doctor	optometrist	social worker
electrocardiograph	osteopathy	surgeon
electroencephalographic	orthodontics	surgical technician
emergency medical	paramedic	urologist
endodontics	pathologist	veterinarian
geriatric aide	pediatrician	ward clerk
gynecologist		

```
O R T H O D O N T I C S Z X E W P T V B P H Y S I C A L T H E R A P I S T X M N E C I D
C X V E T E R I N A R I A N O P C M I D W Q T Y P X B N N A I C I N H C E T L A M I N A
C E W I O N G H T S I G O L O N H C E T C I G O L O I D A R X B N M N I U T Y E M C T V
U M K I J T V E P B I U N J X U T Y O P H Y E P I U O P T O M E T R I S T X V M E K E L
P C V I E I T R O J K L I M U R O L O G I S T T X E M K U L I E R H W E S E S Q D X R L
A A S E T S I E D V B N T U E S M O P I E T H I R O E V U I S E D P A R A M E D I C N X
T L I E K T E R I L K E R N O E G R U S Y U R C E I D Z Q C W E A A T R G E U O C H I O
I T L M I D I C A I N E A R O T C O D T H E R I P H I X E E O R T R H E P R I K I I S L
O B O A T H L E T I C T R A I N E R E M U W T A I N C P I N C H I G R S O G P R N R T A
N P A T H E R O R G Y N P E D O D O N T I C S N P E A D O S D O N O T P I E C S E O D E
A N T I N A I T I T E I D S T N U R T H E A L T A I L Y U E R E S I P I R N A P T P R Y
L R E C G Y N E C O L O G I S T R E A A W A R D C L E R K D X T I D O R N C A E L R A I
T D P H Y S I C I A N E R N E U R O L O G I S T X Y Q R A P D I O R L A O Y G D M A I S
H N S S E U R S E X O S T E O P A T H Y O S T I O P U A T R H Y X A R T O M P I U C M N
E X Y Z W S C E N T R A L S U P P L Y S A N I T A T I J K A H O M C R O E E T A S T L S
R E C B N R T S I C A M R A H P Y O G G R O S T I E P O U C I E T O B R N D M T I I W E
A T H H E L P M E E D I A C I R T A I R E G R I G H M T O T N T O R R Y U I P R C C B O
P H O M E H E A L T H C A R E T I E E S C H O H L R E J U I T O E T M T N C C I T O I P
I X L Y O U S U R G I C A L T E C H N I C I A N F O N I U C N C S C X H P A M C H W Q R
S P O R E C E P T R E C I F F O G N I T T I M D A X T I O A Y Z D E T E C L G I E R U N
T O G E T H I E W A R D I A L Y S I S T E C H N I C I A N L M O M L R R I O P A R U R O
B N I Z Y M E D I C A L L A B O R A T O R Y T E A C H U R N V O W E X A E L M N A S E T
C X S O C I A L W O R K E R R I T W Q Y C V T S I N O I S U F R E P X P L O V I P K E N
F E T H E R B I R T S I P A R E H T L A N O I T A E R C E R E A G L O Y R E T C I H I C
A B X E N D O D O N T I C S H Y G I E N P A T H O L O G I S T V E T E R A M I X S M A L
E L E C T R O C I H P A R G O L A H P E C N E O R T C E L E X E N C A R D G R A T H I C
```

B. Matching: Place the letter of the abbreviation in Column B in the space provided by the career it represents in Column A.

Column A		Column B	
____	1. Occupational Therapist	A.	ATR
____	2. Certified Medical Technologist	B.	CBET
____	3. Nurse Midwife	C.	CLT
____	4. Doctor of Dental Medicine	D.	CMA
____	5. Emergency Medical Technician	E.	CMT
____	6. Doctor of Osteopathy	F.	CNM
____	7. Certified Biomedical Equipment Technician	G.	CRNP
____	8. Registered Nurse	H.	DC
____	9. Optometrist	I.	DMD
____	10. Registered Dietitian	J.	DDS
____	11. Doctor of Dental Surgery	K.	DO
____	12. Registered Animal Technician	L.	DPM
____	13. Doctor of Podiatric Medicine	M.	DVM or VMD
____	14. Certified Medical Assistant	N.	ECG or EKG
____	15. Electrocardiograph Technician	O.	EEG
____	16. Physical Therapist	P.	EMT
____	17. Doctor of Chiropractic	Q.	LPN or LVN
____	18. Licensed Practical/Vocational Nurse	R.	MD
____	19. Doctor of Medicine	S.	OD
____	20. Nurse Practitioner	T.	OT
____	21. Certified Laboratory Technician	U.	PT
____	22. Veterinarian	V.	RD
____	23. Electroencelphalographic Technician	W.	RN
____	24. Respiratory Therapist	X.	RT

C. Completion or Short Answer: In the space provided, print the word(s) that best complete the statement or answer the question.

1. Briefly describe the educational requirements for the following degrees.

Associate's:

Bachelor's:

Master's:

9

2. Identify the following methods used to ensure the skill and competency of health care workers:

   a. An association regulating a particular health career issues a statement that a person has fulfilled the requirements of education and performance and meets the standards:

   b. A government agency authorizes an individual to work in a given occupation after the individual has completed an approved education program and passed a state board test:

   c. A regulatory body in a health care area administers examinations and maintains a list of qualified personnel:

3. What is the difference between a technician and a technologist?

4. Who are multi-competent or multi-skilled workers?

   Why do smaller facilities and rural areas hire these workers?

5. Define *entrepreneur.*

   List three (3) characteristics of a person who is an entrepreneur.

6. The following statements describe medical or dental specialities. Print the correct name of the specialty or specialist in the space provided.

   a. _____ alignment or straightening of the teeth
   b. _____ diseases and disorders of the eye
   c. _____ diseases and disorders of the mind
   d. _____ surgery on the teeth, mouth, and jaw
   e. _____ disorders of the brain and nervous system
   f. _____ diseases of the female reproductive system
   g. _____ diseases of the kidney, bladder, or urinary system
   h. _____ illness or injury in all age groups
   i. _____ treatment and prevention of diseases of the gums
   j. _____ diagnosis and treatment of tumors

7. The following statements describe health careers. Print the correct name of the career in the space provided.

    a. _____ works under supervision of a dentist to remove stains and deposits from the teeth, expose and develop X rays

    b. _____ operates machine to record electrical activity in brain

    c. _____ work with X rays, radiation, nuclear medicine, ultrasound

    d. _____ provide basic care for medical emergencies, illness, injury

    e. _____ organize and code patient records, gather statistical data

    f. _____ manage the operation of a health care facility

    g. _____ nurse assistant who works with elderly individuals

    h. _____ dispense medications on written orders from others who are authorized to prescribe medications

    i. _____ use recreational and leisure activities as form of treatment

    j. _____ examine eyes for vision problems and defects, not an MD

    k. _____ prepare a body for interment

8. Review the different health careers and find at least three careers that interest you. List the three careers and include a brief description of the duties and educational requirements of each. Also include a brief statement about why you might like to work in each career.

9. Choose one of the careers listed previously and write to an organization that will provide additional information about the career. Let your instructor check your letter before you mail it. Organizations and addresses are provided after each career cluster in the textbook. If you have access to the Internet, contact the organization by using the Internet address provided or by doing an Internet search. This will allow you to read or print a hard copy of information on the career.

UNIT 3 PERSONAL QUALITIES OF A HEALTH CARE WORKER

ASSIGNMENT SHEET

Grade _____   Name _____

INTRODUCTION: Certain personal characteristics, attitudes, and rules of appearance apply to all health care workers even though they may be employed in many different careers. This assignment will help you review these basic requirements.

INSTRUCTIONS: Read the information on Personal Qualities of a Health Care Worker. Then follow the instructions by each section and complete this assignment.

A. Use the Key Terms for personal characteristics of a health care worker to complete the crossword puzzle.

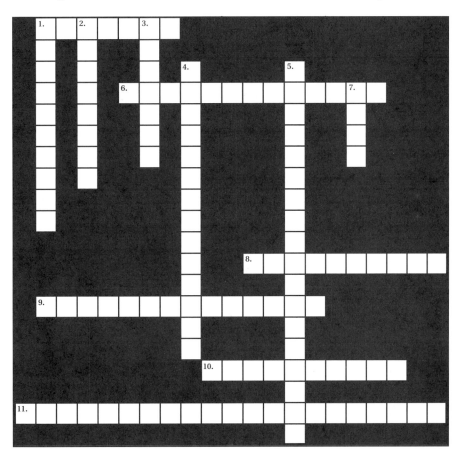

ACROSS

1. Identify with and understand another's feelings
6. Accept responsibility because others rely on you
8. Use good judgment in what you say and do
9. Willing to be held accountable for your actions
10. Qualified and capable of performing a task
11. Accept opinions of others and learn from them

DOWN

1. Display a positive attitude and enjoy work
2. Tolerant and understanding
3. Show truthfulness and integrity
4. Ability to begin or follow through with a task
5. Adapt to changes and learn new things
7. Say or do the kindest or most fitting thing

B. Characteristic Profile: Write a characteristic profile of yourself as a health care worker that describes at least eight (8) of the personal characteristics without using the actual words. A sentence describing empathy is shown as an example.

As a health worker, I must have a sincere interest in people, and I must be able to identify with and understand another person's feelings, situation, and motives.

C. Completion and Short Answer: In the space provided, print the answer to the question or complete the statement.

1. List five (5) factors that contribute to good health and briefly describe why each factor is beneficial.

2. Identify three (3) basic requirements for the appearance of uniforms.

3. How do you determine which type and color of uniform to wear in your place of employment?

4. List three (3) basic rules to observe in regard to shoes worn in a health career.

5. List three (3) ways to control body odor.

6. List three (3) reasons why the nails must be kept short and clean.

7. What can be used to keep the hands from becoming chapped and dry due to frequent handwashing?

8. Why is it important to keep long hair pinned back and off the collar when a job requires close patient contact?

9. What jewelry can be worn with a uniform?

   Why should excessive jewelry be avoided?

10. What is the purpose of makeup?

UNIT 4 LEGAL AND ETHICAL RESPONSIBILITIES

ASSIGNMENT SHEET

Grade _____ Name _____

INTRODUCTION: All health care workers must understand the legal and ethical responsibilities of their particular health career. This assignment will help you review the basic facts on legal and ethical responsibilities.

INSTRUCTIONS: Read the information on Legal and Ethical Responsibilities. In the space provided, print the word(s) that best completes the statement or answers the question.

1. Use the Key Terms to fill in the blanks.

   a.   C _ _ _ _ _ _ _ (agreement between two or more parties)

   b.   _ O _ _ (wrongful acts that do not involve contracts)

   c.   _ _ _ N _ _ _ (spoken defamation)

   d.   _ _ F _ _ _ _ _ _ _ (a false statement)

   e.   _ I _ _ _ (written defamation)

   f.   _ _ _ _ _ D _ _ _ _ _ _ _ _ _ (without legal capacity)

   g.   _ E _ _ _ (authorized or based on law)

   h.   _ _ _ N _ (person working under principal's direction)

   i.   _ T _ _ _ _ (principles morally right or wrong)

   j.   _ _ _ _ _ I _ _ _ _ _ _ _ _ _ _ _ (restricting an individual's freedom)

   k.   _ _ _ _ _ A _ _ _ _ _ (bad practice)

   l.   _ _ _ _ _ L _ (threat or attempt to injure)

   m.   _ _ _ _ I _ _ _ _ _ (failure to give expected care)

   n.   _ _ _ _ _ _ T _ _ _ _ _ _ (factors of care patients can expect)
                   Y

2. Create a situation that provides an example that could lead to legal action for each of the following torts.

   a. malpractice:

   b. negligence:

c. assault and battery:

d. invasion of privacy:

e. false imprisonment:

f. abuse:

g. defamation:

3. How are slander and libel the same? How are they different?

4. What are the three (3) parts of a contract?

5. What is the difference between an implied and an expressed contract?

6. List three (3) examples of individuals who have legal disabilities.

7. What legal mandate must be followed when a contract is explained to a non-English-speaking individual?

8. Why is it important for a health care worker to be aware of his/her role as an agent? Who is responsible for the actions of the agent?

9. What are privileged communications?

What is required before privileged communications can be told to anyone else?

10. List three (3) examples of information that is exempt by law and not considered to be privileged communications.

11. Who has ownership of health care records?

What rights do patients have in regard to their health care records?

12. What should you do if you make an error while recording information on health care records?

13. List three (3) ways health care facilities create safeguards to maintain computer confidentiality.

14. What are ethics?

15. What should you do in the following situations to maintain your legal/ethical responsibilities?

 a. A patient dying of cancer tells you he has saved a supply of sleeping pills and intends to commit suicide.

 b. You work in a nursing home and see a coworker shove a patient into a chair and then slap the patient in the face.

 c. You work as a dental assistant and a patient asks you "Will the doctor be able to save this tooth or will it have to be pulled?"

 d. A patient has just been admitted to an assisted care facility. As you are helping the patient undress and get ready for bed, you notice numerous bruises and scratches on both arms.

16. The factors of care that patients can expect to receive are frequently called _____. These state in part that a patient has the right to _____ and _____ care, receive _____ necessary to give his or her _____ consent, refuse _____ to the extent permitted by law, _____ treatment of all records, reasonable _____ to request for services, _____ the bill and receive a/an _____ of all charges, refuse to _____ in any research project, and expect reasonable _____ of care.

17. What is the name of the act that guarantees certain rights to residents in long-term care facilities?

18. What is the purpose for each of the following advance directives for health care?
 a. Living will:

 b. Durable Power of Attorney (POA):

19. What is the purpose of the Patient Self-Determination Act (PSDA)?

20. Describe two (2) ways you can identify a patient.

21. What should you do in the following situations to maintain professional standards?

a. The doctor you work for asks you to give a patient an allergy shot, but you are not qualified to give injections.

b. An elderly patient, who is frequently confused and disoriented, refuses to let you take his temperature.

c. You work in a medical laboratory. A patient's wife asks you if her husband's blood test was positive for an infectious disease.

UNIT 5:1 USING MEDICAL ABBREVIATIONS

ASSIGNMENT SHEET

Grade _____   Name _____

INTRODUCTION: Shortened forms of words (often just letters) are called abbreviations. You are probably familiar with some such as AM, which means morning, and PM, which means afternoon or evening.

   The world of medicine has many of its own abbreviations. At times they are used by themselves. At other times, several abbreviations are used together to give orders or directions.

   As a health worker, many directions will be given to you in abbreviated form. You will be expected to know their meaning. The following assignment will assist you in starting to see how these abbreviations are used, and how you must translate them to understand them.

INSTRUCTIONS: Review the information on standard medical abbreviations. Try to recall the meanings of the following terms before using them as references to complete the exercises.

A. Print the meanings of the following abbreviations.

   1. D/C _____

   2. OR _____

   3. prn _____

   4. ac _____

   5. stat _____

   6. RN _____

   7. wt _____

   8. Cl _____

   9. Rx _____

  10. AP _____

  11. T _____

  12. NPO _____

  13. spec _____

  14. $\bar{c}$ _____

  15. $\bar{\bar{ss}}$ _____

  16. $\bar{s}$ _____

  17. pt _____

  18. BP _____

  19. R _____

  20. Na _____

  21. CDC _____

  22. DRG _____

  23. LMP _____

24. ↑ _____

25. ♀ _____

B. Look up the meanings of the following combinations to interpret the orders. Print your answers.

1. TPR qid _____

_____

2. 2 gtts bid _____

_____

3. 1 cc IM _____

_____

4. BP q 4 h _____

_____

5. 2 oz OJ qid ac and HS _____

_____

6. Wt and Ht qod in AM _____

_____

7. BR c̄ BRP only _____

_____

8. 1000 cc N/S IV _____

_____

9. Do ECG in CCU _____

_____

10. Dissolve 2 tsp NaCl in 1 qt H_2O _____

_____

11. 1000 cc SSE at HS _____

12. Schedule B1 Wk in AM including CBC, BUN, and FBS _____

_____

13. Dilute 1 tab in 1 pt H_2O _____

_____

14. 1 tab qid pc and HS _____

_____

15. BP is measured in mm of Hg _____

_____

16. NPO pre-op _____

_____

17. Do EENT exam in OPD _____

_____

Name _____

18. Ob-Gyn _____

    _____

19. 500 mg qod 8 AM _____

    _____

20. VS stat and q2 h _____

    _____

21. To PT by w/c for ROMs and ADL bid _____

    _____

22. FF1 cl liq to 240 cc q2h _____

    _____

23. 2 gtts OU qid q6h _____

    _____

24. Dx: COPD, O_2 prn, IPPB bid ql2h _____

    _____

25. Sig: $\ddot{\pi}$ Cap po tid $\bar{c}$ food or milk _____

    _____

UNIT 5:1 Evaluation Sheet

Name _____ Date _____

Evaluated by _____

DIRECTIONS: Read the case history aloud, using words instead of the abbreviations. Each abbreviation has a value of 5 points.

PROFICIENT

Using Medical Abbreviations	Points Possible	Peer Check		Final Check*		Points Earned**	Comments
		Yes	No	Yes	No		
1. Mary was taking medicine *ac* because the *Dr* ordered it. She was complaining of not feeling well so the orders included tests to find out the reason: a *CBC* was done and also a *FBS*. When he received the results, Dr. Pierce made a *dx* of diabetes and asked the *RN* to give Mary insulin. Mary now has to take insulin *qd* by *sc inj* and is on a *low cal* diet.	45						
2. A man was brought into the *ER* but he was *DOA*. The ambulance attendant said that the man had complained of headache, his *BP* was very high, and he may have had a *CVA*.	20						
3. John Smith was taken to the *Orth Dept* after a fall. He had a *Fr* of the knee that required surgery. After going to the *OR*, John was given medication *prn* for pain and was scheduled for *PT* to start next week for *ROM* exercises and *ADL*.	35						
Totals	100						

* Final Check: Instructor or authorized person evaluates.
** Points Earned: Points possible times each "yes" check.

UNIT 5:2 INTERPRETING WORD PARTS

ASSIGNMENT SHEET

Grade _____   Name _____

INTRODUCTION: Special words used in medicine are called medical terminology. Many of these words have common beginnings (prefixes), common endings (suffixes), and common parts (word roots). By learning the main prefixes, suffixes, and word roots, it is possible to put together many new words or to break apart a medical term to understand its meaning.

In the health fields, you will be required to know and understand medical terminology. Even if you have never come into contact with a medical word before, by breaking it down into its parts, you will usually be able to figure out the meaning of the word. This assignment sheet will show you the process.

INSTRUCTIONS: Review the information sheet on prefixes, suffixes, and word roots.

Study the following examples of breaking a word into parts.

Example 1: *erythrocyte:* erythro / cyte

　　　　　　erythro means red

　　　　　　cyte means cell

　　　　　　erythrocyte means red cell

Example 2: *hyperadenosis:* hyper / aden / osis

　　　　　　hyper means increased

　　　　　　aden means gland

　　　　　　osis means condition, state, or process

　　　　　　hyperadenosis means increased glandular condition

A. Determine the meanings of the following words. Print your answers in the spaces provided. The words have been separated to help you do this exercise.

1. crani / otomy _____

　　crani _____

　　otomy _____

2. dys / uria _____

　　dys _____

　　uria _____

3. hyster / ectomy _____

　　hyster _____

　　ectomy _____

4. hemo / toxic _____

　　hemo _____

　　toxic _____

5. peri / card / itis _____

    peri _____

    card _____

    itis _____

6. leuko / cyte _____

    leuko _____

    cyte _____

7. chole / cyst / itis _____

    chole _____

    cyst _____

    itis _____

8. tachy / cardia _____

    tachy _____

    cardia _____

9. neur / algia _____

    neur _____

    algia _____

10. poly / cyt / emia _____

    poly _____

    cyt _____

    emia _____

11. brady / cardia _____

    _____

    _____

12. gastr / ectomy _____

    _____

    _____

13. mening / itis _____

    _____

    _____

14. neo / pathy _____

    _____

    _____

15. dermat / ologist _____

    _____

    _____

16. procto / scope _____

    _____

    _____

28

17. carcin / oma _____

_____

_____

18. electro / encephalo / graph _____

_____

_____

_____

19. osteo / malacia _____

_____

_____

20. para / plegia _____

_____

_____

21. py / uria _____

_____

_____

22. acro / megaly _____

_____

_____

23. geront / ology _____

_____

_____

24. dys / phagia _____

_____

_____

25. hydro / cele _____

_____

_____

B. Analyze each word to determine the breaking-off point. Mentally separate them into word elements. Print the meaning of the word.

1. adenoma _____

_____

_____

2. antitoxic _____

_____

_____

3. ophthalmology _____

_____

_____

4. cholecystectomy _____

_____

_____

5. endocarditis _____

_____

_____

6. gastroenteritis _____

_____

_____

7. hypoglycemia _____

_____

_____

8. septicemia _____

_____

_____

9. oliguria _____

_____

_____

10. bronchitis _____

_____

_____

11. homogenous _____

_____

_____

12. arteriosclerosis _____

_____

_____

13. dysmenorrhea _____

_____

_____

14. angiopathy _____

_____

_____

15. blepharorrhaphy _____

_____

_____

16. urethrocystitis _____

_____

_____

17. pneumonomelanosis _____

_____

_____

18. paraosteoarthropathy _____

_____

_____

19. salpingo-oophorocele _____

_____

_____

20. idiopathic thrombocytopenia _____

_____

_____

21. narcoepilepsy _____

_____

_____

22. postpartum _____

_____

_____

23. herniorrhaphy _____

_____

_____

24. dermacyanosis _____

_____

_____

25. thoracentesis _____

_____

_____

Name _____   Date _____

Evaluated by _____

DIRECTIONS: Be able to tell your instructor the meaning of the underlined sentences. Pronunciation, spelling, and definition of the medical term will be evaluated. Be prepared to spell the word without looking at the term.

PROFICIENT

Prefixes, Suffixes, and Word Roots	Points Possible	Peer Check Yes	No	Final Check* Yes	No	Points Earned**	Comments
1. Mary had *dermalgia* that was due to a rash.	10						
2. Mary's friend had *thrombophlebitis.*	10						
3. *Anuria* may be a sign of kidney disease.	10						
4. A *nephrectomy* requires a surgeon's skill.	10						
5. The *gastric* secretions were high in acid content.	10						
6. A *hysterectomy* was done to remove the tumor.	10						
7. *Hyperglycemia* may be a sign of diabetes.	10						
8. *Cholecystitis* may be caused by eating large quantities of undigestible fats.	10						
9. A fractured neck can cause *quadriplegia.*	10						
10. *Hepatitis* can produce a yellow tinge to the skin.	10						
Totals	100						

* Final Check: Instructor or authorized person evaluates.
** Points Earned: Points possible times each "yes" check.

UNIT 6:1 BASIC STRUCTURE OF THE HUMAN BODY

ASSIGNMENT SHEET

Grade _____   Name _____

INTRODUCTION: A basic understanding of the structure of the human body will help a health care worker understand the total function of the body. This assignment will help you review the main facts.

INSTRUCTIONS: Read the information on Basic Structure of the Human Body. In the space provided, print the word(s) that best completes the statement or answers the question.

1. Label the parts of the cell on the following illustration. Briefly state the function of each part.

A.   F.

B.   G.

C.   H.

D.   I.

E.   J.

33

2. The study of the form and structure of an organism is _____. The study of the processes of living organisms is _____. The study of how disease occurs is _____.

3. What is the basic unit of structure and function in all living things?

4. List four (4) functions of cells.

5. What is the form of asexual reproduction used by cells?

   Briefly sketch this process and state what occurs in each step.

6. What condition results from an insufficient amount of tissue fluid?

   What condition results from an excess amount of tissue fluid?

7. List the four (4) main types of tissues and state the function of each type.

8. What is the proper name for fatty tissue?

   List three (3) functions of fatty tissue.

9. How does bone tissue differ from cartilage?

10. List the three (3) main types of muscle tissue and state the function of each type.

11. When two or more tissues join together for a specific function, they form a/an _____. Examples include _____, _____, and _____.

12. Name ten (10) body systems.

UNIT 6:2 BODY PLANES, DIRECTIONS, AND CAVITIES

ASSIGNMENT SHEET

Grade _____   Name _____

INTRODUCTION: Directional terms are used to describe the relationship of one part of the body to another part. This assignment will help you review the main terms used.

INSTRUCTIONS: Read the information on Body Planes, Directions, and Cavities. In the space provided, print the word(s) that best completes the statement or answers the question.

1. Place the letter of the correct term in Column B in the space provided by a description of the term in Column A.

Column A	Column B
1. _____ Body parts away from the point of reference	A. Caudal
2. _____ Horizontal plane that divides the body into a top and bottom half	B. Cranial
3. _____ Body parts away from the midline	C. Distal
4. _____ Body parts below the transverse plane	D. Dorsal or posterior
5. _____ Body parts on the front of the body	E. Frontal
6. _____ Plane that divides the body into a right and left side	F. Inferior
7. _____ Body parts close to the point of reference	G. Lateral
8. _____ Body parts located near the head	H. Medial
9. _____ Body parts above the transverse plane	I. Midsaggital
10. _____ Body parts on the back of the body	J. Proximal
11. _____ Body parts close to the midline	K. Superior
12. _____ Body parts located near sacral region or "tail"	L. Transverse
13. _____ Plane that divides body into front and back section	M. Ventral or anterior

2. Identify the body cavities in the following illustration.

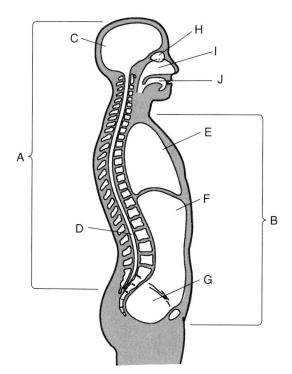

A.

B.

C.

D.

E.

F.

G.

H.

I.

J.

3. List the organs located in each of the following body cavities.

cranial:

spinal:

thoracic:

upper abdominal:

pelvic:

4. The abdominal cavity can be divided into quadrants or four (4) main sections. Name these sections and the proper abbreviation for each section.

5. Identify the abdominal region for each of the following descriptions.

a. _____ region above the stomach

b. _____ region on the right side by the groin

c. _____ region on the left side below the ribs

d. _____ region by the umbilicus or belly-button

e. _____ region on the right side by the large bones of the spinal cord

f. _____ region below the stomach

UNIT 6:3 INTEGUMENTARY SYSTEM

ASSIGNMENT SHEET

Grade _____ Name _____

INTRODUCTION: The integumentary system consists of the skin and all of its parts. This assignment will help you review the main facts of this system.

INSTRUCTIONS: Read the information on the Integumentary System. In the space provided, print the word(s) that best completes the statement or answers the question.

1. Label the following diagram of a cross section of the skin.

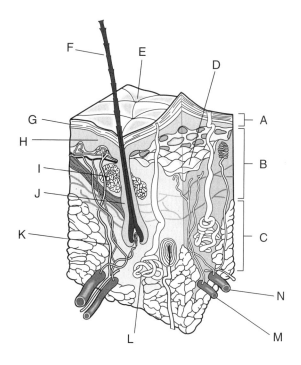

A.	H.
B.	I.
C.	J.
D.	K.
E.	L.
F.	M.
G.	N.

39

2. What are papillae?

   How do they provide a method of identification?

3. What is the proper name for sweat glands?
   Name three (3) substances found in perspiration.

4. What is the proper name for oil glands?
   What is the function of oil glands?

5. What is alopecia?

6. List seven (7) functions of the skin.

7. What happens when blood vessels dilate? How does this regulate temperature?

   What happens when blood vessels constrict? How does this regulate temperature?

8. Define the following words, and give one cause for each discoloration.
   a. erythema:

   b. jaundice:

   c. cyanosis:

9. Identify the following skin eruptions.

   a. blisters or sacs full of fluid:

   b. firm raised areas on the skin:

   c. areas of dried pus and blood:

   d. sacs filled with pus:

   e. flat spots on the skin:

   f. itchy, elevated areas with an irregular shape:

   g. deep loss of skin surface that may extend into dermis:

10. Briefly describe the following skin diseases.

   a. impetigo:

   b. warts or verrucae:

   c. dermatitis:

   d. acne vulgaris:

   e. athlete's foot:

   f. psoriasis:

   g. ringworm:

UNIT 6:4 SKELETAL SYSTEM

ASSIGNMENT SHEET

Grade _____   Name _____

INTRODUCTION: The skeletal system forms the framework of the entire body. This assignment will help you review the main facts about this system.

INSTRUCTIONS: Read the information on the Skeletal System. In the space provided, print the word(s) that best completes the statement or answers the question.

1. Use the Key Terms to complete the following crossword puzzle.

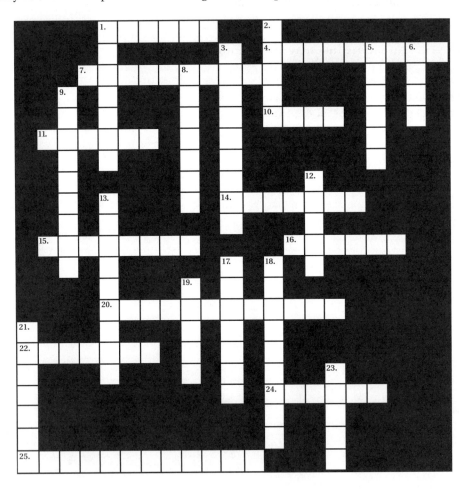

ACROSS

1. Area where cranial bones have joined together

4. Membrane that lines the medullary canal

7. Tough membrane on the outside of bone

10. Twelve pairs of bones that surround the heart and lungs

11. Lateral bone of the lower leg

14. Two bones that form the pelvic girdle

15. Connective tissue band that holds bones together

16. Wrist bone

20. Material inside the medullary canal

22. Eight bones that surround and protect the brain

24. Lower arm bone on thumb side

25. Bones that form the extremities

DOWN

1. Breastbone

2. Thigh bone

3. Material found in some bones that produces blood cells

5. Anklebone

6. Larger bone of lower arm

8. Air spaces in the bones of the skull

9. An extremity or end of bone

12. Bones that form the main trunk of the body

13. Long shaft of bones

17. Upper arm bone

18. Twenty-six bones of the spinal column

19. Area where two or more bones join together

21. Shoulder bone or shoulder blade

23. Medial bone of the lower leg

2. List five (5) functions of bones.

3. Name the eight (8) bones that form the cranium.

4. Name the twenty-six (26) vertebrae.

5. What is the difference between true ribs, false ribs, and floating ribs?

6. What is the name of the small piece of cartilage at the bottom of the sternum?

7. What are the three (3) regions on each os coxae?

8. Name the three (3) main types of joints. Describe the degree of movement, and give an example for each type.

9. What is the purpose of ligaments?

10. Briefly describe the following diseases or disorders of the skeletal system.
    a. arthritis:

    b. fractures:

    c. osteomyelitis:

    d. osteoporosis:

    e. sprain:

    f. bursitis:

    g. dislocation:

    h. scoliosis:

Name _____

11. Label the skeleton with the correct names for all of the bones.

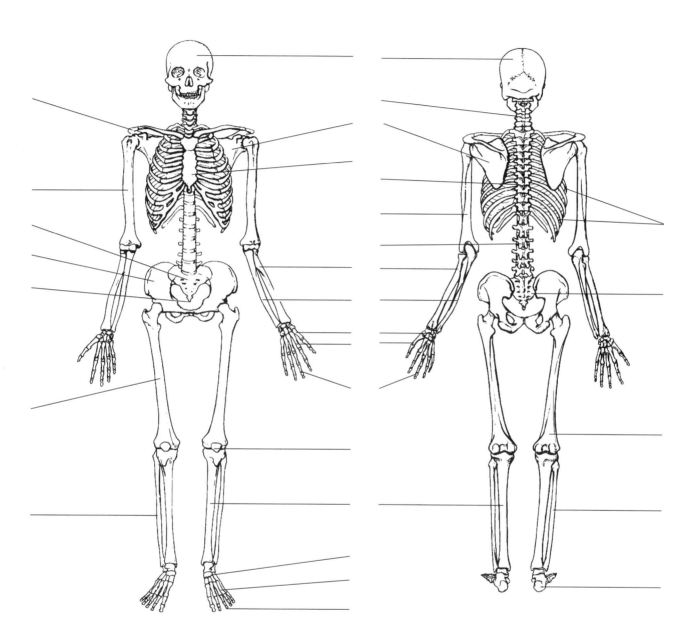

45

ASSIGNMENT SHEET

Grade _____ Name _____

INTRODUCTION: The muscular system provides movement for the body. This assignment will help you review the main facts about this system.

INSTRUCTIONS: Read the information on the Muscular System. In the space provided, print the word(s) that best completes the statement or answers the question.

1. Identify each of the following properties or characteristics of muscles.

    a. ability to respond to a stimulus:

    b. ability to be stretched:

    c. ability to become short and thick:

    d. ability to return to its original shape:

2. List the three (3) main kinds of muscles and the main function of each kind.

3. What is the difference between voluntary and involuntary muscles?

4. List four (4) functions of skeletal muscles.

5. Name two (2) ways skeletal muscles attach to bones.

6. Identify the following action or movement performed by muscles.

    a. decreasing the angle between two bones:

    b. swinging the arm around in a circle:

    c. moving a body part toward the midline:

    d. bending the lower arm up towards the upper arm:

    e. moving the arm away from the side of the body:

    f. straightening the lower leg away from the upper leg:

    g. increasing the angle between two bones:

    h. turning a body part on its own axis:

    i. moving the leg in toward the body:

    j. turning the head from side to side:

7. What is muscle tone?

8. What occurs when muscles atrophy? What causes muscles to atrophy?

9. What is a contracture?

   Name the joints affected most frequently by contractures.

10. Name the following muscles.
    a. muscle of upper arm that flexes lower arm:
    b. muscle on front of thigh that abducts and flexes leg:
    c. muscle on upper back and neck that extends head and moves shoulder:
    d. muscles between ribs used for breathing:
    e. muscle on front of lower leg that flexes and inverts the foot:
    f. two muscles that can be used as injection sites:
    g. muscle that compresses the abdomen:
    h. muscle on upper chest that adducts upper arm:
    i. muscle on side of neck that turns and flexes head:
    j. muscle on front of thigh that extends leg:

11. Unscramble the following words to identify some diseases of the muscular system. Then give a brief description of each disease.
    a. LUMCSE PASMSS:

    b. CASMULRU PTSDOHYRY:

    c. YAHMTNSIEA RVGISA:

    d. RISATN:

    e. GIBOYLFIRAMA:

UNIT 6:6 NERVOUS SYSTEM

ASSIGNMENT SHEET

Grade _____   Name _____

INTRODUCTION: The nervous system coordinates all of the activities of the body. This assignment will help you review the main facts about this system.

INSTRUCTIONS: Read the information on the Nervous System. In the space provided, print the word(s) that best completes the statement or answers the question.

1. Some of the Key Terms are hidden in the following puzzle. Can you find the following terms?

autonomic nervous system	nerve
brain	neuron
central nervous system	parasympathetic
cerebellum	peripheral nervous system
cerebrospinal fluid	pons
cerebrum	spinal cord
medulla oblongata	sympathetic
meninge	ventricle
midbrain	

```
S E T P A R A S Y M P A T H E T I C M I U B E M S D
A V N E M R U R E N T H E C M R S E D T I C E I L W
T X Q R Z D E I U T E L C I R T N E V X L O V D E S
A I D I U L F L A N I P S O R B E R E C M M E B R F
G L O P Y D J O S E S H A R O L U O U I S E X R W T
N A N H N I A M A R K A R E C E R E B R U M C A E R
O E C E R E B E L L U M B R U M O S Y S T O M I T H
L I S R I S C R A Z E N A N D I N A M N O T S N U R
B E W A H Y I A M D O E I M G I D R O C L A N I P S
O T B L U T Y G U E S R S H A V U N R I C T K E O X
A C E N T R A L N E R V O U S S Y S T E M W O G N U
L L D E U N D E R B L E O O D L Y M P H E R Y N S P
L S B R A I N P I C I T E H T A P M Y S N A L I C O
U R D V N A T O P H Y S I O L E G E E R T S D N M I
D D I O V E R S I O C C F E D I P A Y T I O N E L J
E X A U T O N O M I C N E R V O U S S Y S T E M M H
M C A S Y S T E M N Y O U F I N D T H E W O R D S I
```

2. The basic structural unit of the nervous system is the _____. It consists of a cell body that contains the _____, nerve fibers called _____, which carry impulses toward the cell body, and a single nerve fiber called a/an _____, which carries impulses away from the cell body. Many axons have a lipid covering called a/an _____, which increases the rate of transmission of a/an _____, and _____ and _____ the axon.

3. What is a synapse?

4. Identify all of the parts of the brain shown on the diagram. Briefly state the function of each part.

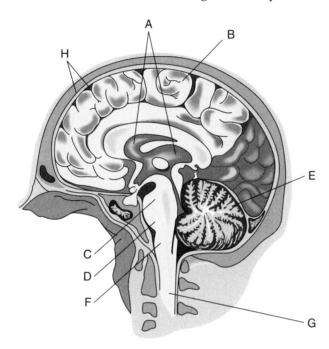

A.

B.

C.

D.

E.

F.

G.

H.

5. Name the three (3) layers of the meninges.

   What is the function of the meninges?

6. List two (2) functions of cerebrospinal fluid.

7. The peripheral nervous system consists of the _____ and the _____ nervous systems. The somatic nervous system consists of 12 pairs of _____ and 31 pairs of _____.

8. State the actions that the sympathetic and parasympathetic nervous systems have on the following functions of the body.

	Sympathetic	Parasympathetic
heart rate		
respirations		
blood pressure		
digestive activity		

9. What is homeostasis?

10. Briefly describe the following diseases of the nervous system.

   a. paraplegia:

   b. encephalitis:

   c. hydrocephalus:

   d. neuralgia:

   e. cerebrovascular accident:

   f. epilepsy:

   g. cerebral palsy:

   h. Parkinson's disease:

ASSIGNMENT SHEET

Grade _____ Name _____

INTRODUCTION: Special senses allow the human body to react to the environment. This assignment will help you review the main facts about these senses.

INSTRUCTIONS: Read the information on Special Senses. In the space provided, print the word(s) that best completes the statement or answers the question.

1. Special senses occur because the body has organs that receive _____, nerves that carry the message to the _____, and a brain that _____ and _____ to the message.

2. Label the following diagram of the eye and briefly state the function of each part.

Ciliary muscle

Muscles of eyeball

D

G

H

Path of Light

F

E

I

J

C

Retinal Arteries and Veins

Optic Nerve

B

A

A.   F.

B.   G.

C.   H.

D.   I.

E.   J.

3. List four (4) things that protect the eye.

4. Name five (5) parts of the eye that light rays pass through to focus on the retina.

   What happens if these parts do not refract the light rays correctly?

5. Name the following eye diseases.
   a. blurred vision due to an abnormal shape or curvature in the cornea:
   b. excess pressure in the eye due to an excess amount of aqueous humor:
   c. nearsightedness:
   d. crossed eyes due to a lack of coordination in eye muscles:
   e. lens become cloudy or opaque:
   f. contagious inflammation of conjunctiva:
   g. farsightedness caused by a loss of elasticity in lens:

6. What is cerumen? What is its function?

7. What is the correct name for the eardrum? What does it do?

8. Name the three (3) bones or ossicles of the middle ear.

9. What is the auditory (eustachian) tube? What does it do?

10. State the function of the following parts of the inner ear.
    a. vestibule:

    b. cochlea:

    c. organ of Corti:

    d. semicircular canals:

Name _____

11. An infection of the middle ear is _____. A hearing loss due to lack of movement of the stapes is _____. If sound waves are not being conducted to the inner ear, this causes a/an _____ hearing loss or deafness. Damage to the inner ear or auditory nerve causes a/an _____ hearing loss or deafness.

12. List the four (4) main tastes. Where are they located on the tongue?

13. What determines the sense of smell?

14. Name four (4) general sense receptors located throughout the body.

ASSIGNMENT SHEET

Grade _____ Name _____

INTRODUCTION: The circulatory system is often called the transportation system of the body. This assignment will help you review the main facts on this system.

INSTRUCTIONS: Read the information on the Circulatory System. In the space provided, print the word(s) that best answers the question or completes the statement.

1. Use the Key Terms to complete the crossword puzzle.

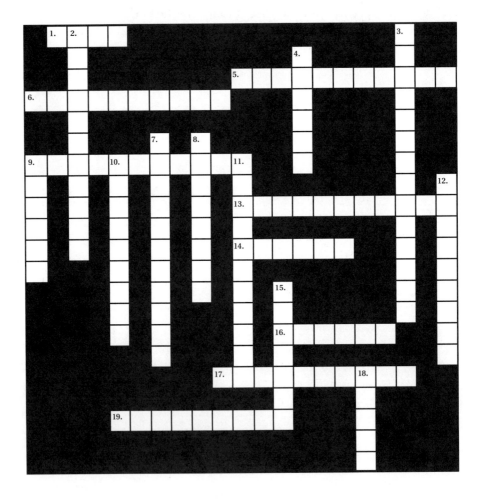

ACROSS

1. Blood vessel that carries blood back to the heart

5. Valve between the left ventricle and aorta

6. Muscular middle layer of the heart

9. Double-layered membrane on the outside of the heart

13. Blood cell required for the clotting process

14. Blood vessel that carries blood away from the heart

16. Muscular wall that separates the heart into a right and left side

17. Complex protein on red blood cells

19. Lower chamber of the heart

DOWN

2. Smooth layer of cells lining the inside of the heart

3. Valve between the right ventricle and pulmonary artery

4. Upper chamber of the heart

7. Blood cell that carries oxygen and carbon dioxide

8. Brief period of rest in the heart

9. Fluid portion of blood

10. Blood vessel that connects arterioles with venules

11. Valve between the left atrium and left ventricle

12. Blood cell that helps fight infection

15. Period of ventricular contraction in the heart

18. Tissue that flows through the circulatory system

2. Label the following diagram of the heart.

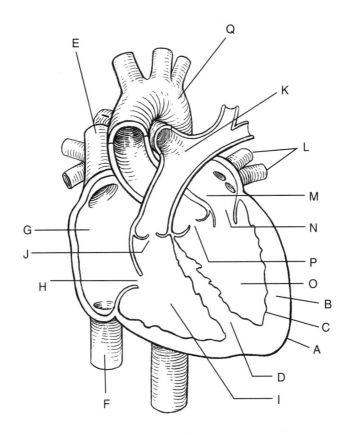

A.   J.

B.   K.

C.   L.

D.   M.

E.   N.

F.   O.

G.   P.

H.   Q.

I.

3. Describe what happens in the heart during diastole.

4. Describe what happens in the heart during systole. State where each ventricle sends the blood.

5. List the parts of the conductive pathway for electrical impulses in the heart. List the parts in correct order.

6. What is arrhythmia? How is it diagnosed?

7. Identify the following blood vessels:

   a. blood vessels that carry blood away from the heart:

   b. blood vessels that carry blood back to the heart:

   c. blood vessels that connect arterioles with venules:

   d. largest artery in the body:

   e. two largest veins in the body:

   f. vessels that allow oxygen and nutrients to pass through to cells:

   g. smallest branches of arteries:

   h. smallest branches of veins:

   i. vessels that contain valves to prevent backflow of blood:

   j. most muscular and elastic blood vessels:

8. List five (5) substances transported by the blood.

9. List five (5) substances that are dissolved or suspended in plasma.

10. Name the three (3) main types of blood cells. State the normal count and the function of each type.

Blood Cell	Normal Count Per Cubic Millimeter of Blood	Function

11. What gives blood its characteristic red color?

12. What is hemoglobin? What is its function?

13. Identify the type of leukocyte(s) that performs the following function.

    a. phagocytize bacteria:

    b. provide immunity for the body by developing antibodies:

    c. defend the body from allergic reactions:

    d. produce histamine and heparin:

14. Name the following diseases of the circulatory system.

    a. saclike formation in the wall of an artery:

    b. inadequate number of red blood cells, hemoglobin, or both:

    c. dilated swollen veins:

    d. a fatty deposit on the walls of arteries:

    e. disease characterized by failure of the blood to clot:

    f. high blood pressure:

    g. inflammation of the veins with formation of a clot:

    h. blockage in the coronary arteries of the heart:

    i. foreign substance circulating in the blood stream:

    j. malignant disease with large numbers of immature white blood cells:

UNIT 6:9 LYMPHATIC SYSTEM

ASSIGNMENT SHEET

Grade _____   Name _____

INTRODUCTION: The lymphatic system works with the circulatory system to remove waste and excess fluid from the tissues. This assignment will help you review the main facts about this system.

INSTRUCTIONS: Read the information on the Lymphatic System. In the space provided, print the word(s) that best completes the statement or answers the question.

1. What is lymph? Of what is it composed?

2. Small, open-ended lymph vessels called _____ pick up _____ at tissues throughout the body. They join together to form larger _____, which pass through _____.

3. What keeps the lymph flowing in a one-way direction while it is in the lymphatic vessels?

4. What are lacteals? What do they do?

5. Name four (4) substances that are filtered from the lymph while it is in lymph nodes.

6. Name two (2) things produced by the lymph tissues in lymph nodes.

7. Name the two (2) lymphatic ducts and the areas of the body that they drain.

8. What is the cisterni chyli? Where is it located?

9. The purified lymph, with lymphocytes and antibodies added, returns to the _____ when it leaves the lymphatic ducts. The right lymphatic duct empties the purified lymph into the _____, and the thoracic duct empties into the _____.

10. List the three (3) types of tonsils and state where they are located.

11. List four (4) functions of the spleen.

12. What is the thymus? What happens to it at puberty?

13. Name the following diseases of the lymphatic system.
   a. inflammation or infection of the lymph nodes or glands:
   b. chronic malignant condition with enlargement of lymph nodes:
   c. enlargement of the spleen:
   d. inflammation of the tonsils:
   e. inflammation of lymphatic vessels:

UNIT 6:10 RESPIRATORY SYSTEM

ASSIGNMENT SHEET

Grade _____ Name _____

INTRODUCTION: The respiratory system is responsible for taking in oxygen and removing carbon dioxide from the body. This assignment will help you review the main facts about this system.

INSTRUCTIONS: Read the information on the Respiratory System. In the space provided, print the word(s) that best completes the statement or answers the question.

1. Label the following diagram of the respiratory system.

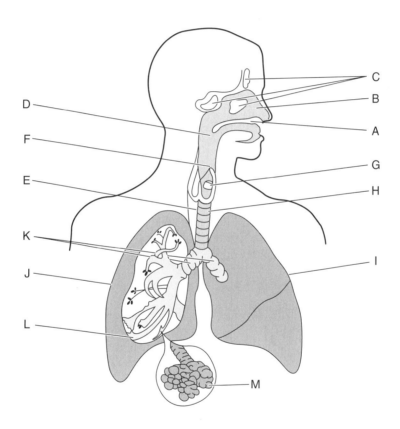

A.

B.

C.

D.

E.

F.

G.

H.

I.

J.

K.

L.

M.

2. List three (3) things that happen to air when it enters the nasal cavity.

3. What are cilia? What do they do?

4. Name the three (3) sections of the pharynx.

5. How is sound or speech produced?

6. What prevents food and liquids from entering the respiratory tract?

7. The alveoli contains a rich network of _____. They allow for the exchange of _____ and _____ between the bloodstream and the lungs. The inner surfaces of the alveoli are covered with a lipid substance called _____ to help prevent the alveoli from collapsing.

8. Why is the left lung smaller than the right lung?

9. Describe what is happening during each of the following phases of respiration. Be sure to include the actions of the muscles during each phase.

    a. inspiration:

    b. expiration:

10. How does external respiration differ from internal respiration?

11. What causes the respiratory center in the medulla oblongata of the brain to increase the rate of respirations?

12. Use the names of respiratory diseases to fill in the blanks.

_ R _ _ _ _ _ _ _ (inflammation of bronchi and bronchial tubes)

_ _ _ _ _ E _ _ _ (highly contagious viral infection)

_ _ _ _ S _ _ _ _ (inflammation of mucous membrane lining sinuses)

_ _ P _ _ _ _ _ (walls of alveoli deteriorate and lose their elasticity)

_ _ I _ _ _ _ _ _ (a nosebleed)

_ _ _ _ R _ _ _ _ _ _ _ (infectious lung disease caused by bacteria)

_ _ _ _ _ A (bronchospasms narrow the openings of the bronchioles)

_ _ _ _ _ T _ _ (inflammation of nasal mucous membranes)

_ O _ _ (any chronic lung disease that results in obstruction of the airways)

_ _ _ _ R _ _ _ (inflammation of membranes of the lungs)

_ _ _ Y _ _ _ _ _ _ (inflammation of the voicebox and vocal cords)

UNIT 6:11 DIGESTIVE SYSTEM

ASSIGNMENT SHEET

Grade _____   Name _____

INTRODUCTION: The digestive system is responsible for the breakdown of food so it can be taken into the blood-stream and used by body cells and tissues. This assignment will help you review the main facts about this system.

INSTRUCTIONS: Read the information on the Digestive System. In the space provided, print the word(s) that best completes the statement or answers the question.

1. Label the diagram of the digestive system.

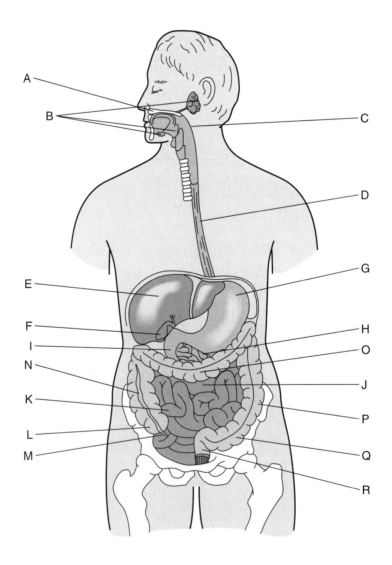

A.   J.

B.   K.

C.   L.

D.   M.

E.   N.

F.   O.

G.   P.

H.   Q.

I.   R.

2. List two (2) functions of the tongue.

3. What is mastication?

4. Three pairs of salivary glands, the _____, _____, and the _____ produce saliva that _____ the mouth during speech and chewing and _____ food so
   it can be swallowed easily. Saliva also contains an enzyme called _____, which begins the
   chemical breakdown of _____ or _____. After the food is chewed and mixed with
   saliva, it is called a _____.

5. What is the wavelike involuntary movement of muscles that causes the food to move in a
   forward direction through the digestive tract?

6. List four (4) things that happen in the stomach during digestion.

7. What do the following digestive juices or enzymes do to food while it is in the small intestine?

   a. maltase:

   b. sucrase:

   c. peptidases:

   d. bile:

   e. pancreatic amylase:

   f. trypsin:

   g. lipase:

8. Fingerlike projections in the small intestine, called _____, contain _____ and _____. The blood capillaries absorb most of the _____, while the lacteals absorb most of the digested _____.

9. List three (3) functions of the large intestine.

10. Name the four (4) divisions of the colon.

11. List five (5) functions of the liver.

12. What is the function of the gallbladder?

13. What is the glandular organ behind the stomach?

    What two (2) secretions does it produce?

14. Name the following diseases of the digestive system.
    a. inflammation of the liver usually caused by a virus:
    b. condition characterized by frequent watery stools:
    c. presence of stones in the gallbladder:
    d. chronic disease of the liver in which scar tissue replaces liver cells:
    e. dilated or varicose veins in the rectal or anal area:
    f. inflammatory disease of the colon with formation of ulcers and abscesses:
    g. inflammation of mucous membrane of stomach and intestines:
    h. stomach protrudes through the diaphragm by opening for esophagus:

UNIT 6:12 URINARY SYSTEM

ASSIGNMENT SHEET

Grade _____   Name _____

INTRODUCTION: The urinary system is responsible for removing certain wastes and excess water from the body. This assignment will help you review the main facts about this system.

INSTRUCTIONS: Read the information on the Urinary System. In the space provided, print the word(s) that best completes the statement or answers the question.

1. Label the diagram of the urinary system.

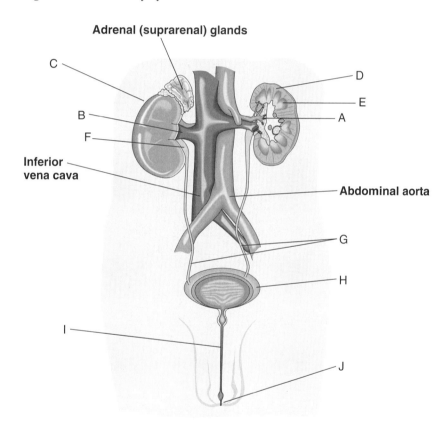

A.	F.
B.	G.
C.	H.
D.	I.
E.	J.

2. Microscopic filtering units in the kidney are called _____. The _____ artery carries blood to the kidney and branches of this artery carry this blood to the first part of the nephron, the _____. As blood passes through this cluster of capillaries, _____, _____, _____, _____ and other substances are filtered out of the blood. The substances filtered out enter the next section of the nephron, _____, which passes the substances into the _____. As these substances pass through various sections of the tubule, substances needed by the body are _____ and returned to blood _____. Excess products such as _____ and _____, some _____, and _____ remain in the tubule and become known as the concentrated waste liquid called _____.

3. What is the rhythmic wavelike motion of the involuntary muscle of the ureter called? What does it do?

4. What are rugae? What is their function?

5. How is the urethra different in males and females?

6. List five (5) waste products found in urine.

7. Define the following terms.

   a. polyuria:

   b. oliguria:

   c. anuria:

   d. hematuria:

   e. nocturia:

   f. dysuria:

   g. retention:

   h. incontinence:

8. An inflammation of the kidney and renal pelvis is called _____. An inflammation of the bladder is _____. The formation of stones is _____. An accumulation of urinary wastes in the blood due to kidney failure is _____.

UNIT 6:13 ENDOCRINE SYSTEM

ASSIGNMENT SHEET

Grade _____ Name _____

INTRODUCTION: The endocrine system is composed of a group of glands that secrete substances that control many body activities. This assignment will help you review the main facts about this system.

INSTRUCTIONS: Read the information on the Endocrine System. In the space provided, print the word(s) that best completes the statement or answers the question.

1. What are hormones?

   How are they transported through the body?

2. List five (5) functions of hormones.

3. Name the endocrine glands located in the following areas of the body.
   a. above each kidney:
   b. on each side of the uterus in the female:
   c. under the brain in the sella turcica:
   d. in front of the upper part of the trachea:
   e. in the scrotal sac of the male:
   f. behind and attached to the thyroid:
   g. glandular organ behind the stomach:

4. Name the hormone that performs the following function.
   a. used in metabolism of glucose:
   b. stimulates secretion of milk:
   c. growth hormone, stimulates normal body growth:
   d. regulates amount of calcium in the blood:
   e. stimulates growth and development of sex organs in male:
   f. increases metabolic rate, stimulates physical and mental growth:
   g. stimulates growth and secretion of the thyroid gland:

h. activates the sympathetic nervous system:

i. antidiuretic, promotes reabsorption of water in kidneys:

j. regulates reabsorption of sodium in kidney and elimination of potassium:

k. promotes growth and development of sex organs in female:

l. maintains lining of uterus:

5. Various diseases are listed below. Place the letter of the endocrine gland in Column B that is affected by each disease in the space provided by the disease in Column A.

Column A

1. _____ Diabetes mellitus

2. _____ Cushing's syndrome

3. _____ Giantism

4. _____ Hyperthyroidism

5. _____ Addison's disease

6. _____ Acromegaly

7. _____ Hypoparathyroidism

8. _____ Cretinism

9. _____ Dwarfism

10. _____ Goiter

Column B

A. Adrenal

B. Pancreas

C. Parathyroid

D. Pituitary

E. Thyroid

6. What is the thymus? What is its function?

7. What is the name of the temporary endocrine gland produced during pregnancy? What happens to it after the birth of the child?

8. What is the pineal body? What is its function?

9. What are the gonads or sex glands of the male?

What are the gonads of the female?

10. List six (6) symptoms of diabetes mellitus.

UNIT 6:14 REPRODUCTIVE SYSTEM

ASSIGNMENT SHEET

Grade _____   Name _____

INTRODUCTION: The reproductive system is responsible for the creation of new life. This assignment will help you review the main facts about this system.

INSTRUCTIONS: Read the information on the Reproductive System. In the space provided, print the word(s) that best completes the statement or answers the question.

1. Label the parts of the male reproductive system. Briefly state the function of each part.

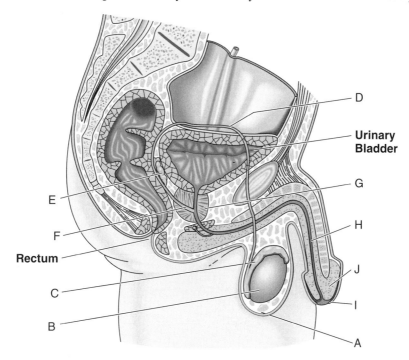

A.

B.

C.

D.

E.

F.

G.

H.

I.

J.

2. Why are the testes suspended outside the body in the scrotal sac?

3. List four (4) organs that produce a secretion that becomes a part of the semen.

4. Which tube is cut to produce sterility in the male?

5. A surgical removal of the prepuce is called a/an _____.

6. Why is testicular self-examination important for all males? How frequently should it be done?

7. Label the parts of the female reproductive system. Briefly state the function of each part.

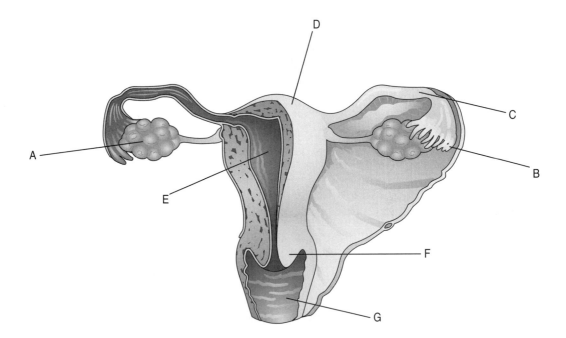

A.

B.

C.

D.

E.

F.

G.

8. What is fertilization? Where does it take place?

9. What two (2) factors keep the ovum moving through the fallopian tube toward the uterus?

10. What is the inner layer of the uterus called?

What happens to this layer if fertilization does not occur?

11. The structures that form the external female genital area are the _____.
The _____ are two folds of fatty tissue covered with hair that
_____ and _____ the vagina. Two smaller folds of
tissue located within the labia majora are the _____. An area of erectile
tissue called the _____ is located at the junction of the labia minora.

12. Why is it important for women to perform breast self-examinations (BSEs)? How frequently and when should a woman do a BSE?

13. List four (4) ways to prevent contracting the human immunodeficiency virus (HIV) that causes acquired immune deficiency syndrome (AIDS).

14. Use the names of diseases of the reproductive systems to complete the crossword puzzle.

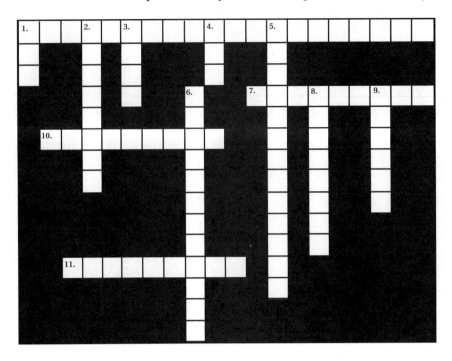

ACROSS

1. Enlargement of the prostate gland

7. STD that produces a greenish-yellow discharge in males

10. STD caused by a bacteria that lives as an intracellular parasite

11. Parasites that are transmitted sexually

DOWN

1. Abbreviation for inflammation of the cervix, endometrium, fallopian tubes, and, at times, ovaries

2. STD caused by a spirochete bacteria

3. Abbreviation for acquired immune deficiency syndrome

4. Abbreviation for the virus that causes AIDS

5. Growth of endometrial tissue outside the uterus

6. Inflammation of the epididymis

8. Inflammation of the testes

9. STD caused by a virus and characterized by fluid-filled vesicles and ulcers

UNIT 7:1 LIFE STAGES

ASSIGNMENT SHEET

Grade _____ Name _____

INTRODUCTION: An understanding of life stages allows a health care worker to meet individual needs and provide quality health care. This assignment will help you gain this understanding.

INSTRUCTIONS: Read the information on Life Stages. In the space provided, print the word(s) that best completes the statement or answers the question.

1. Briefly describe the four main types of growth and development that occur during each of the life stages.

   a. physical:

   b. mental:

   c. emotional:

   d. social:

2. Name the following reflex actions that allow an infant to respond to the environment.

   a. response to a loud noise or sudden movement:

   b. response to a slight touch on the cheek:

   c. response to a slight touch on the lips:

   d. response when an object is placed in the hand:

3. The following developments occur during an infant's first year of life. Put the approximate age at which they occur by the event.

   a. roll from side to back:

   b. sit unsupported for several minutes:

   c. walk without assistance:

   d. understand some words and make basic sounds:

   e. show distress, delight, anger, disgust, and fear:

   f. become shy and withdraw from strangers:

   g. mimic and imitate gestures and facial expressions:

4. The following changes occur during early childhood. List the approximate ages at which they occur.

   a. learn bladder and bowel control:

   b. make decisions based on logic instead of trial and error:

   c. make decisions based on past and present experiences:

   d. display frequent temper tantrums:

   e. show less anxiety when faced with new experiences:

   f. friends of their own age become important:

5. When a two-year-old is admitted to a hospital, why is it important to encourage the parent(s) to bring a familiar object, such as a blanket or favorite toy, with the child?

6. Identify four (4) abstract concepts that children begin to understand in late childhood.

7. What is puberty?

8. List at least three (3) causes of conflict during the emotional development of adolescents.

9. Identify the following eating disorders.
   a. person drastically reduces food intake or refuses to eat:
   b. person alternately eats excessively or refuses to eat:
   c. person uses laxatives or induces vomiting:

10. Identify at least four (4) reasons why people use chemicals or become involved in chemical abuse.

11. A friend says, "I'd rather be dead!" Should you ignore him/her? Why or why not?

12. List at least five (5) major changes or decisions that individuals must make during early adulthood.

13. During middle adulthood, an individual can experience satisfaction or stress. List at least (3) factors that could provide satisfaction and three (3) factors that could produce stress.

<table>
<tr><td>Satisfaction</td><td>Stress</td></tr>
</table>

14. List eight (8) physical changes that might occur during late adulthood.

15. Do all individuals show physical changes of aging in their sixties and seventies? Why or why not?

16. List four (4) events that require emotional adjustment during late adulthood.

UNIT 7:2 DEATH AND DYING

ASSIGNMENT SHEET

Grade _____   Name _____

INTRODUCTION: Death is a part of life, and health care workers must deal with death and dying patients. This assignment will help provide some understanding about death.

INSTRUCTIONS: Read the information on Death and Dying. In the space provided, print the word(s) that best answers the question or completes the statement.

1. What is a terminal illness?

2. Identify three (3) fears that a person with a terminal illness might have.

3. Most medical personnel now feel that a patient _____ be told of his/her approaching death. However, the patient should be left with _____ and the knowledge that they will _____.

4. Identify the stage of dying a person is experiencing with the following statements or behaviors. Place the letter or letters of the stage from Column B in the space provided in Column A.

    Column A   Column B

    1. _____ "No, not me."   A. Acceptance

    2. _____ Promises made to God   B. Anger

    3. _____ Hostile and bitter   C. Bargaining

    4. _____ At peace and ready for death   D. Denial

    5. _____ Experiencing sadness and despair   E. Depression

    6. _____ "I don't believe the doctor."

    7. _____ Needs support and the presence of others

    8. _____ "Just let me live until my grandchild is born."

    9. _____ Withdraw from others

    10. _____ Refuses to discuss illness

    11. _____ Crying frequently

    12. _____ "If my husband would help more, I wouldn't be sick."

5. Do all dying patients progress through the five stages of grieving? Why or why not?

6. Before health care workers can provide care to dying patients, they must first understand their own _____ about death and come to _____ with these feelings.

7. What is the philosophy behind hospice care?

8. List three (3) types of care provided by hospice.

9. What legal documents allow a dying patient to instruct the doctor to withhold treatments that might prolong life?

10. Do you believe in the "right to die"? Why or why not?

UNIT 7:3 HUMAN NEEDS

ASSIGNMENT SHEET

Grade _____ Name _____

INTRODUCTION: It is important for health care workers to be aware of both their own needs and the needs of patients. This assignment will help provide an understanding of basic human needs.

INSTRUCTIONS: Read the information on Human Needs. In the space provided, print the word(s) that completes the statement or answers the question.

1. Explain what is meant by a hierarchy of needs.

2. List six (6) physiological needs.

3. Identify three (3) events that might threaten an individual's safety.

4. Why might a person hesitate to take a job with prestige and a high salary in a hospital located in an area with a high crime rate?

5. Individuals who feel safe and secure are more willing to _____ to change and more willing to face _____.

6. Identify three (3) ways in which the need for affection is satisfied.

7. Define *sexuality*.

8. What policy of long-term care facilities recognizes the fact that sexuality needs do not cease in late adulthood?

9. When does an individual begin to feel esteem and gain self-respect?

10. What is meant by self-actualization?

11. When needs are felt, individuals are _____ to act. If the need is met, _____ occurs. If the need is not met, _____ occurs.

12. A student, currently in the 10th grade, wants to become a respiratory therapist. The student wants to attend a private school that is very expensive. However, money is limited and the tuition is too high for her parents. List the four (4) direct methods of meeting needs and explain how this student could work to become a respiratory therapist by each method.

13. Is the use of defense mechanisms healthy or unhealthy? Why?

14. Create a situation that shows the use of each of the following defense mechanisms.

   a. rationalization:

   b. projection:

   c. displacement:

   d. compensation:

   e. daydreaming:

   f. repression:

   g. suppression:

   h. denial:

   i. withdrawal:

15. You work in a medical laboratory. Mr. Brown is scheduled for a Glucose Tolerance Test that takes three hours to complete and requires that the patient not eat or drink anything after 12 midnight. When Mr. Brown arrives at 9:00 AM for the test, he seems angry and says, "I can't believe this stupid test is going to take three hours. Why does it take so long?"

    a. Why do you think Mr. Brown is angry?

    b. What would you do in this situation?

UNIT 7:4 EFFECTIVE COMMUNICATIONS

ASSIGNMENT SHEET

Grade _____ Name _____

INTRODUCTION: Communicating effectively with others is an important part of any health care. This assignment will help you review the main facts on effective communications.

INSTRUCTIONS: Read the information on Effective Communications. In the space provided, print the word(s) that completes the statement or answers the question.

1. Communication is the exchange of _____, _____, _____, and _____.

2. List four (4) factors that must be met to avoid interfering with the communication process.

3. What is wrong with the following communication processes as they relate to patients?

   a. "I think your problem is cholelithiasis."

   b. Speaking in a very soft, muted tone

   c. Radio playing loudly while pre-operative care is discussed

   d. "I don't got any appointments at that time."

   e. "I don't know. Who cares?"

   f. Interrupting before the patient has finished speaking

4. Define *listening.*

5. Why does reflecting statements back to the speaker help in the communication process?

6. Nonverbal communication involves the use of _____, _____, and _____ to convey messages or ideas.

7. Why is it important to observe a person's nonverbal behavior?

8. Identify three (3) nonverbal ways a person can convey interest and caring.

9. List three (3) common causes of communication barriers.

10. Identify four (4) ways to improve communications with a person who is blind or visually impaired.

11. What is a common cause of anger or a negative attitude?

    List four (4) ways you can deal with an angry patient.

12. What is culture?

13. How can you deal with or react to the following situations?
    a. You are preparing a patient for surgery and all jewelry must be removed. A patient refuses to remove a religious neck chain.

    b. A patient tells you, "I don't believe in God."

    c. A patient constantly avoids eye contact while you are talking to her.

d. A patient with limited English nods his head but still seems confused as you explain a procedure.

14. Identify three (3) main barriers created by cultural diversity.

15. List four (4) senses a health care worker can use to make observations.

16. Differentiate between subjective and objective observations.

17. How should an error on a health care record be corrected?

18. Identify four (4) benefits patients experience when health care workers have effective communication skills.

UNIT 8 CULTURAL DIVERSITY

ASSIGNMENT SHEET

Grade _____ Name _____

INTRODUCTION: Every health care provider must be aware of the factors that cause each individual to be unique. This assignment will help you learn these factors.

INSTRUCTIONS: Read the information on Cultural Diversity. In the space provided, print the word(s) that best completes the statement or answers the question.

1. Define *culture*.

2. List the four (4) basic characteristics of culture.

3. A classification of people based on national origin and/or culture is _____. A classification of people based on physical or biological characteristics is _____. The differences among people resulting from cultural, ethnic, and racial factors is_____.

4. Do you think the United States is a "multicultural" society? Why or why not?

5. Label each of the following statements as a bias, prejudice, or stereotype.

   a. All fat people are lazy.

   b. Chemotherapy is much better than radiation to treat cancer.

c. Herbal remedies are a waste of money.

d. All teenagers are reckless drivers.

e. He must be really stupid because he does not know how to use the Internet.

f. Baptists are better Christians than Lutherans.

6. Identify six (6) ways to avoid bias, prejudice, and stereotyping.

7. What is holistic care?

8. Identify five (5) areas of cultural diversity.

9. Identify the following types of family organization.

   a. father is the authority figure:

   b. family consists of mother, father, and two children:

   c. parents, children, and grandparents all live in one home:

   d. mother is the authority figure:

10. Identify the culture(s) that may have the following health care beliefs.

   a. illness is caused by an imbalance between yin and yang:

   b. wearing an Azabache will treat disease:

   c. health is harmony between man and nature:

   d. health is a balance between "hot and cold" forces:

   e. evil spirits or evil "eye" cause illness:

   f. lack of cleanliness causes illness:

   g. pain must be accepted and endured silently:

   h. tolerating pain is a sign of strength:

   i. males make decisions on the health care of the family:

   j. shaman or medicine man is the traditional healer:

   k. health can be maintained by diet, rest, and exercise:

11. Are spirituality and religion the same? Why or why not?

12. Why is it important for a health care provider to be aware of the beliefs about death in different religions?

13. Name two (2) religions that may prohibit blood transfusions.

14. A person who does not believe in any deity is a/an _____. A person who believes the existence of God cannot be proved or disproved is a/an _____.

15. List eight (8) ways to respect cultural diversity by appreciating and respecting the personal characteristics of others.

16. How would you respond to the following situations?

    a. You work as a dental assistant and attempt to explain pre-operative instructions to a patient who is scheduled for oral surgery. He has limited English-speaking abilities and is nodding his head yes, but he does not seem to understand the instructions.

    b. You work as a medical assistant and prepare a patient for a gynecological exam. She insists her husband must be in the room and states she will not undress until her husband is present.

    c. You work as a surgical technician and prepare a patient for surgery. When you tell her she must remove all jewelry, she says she never removes her cross necklace.

    d. You work as an electrocardiograph technician and a patient has given you permission to perform an electrocardiogram. As you start to position the electrodes for each of the leads, the patient becomes very tense, pulls his arm away, and appears anxious and very nervous.

    e. You have just started working as a geriatric assistant. As you prepare to bathe a patient, she tells you that she will wait until her daughter arrives and that her daughter will help her with her bath.

UNIT 9:1 MYTHS ON AGING

ASSIGNMENT SHEET

Grade _____ Name _____

INTRODUCTION: There are many myths about aging and elderly individuals. This assignment will help you distinguish between myths and facts.

INSTRUCTIONS: Read the information on Myths on Aging. Then read the statements below. If the statement is a fact, put a check in the "Fact" column. If the statement is a myth, put a check in the "Myth" column. Then write why the statement is a myth in the space provided.

Fact   Myth

_____   _____   1. Aging is a normal process that leads to normal changes in body structure and function.

_____   _____   2. Most elderly individuals experience confusion and disorientation.

_____   _____   3. Over 2 million people will be cared for in long-term care facilities by the year 2005.

_____   _____   4. Many individuals are active, productive, and self-sufficient into their eighties and nineties.

_____   _____   5. The majority of the elderly live in poverty.

_____   _____   6. Older people are usually lonely and unhappy.

_____   _____   7. Most individuals lose interest in work at age 60 and make plans to retire.

_____   _____   8. Old age begins at age 65.

_____   _____   9. Most elderly individuals live in their own home or apartment or with other family members.

_____   _____   10. Retired people are usually bored and have nothing to do with their lives.

UNIT 9:2 PHYSICAL CHANGES OF AGING

ASSIGNMENT SHEET

Grade _____   Name _____

INTRODUCTION: Physical changes are a normal part of the aging process. This assignment will help you learn the main physical changes.

INSTRUCTIONS: Read the information on Physical Changes of Aging. In the space provided, print the word(s) that best completes the statement or answers the question.

1. Most physical changes that occur with aging are _____ and take place over a/an _____ of time. In addition, the _____ and _____ of change varies with different individuals. Previous _____, _____, _____ status, and _____ environment can also have an effect. If an individual can recognize the changes as a/an _____ part of aging, the individual can usually learn to _____ and _____ with the changes.

2. List three (3) physical changes that may occur in each of the following systems.

   a. integumentary:

   b. musculoskeletal:

   c. circulatory:

   d. respiratory:

   e. nervous:

   f. digestive:

   g. urinary:

   h. endocrine:

   i. reproductive:

3. Identify the following common diseases or conditions in the elderly.

   a. calcium and minerals are lost from bones and bones become brittle and more likely to fracture:

   b. inflammation of the joints:

   c. formation of a blood clot:

   d. alveoli lose their elasticity:

   e. lens of eye becomes cloudy or opague:

   f. increased intraocular pressure in the eye:

   g. difficulty in swallowing:

   h. inability to control urination:

   i. dark yellow or brown colored spots on the skin:

4. In each of the following situations, a physical change of aging has occurred. Briefly describe how a health care worker can assist the individual in learning how to cope or adapt to the change.

   a. Mrs. Darbey complains of dry and itchy skin.

   b. Mr. Polinski constantly complains of feeling cold.

   c. Mr. Stark is irritable and tired during the day because he gets up three or four times at night to urinate.

   d. Because of arthritis, Mrs. Mendosa is unable to button her blouses. However, she insists on dressing herself.

   e. Mr. Pease lives at home but refuses to take a bath. He is afraid of falling in the tub.

   f. Mrs. Webber refuses to sleep in a bed because she becomes short of breath while lying down.

   g. Mr. Chang uses excessive salt, pepper, and sugar on all of his food but still complains that the food has no taste.

   h. Mrs. Pearce wants to exercise and walk two miles each day, but she gets very tired and short of breath.

   i. Mr. Mende constantly talks very loudly and asks everyone to speak up or repeat what has been said.

   j. Mrs. Valentino refuses to leave her room because she says, "I have been wetting my pants, and it is embarrassing."

UNIT 9:3 PSYCHOSOCIAL CHANGES OF AGING

ASSIGNMENT SHEET

Grade _____ Name _____

INTRODUCTION: Elderly individuals experience psychological and social changes along with physical changes. This assignment will help provide an understanding of these changes.

INSTRUCTIONS: Read the information on Psychosocial Changes in Aging. In the space provided, print the word(s) that best completes the statement or answers the question.

1. Some individuals cope with psychosocial changes, and others experience extreme
   _____ and _____.

2. List two (2) things a person might do after retirement to find a satisfactory replacement for the role their job played.

3. List three (3) causes for the sense of loss some individuals feel at retirement.

4. Identify two (2) factors that can cause a change in social relationships for an elderly individual.

5. Identify two (2) ways an individual can adjust to social changes when a spouse and friends die.

6. Why does a move to a long-term care facility usually create stress in elderly individuals?

7. Identify two (2) ways an individual can be given the opportunity to create a "home" environment in a long-term care facility.

8. List three (3) factors that can lead to a loss of independence in the elderly.

Name _____

9. How can a health care worker allow an elderly individual as much independence as possible?

10. How does a disease differ from a disability?

11. Identify four (4) fears experienced by a sick person.

12. Identify two (2) ways a health care worker can help an individual deal with the fears created by an illness.

UNIT 9:4 CONFUSION AND DISORIENTATION IN THE ELDERLY

ASSIGNMENT SHEET

Grade _____ Name _____

INTRODUCTION: This assignment will help you gain an understanding of how to care for a confused or disorientated individual.

INSTRUCTIONS: Read the information on Confusion and Disorientation in the Elderly. In the space provided, print the word(s) that best completes the statement or answers the question.

1. List six (6) signs of confusion or disorientation.

2. Name six (6) causes of temporary confusion or disorientation.

3. Name the following diseases that can cause chronic confusion or disorientation.

   a. blood clot obstructs blood flow to brain:

   b. walls of blood vessels become thick and lose elasticity:

   c. walls of blood vessels become narrow due to deposits of fat and minerals:

4. How does acute dementia differ from chronic dementia?

5. Each of the following changes can occur in a patient with Alzheimer's disease. Identify the stage at which the change occurs by putting "early," "middle," or "terminal" by each symptom.

   a. paranoia and hallucinations increase:

   b. incoherent and not able to communicate with words:

   c. total disorientation regarding person, time, and place:

   d. inability to plan and follow through with activities of daily living:

   e. restlessness at night:

   f. loses control of bladder and bowel function:

g. mood and personality changes:

h. personal hygiene ignored:

6. Certain aspects of care should be followed with any confused or disorientated individual. Provide a/an _____ and _____ environment, follow the same _____, keep activities _____, and avoid loud _____, _____ rooms, and excessive _____. Promote awareness of person, time, and place by providing _____.

7. How can a health care worker use reality orientation to correct or improve the following situations?

a. Mrs. Kupin is confused about time and cannot read her watch.

b. Mrs. Mendez wants to sleep all day and wander all night.

c. Many assistants call Mr. Blanton "Grandpa," and he does not know his name.

d. Mr. Pearson keeps calling you "Janet," which is his wife's name.

e. Mrs. Handwork likes to walk in the hall but cannot find her own room. She does recognize pictures of herself.

f. Mrs. Zimmerman wears a hearing aid but does not appear to hear most conversations.

8. True-False: Circle the T if the statement is true. Circle the F if the statement is false.

T   F   a. Caring for a confused or disoriented individual can be frustrating and even frightening.

T   F   b. Transient ischemic attacks (TIAs) cause a temporary period of diminished blood flow to the brain.

T   F   c. Elderly individuals are more sensitive to medications.

T   F   d. A high fever can cause chronic dementia.

T   F   e. Alzheimer's disease is caused by a genetic defect.

T   F   f. Bingo games and large group activities help a confused individual by providing mental stimulation.

T   F   g. When a disoriented patient makes an incorrect statement, agree with the patient.

T   F   h. Patience, consistency, and sincere caring are essential when dealing with confusion and disorientation.

UNIT 9:5 MEETING THE NEEDS OF THE ELDERLY

ASSIGNMENT SHEET

Grade _____ Name _____

INTRODUCTION: This assignment will help you to identify and learn how to meet the needs of an elderly individual.

INSTRUCTIONS: Read the information on Meeting the Needs of the Elderly. In the space provided, print the word(s) that best completes the statement or answers the question.

1. Elderly individuals have the same _____ and _____ needs of any person at any age. However, these needs are sometimes intensified by _____ or _____ changes that disrupt the normal life pattern.

2. List six (6) areas that can be affected by an individual's culture.

3. The spiritual beliefs and practices of an individual are called their _____. It is important to accept an individual's belief without _____, and that health care workers not force their own _____ on the individuals they are caring for.

4. List three (3) ways a health care worker can show respect and consideration of a person's religious beliefs.

5. Identify four (4) types of abuse.

6. You see a fellow worker push Mr. Davis into a chair and say, "I am sick and tired of your wandering outside. You stay in this chair until I get back or I'll tie you in."

   What type(s) of abuse might this represent?

   What should you do?

7. You work as a medical assistant. A daughter, who brings her mother, Mrs. Kupin, to the office says, "She wets the bed constantly, and I can't stand it any more." Mrs. Kupin is 92 years old and lives with her daughter. As you help prepare her for an examination, you observe that she is very thin, has bruises and scratches on her arms and legs, and seems confused. Mrs. Kupin asks, "Where am I? Is this a nursing home?"

What type(s) of abuse might this represent?

What should you do?

8. Why do elderly individuals who are abused hesitate or refuse to report abuse?

9. Why are patients' rights important?

10. In its Older Americans Act, the federal government established a/an _____ Program. This is a specially trained individual who may _____ and try to _____ complaints, suggest _____ for health care, _____ and _____ state and/or federal regulations, report _____ to the correct agency, and provide _____ for individuals involved in the care of the elderly.

ASSIGNMENT SHEET

Grade _____   Name _____

INTRODUCTION: A solid understanding of basic nutrition is essential for a health care worker. This assignment will help you review the main facts about proper nutrition and its relationship to good health.

INSTRUCTIONS: Read the information on Nutrition and Diets. Then follow the directions by each section to complete this assignment.

A. Matching: Place the letter of the correct word in Column B in the space provided by the definitions in Column A.

Column A	Column B
____ 1. state or condition of one's nutrition	A. absorption
____ 2. high blood pressure	B anorexia
____ 3. state of poor nutrition caused by diet or illness	C. atherosclerosis
____ 4. commonly called starches or sugars, major source of energy	D. carbohydrates
____ 5. fatty substance found in body cells and animal fats	E. cholesterol
____ 6. essential nutrients that build and repair tissue and provide heat or energy	F. digestion
____ 7. process of breaking down food into smaller parts and changing it chemically	G. fats
____ 8. process where blood capillaries pick up digested nutrients	H. hypertension
____ 9. loss of appetite	I. hypotension
____ 10. modifications of normal diet used to improve specific health conditions	J. malnutrition
	K. metabolism
	L. minerals
	M. nutritional status
	N. proteins
	O. regular diet
	P. therapeutic diet

B. Completion and Short Answer: In the space provided, print the word(s) that best completes the statement or answers the question.

1. List at least four (4) immediate effects of good nutrition.

2. A condition in which bones become porous and break easily is called _____.

3. The fibrous indigestible form of carbohydrate that provides bulk in the digestive tract is
_____.

4. List four (4) functions of fats.

5. What is the difference between saturated and unsaturated fats?

   List four (4) examples of saturated fats.

   List three (3) examples of polyunsaturated fats.

6. List three (3) functions of proteins.

   What is the difference between complete and incomplete proteins?

7. Vitamins that dissolve in water and are easily destroyed by cooking, air, and light are called
_____. Vitamins that dissolve in fat and are not easily destroyed by cooking, air, and light are called _____.

8. Identify the vitamin that performs the function listed.
   a. aids in wound healing:
   b. normal clotting of the blood:
   c. production of healthy red blood cells and metabolism:
   d. builds and maintains bones and teeth:
   e. healthy mouth tissues and eyes:
   f. structure and function of cells of skin and mucous membrane:
   g. protection of cell structure, especially red blood cells:
   h. production of antibodies:

9. Identify the mineral(s) that performs the function listed.
   a. formation of hemoglobin on red blood cells:
   b. regular heart rhythm:
   c. clotting of the blood:
   d. formation of hormones in thyroid gland:
   e. develop and maintain bones and teeth:

Name _____

    f. healthy muscles and nerves:

    g. formation of hydrochloric acid:

    h. component of enzymes and insulin:

10. Identify four (4) functions of water.

    How many glasses of water should the average person drink per day?

11. What is the difference between digestion and absorption?

12. The unit of measurement used to measure the amount of heat produced during metabolism is a/an _____.

13. List four (4) factors that cause calorie requirements to vary from person to person.

14. An individual who wants to lose weight should increase _____ and decrease _____.

15. Calculate the number of calories your body requires daily to maintain your current weight. To do this, multiply your current weight in pounds by 15 calories.

    To lose one pound a week, you should decrease calorie intake by _____ calories per day. How many calories should you eat per day to lose one pound a week? _____

    To gain one pound a week, you should increase calorie intake by _____ calories per day. How many calories should you eat per day to gain one pound a week? _____

C. Menu Plans: Using the Food Guide Pyramid and five major food groups as a guide, create a day's menus that would fulfill the nutritional requirements of an adolescent.

<u>Breakfast</u>   <u>Lunch</u>   <u>Dinner</u>

<u>Snacks:</u> Include at least three (3).

D. Therapeutic Diets: List at least four (4) foods to limit or avoid in each of the following therapeutic diets.

Diet	Foods to Limit or Avoid
1. Soft	
2. Diabetic	
3. Low Calorie	
4. High Calorie	
5. Low Cholesterol	
6. Fat Restricted	
7. Sodium Restricted	
8. Low Protein	
9. Bland	
10. Low Residue	

UNIT 11 COMPUTERS IN HEALTH CARE

ASSIGNMENT SHEET

Grade _____   Name _____

INTRODUCTION: The computer has become an essential ingredient in almost every aspect of health care. This assignment will help you review the main facts about computers.

INSTRUCTIONS: Read the information on Computers in Health Care. In the space provided, print the word(s) that best completes the statement or answers the question.

1. Name four (4) general areas of health care that use computers.

2. Define *computer literacy.*

3. List at least eight (8) commonly used items that contain computer chips.

4. A computer system is a/an _____ device that can be thought of as a complete
   _____. It can _____, _____, _____,
   _____, _____, _____, _____, and
   _____ data.

5. What is the difference between hardware and software in computer systems?

6. Identify at least six (6) input devices that can be used to enter data into the computer.

7. What is the function of the central processing unit (CPU) of the computer?

8. What is the difference between the read only memory (ROM) and the random access memory (RAM) in the internal memory unit of a computer?

9. What is output?

   Name two (2) output devices.

10. Health care providers use computers to perform many functions. Identify at least five (5) of these functions.

11. How can confidentiality be maintained while using a computer for patient records?

12. What advantage does computerized tomography have over regular X rays?

13. How does ultrasonography create an image of the body part such as a developing fetus?

14. What is the Internet?

    What is a major use for the Internet in health care?

15. The use of computers has introduced many new abbreviations. Identify the following abbreviations as they relate to computers.

    a. CAI

    b. CPU

    c. CRT

    d. CT

    e. HIS

    f. MIS

    g. MRI

    h. PET

    i. RAM

    j. ROM

UNIT 12:1 USING BODY MECHANICS

ASSIGNMENT SHEET

Grade _____ Name _____

INTRODUCTION: The correct use of body mechanics is essential to protect both the worker and the patient. This sheet will allow you to review the main facts.

INSTRUCTIONS: Review the information in the text about Using Body Mechanics. Put the text aside and answer the following questions. Print your answers in the spaces provided.

1. Define body mechanics.

2. List three (3) reasons for using correct body mechanics.

3. In the following diagrams, certain rules for correct body mechanics are not being observed. At least three rules are being broken in each diagram. In the space provided for each diagram, list three rules not being observed.

Diagram 1:

(1)

(2)

(3)

Diagram 2:

(1)

(2)

(3)

Diagram 3:

(1)

(2)

(3)

Name _____ Date _____

Evaluated by _____

DIRECTIONS: Practice body mechanics according to the criteria listed. When you are ready for your final check, give this sheet to your instructor for evaluation.

PROFICIENT

Using Body Mechanics	Points Possible	Peer Check		Final Check*		Points Earned**	Comments
		Yes	No	Yes	No		
1. Demonstrates broad base of support:							
Keeps feet 8 to 10 inches apart	5						
Puts one foot slightly forward	5						
Points toes in direction of movement	5						
Balances weight on both feet	5						
2. Picks up heavy object:							
Gets close to object	6						
Maintains broad base of support	6						
Bends from hips and knees	6						
Uses strongest muscles	6						
3. Pushes heavy object:							
Gets close to object	8						
Maintains broad base of support	8						
Uses weight of body	8						
4. Carries heavy object:							
Keeps object close to body	8						
Uses strongest muscles	8						
5. Changes directions:							
Maintains broad base of support	8						
Turns with feet and entire body	8						
Totals	100						

* Final Check: Instructor or authorized person evaluates.
** Points Earned: Points possible times each "yes" check.

UNIT 12:2 PREVENTING ACCIDENTS AND INJURIES

ASSIGNMENT SHEET

Grade _____   Name _____

INTRODUCTION: Safety standards have been established to protect you and the patient. This sheet will help you to review the main standards.

INSTRUCTIONS: Read the information sheet on Preventing Accidents and Injuries. In the space provided, print the word(s) that best completes the statement or answers the question.

1. What is OSHA? What is its purpose?

2. List four (4) types of information that must be included on Material Safety Data Sheets (MSDSs).

3. What is the hazardous ingredient in Clorox bleach? (Hint: Review the MSDS figure in the textbook.)

4. Identify four (4) body fluids included in the bloodborne pathogen standard.

5. Name the two (2) main diseases that can be contracted by exposure to body fluids.

6. List four (4) rules or standards to observe while working with solutions in the laboratory.

7. List four (4) rules or standards to observe while working with equipment in the laboratory.

8. Before you perform any procedure on patients, there are several standards you must observe. List four (4) of these standards.

9. Identify two (2) ways to show respect for a patient's right to privacy.

10. What are two (2) methods you can use to correctly identify a patient?

11. List five (5) safety checkpoints that should be observed before leaving a patient or resident in a bed.

12. When should hands be washed?

13. When should safety glasses be worn?

14. Briefly state how you should handle the following situations.

    a. You cut your hand slightly on a piece of glass:

    b. You get a particle in your eye:

    c. You turn a piece of equipment on, but it does not run correctly:

    d. You spill an acid solution on the counter:

    e. You start to plug in an electrical cord and notice that the third prong for grounding has been bro-ken off:

UNIT 12:2 Evaluation Sheet

Name _____ Date _____

Evaluated by _____

DIRECTIONS: Practice safety according to the criteria listed. When you are ready for your final check, give this sheet to your instructor. Given simulated situations and using the proper equipment and supplies, you will be expected to respond orally or demonstrate the following safety criteria.

PROFICIENT

Preventing Accidents and Injuries	Points Possible	Peer Check Yes	No	Final Check* Yes	No	Points Earned**	Comments
1. Wears required laboratory uniform	5						
2. Walks in the laboratory area	5						
3. Reports injuries, accidents, and unsafe situations	5						
4. Keeps area clean and replaces supplies	5						
5. Washes hands frequently as needed	5						
6. Dries hands before handling electrical equipment	5						
7. Wears safety glasses	5						
8. Avoids horseplay	5						
9. Flushes solutions out of eyes or off of skin	5						
10. Informs teacher if particle gets in eye	5						
11. Operates equipment only after taught	5						
12. Reads instructions accompanying equipment	5						
13. Reports damaged or malfunctioning equipment	5						
14. Reads Material Safely Data Sheets (MSDSs) provided with hazardous chemicals	5						
15. Reads labels on solution bottles 3 times	5						
16. Handles solutions carefully to avoid contact with skin and eyes	5						
17. Reports broken equipment or spilled solutions	5						
18. Identifies patients in two (2) ways	5						
19. Explains procedures to patients	5						
20. Observes patients closely during any procedure	5						
Totals	100						

* Final Check: Instructor or authorized person evaluates.
** Points Earned: Points possible times each "yes" check.

UNIT 12:3 OBSERVING FIRE SAFETY

ASSIGNMENT SHEET

Grade _____ Name _____

INTRODUCTION: Knowing how to respond to a fire can save your life. This sheet will help you review the main facts of fire safety.

INSTRUCTIONS: Read the text information about Observing Fire Safety. In the space provided, print the word(s) that best completes the statement or answers the question.

1. Fires need three (3) things to start. What are they?

2. List four (4) causes of fires.

3. List three (3) rules for preventing fires.

4. Where is the nearest fire alarm box located?

5. a. What is the location of the nearest fire extinguisher?

   b. What class of fire extinguisher is it? What kind of fire will it extinguish?

6. Fill in the following chart about fire extinguishers.

Class	Contains	Used on what type of fires?
A		
B		
C		
ABC		

7. For what does the acronym RACE stand?

R:

A:

C:

E:

8. List three (3) special precautions that must be observed when a patient is receiving oxygen.

9. Identify three (3) basic principles that must be followed when any type of disaster occurs.

10. Health care workers are _____ responsible for familiarizing themselves with disaster policies so appropriate action can be taken when a disaster strikes.

UNIT 12:3 Evaluation Sheet

Name _____   Date _____

Evaluated by _____

DIRECTIONS: Practice fire safety according to the criteria listed. When you are ready for your final check, give this sheet to your instructor.

PROFICIENT

Observing Fire Safety	Points Possible	Peer Check Yes	No	Final Check* Yes	No	Points Earned**	Comments
1. Identifies nearest alarm box	9						
2. Sounds alarm correctly	9						
3. Points out locations of extinguishers in area	9						
4. Selects correct extinguisher for following types of fires:							
Burning paper	5						
Burning oil	5						
Electrical fire	5						
5. Simulates the operation of an extinguisher:							
Checks type	5						
Releases lock	5						
Holds firmly	5						
Stands 6 to 10 feet away from edge	5						
Aims at fire	5						
Discharges correctly	5						
Uses side-to-side motion	5						
Sprays at near edge at bottom of fire	5						
6. Replaces or has extinguisher recharged after use	9						
7. Evacuates laboratory or clinical area following established policy for fires	9						
Totals	100						

* Final Check: Instructor or authorized person evaluates.
** Points Earned: Points possible times each "yes" check.

UNIT 12 SAFETY EXAMINATION

Grade _____   Name _____

Read all directions carefully. Put your name on all pages of the examination.

Multiple Choice: In the space provided, place the letter of the answer that best completes the statement or answers the question.

_____   1. Operate a piece of equipment only when
   a. you have been instructed on how to use it
   b. you see other students using it
   c. you think you know how to handle it
   d. you have similar equipment in other classes

_____   2. If you find a damaged piece of equipment
   a. dispose of it immediately
   b. report it to the instructor
   c. use it but be very careful
   d. repair it yourself before you use it

_____   3. Solutions that will be used in the laboratory
   a. can be injurious, so avoid eye and skin contact
   b. can be mixed together in most cases
   c. do not always need a label
   d. are all safe for your use

_____   4. When the instructor is out of the room
   a. equipment should not be operated
   b. it is all right to operate equipment
   c. it is a good time to experiment with equipment
   d. be extra careful when using equipment

_____   5. All injuries obtained in the laboratory
   a. should be treated by a fellow student
   b. can be ignored if minor
   c. should be washed with soap and water
   d. should be reported to the instructor

_____   6. If a particle gets in your eye, you should
   a. rub your eye
   b. use cotton to remove it
   c. call the instructor
   d. flush your eye with water to remove it

_____ 7. When handling any electrical equipment, be sure to

     a. wash your hands immediately before handling it

     b. check first for damaged cords or improper grounds

     c. plug equipment carefully into any socket

     d. ask for written instructions on how to use it

_____ 8. Horseplay or practical jokes

     a. are permitted if no one is insulted

     b. may be done during breaks or study time

     c. cause accidents and have no place in the lab

     d. usually do not result in accidents

_____ 9. The major cause of fires is

     a. smoking and matches

     b. defects in heating systems

     c. improper rubbish disposal

     d. misuse of electricity

_____ 10. The three things needed to start a fire are

     a. air, oxygen and fuel

     b. fuel, heat and oxygen

     c. fuel, carbon dioxide and heat

     d. air, carbon dioxide and fuel

_____ 11. Injuries are more likely to happen to persons who

     a. take chances

     b. use equipment properly

     c. practice safety

     d. respect the dangers in using equipment

_____ 12. If your personal safety is in danger because of fire

     a. get the fire extinguisher and put it out

     b. run out of the area as fast as you can

     c. leave the area quietly and in an orderly fashion

     d. open all windows and doors

_____ 13. Wearing safety glasses in a laboratory

     a. is never necessary

     b. should be done if you think it is necessary

     c. is a requirement at all times

     d. is required for certain procedures

True-False: Circle the T if the statement is true. Circle the F if the statement is false.

T   F   14. Carbon dioxide fire extinguishers leave a residue or snow that can cause burns or eye irritations.

T   F   15. Spilled solutions, such as bleach, should be wiped up immediately.

T   F   16. Laboratory uniforms are worn for protection and as a safety measure.

T   F   17. If any solution comes in contact with your skin or eyes, flush the area with water and call the instructor.

T	F	18.	The third prong on an electric plug is important for grounding electrical equipment.
T	F	19.	In case of a fire alarm, avoid panic.
T	F	20.	Correct body mechanics should be used while performing procedures.
T	F	21.	Class A fire extinguishers can be used on electrical fires.
T	F	22.	While using a fire extinguisher, hold the extinguisher firmly and direct it to the middle or main part of the fire.
T	F	23.	Smoke and panic kill more people in fires than the fire itself.
T	F	24.	For your own safety and the safety of a patient, it is important that you wash your hands frequently.
T	F	25.	All waste material should be disposed of in the nearest available container.
T	F	26.	All solutions used in the laboratory are poisonous.
T	F	27.	You should read the bottle label of any solution that you use at least three (3) times.
T	F	28.	All manufacturers must provide a Material Safety Data Sheet (MSDS) with any hazardous product they sell.
T	F	29.	When lifting a patient in bed, a narrow base of support should be maintained.
T	F	30.	Keep the feet apart and the knees flexed when picking up an item from the floor.

31. Fill in the following chart with the indicated information.

Type Fire Extinguisher	Contains	Used on what type of fire?

a. _____

b. _____

c. _____

d. _____

32. List three (3) rules for preventing fires.

33. What is OSHA? What is its purpose?

34. How can you determine precautions that should be followed while using a hazardous chemical?

35. Identify the two (2) main diseases that can be contracted by exposure to body fluids.

UNIT 13:1 UNDERSTANDING THE PRINCIPLES OF INFECTION CONTROL

ASSIGNMENT SHEET

Grade _____ Name _____

INTRODUCTION: This assignment will allow you to gain a basic knowledge of how disease is transmitted and the main ways to prevent it.

INSTRUCTIONS: Read the information on Understanding the Principles of Infection Control. In the space provided, print the word(s) that best completes the statement or answers the question.

1. Use the Key Terms to complete the crossword puzzle.

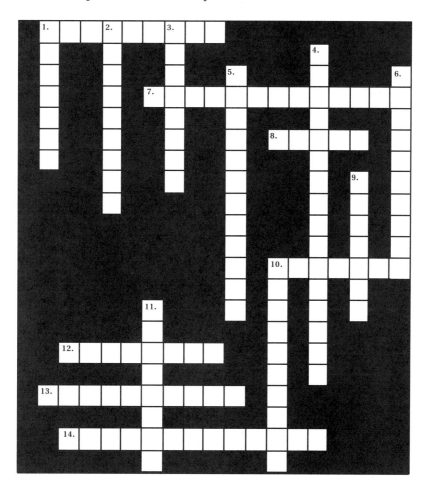

ACROSS

1. Organisms that live and reproduce in the absence of oxygen

7. Process that destroys all microorganisms including spores and viruses

8. Plantlike organisms that live on dead organic matter

10. Absence of pathogens

12. Germ- or disease-producing microorganism
13. Infections acquired in a health care facility
14. Small living plant or animal organism not visible to naked eye

DOWN
1. Organisms that require oxygen to live
2. Disease originates outside the body
3. One-celled plantlike organisms that multiply rapidly
4. Factors that must be present for disease to occur
5. Process that destroys or kills pathogens
6. Disease originates within the body
9. Smallest microorganisms
10. Process that inhibits or prevents the growth of pathogenic organisms
11. One-celled animal organisms found in decayed materials and contaminated water

---

2. How do nonpathogens differ from pathogens?

3. Identify the following shapes of bacteria.
   a. rod shaped:
   b. comma shaped:
   c. round or spherical arranged in a chain:
   d. spiral or corkscrew:
   e. round or spherical arranged in clusters:
4. Identify the class of microorganisms described by the following statements.
   a. smallest microorganisms:
   b. parasitic microorganisms:
   c. one-celled animal organisms found in decayed materials and contaminated water:
   d. plantlike organisms that live on dead organic matter:
   e. microorganisms that live on fleas, lice, ticks, and mites:
   f. cause diseases such as gonorrhea and syphilis:
   g. cause diseases such as measles and mumps:
   h. cause diseases such as ringworm and athlete's foot:
5. What does federal law require of employers in regards to the hepatitis B vaccine?

6. List three (3) things needed for microorganisms to grow and reproduce.

7. Identify two (2) ways pathogenic organisms can cause infection and disease.

8. What is the difference between an endogenous disease and an exogenous disease?

9. Name three (3) common examples of nosocomial infections.

   What do health care facilities do to prevent and deal with nosocomial infections?

10. Identify the part(s) of the chain of infection that has been eliminated by the following actions.
    a. thorough washing of the hands:
    b. intact unbroken skin:
    c. healthy, well rested individual:
    d. cleaning and sterilizing a blood covered instrument:
    e. spraying to destroy mosquitoes:
    f. rapid, accurate identification of organisms:

11. List four (4) common aseptic techniques.

12. Define the following.
    a. antisepsis:

    b. disinfection:

    c. sterilization:

UNIT 13:2 WASHING HANDS

ASSIGNMENT SHEET

Grade _____ Name _____

INTRODUCTION: Handwashing is the most important method used to practice aseptic technique. This assignment will help you review the main facts.

INSTRUCTIONS: Read the information on Washing Hands. In the space provided, print the word(s) that best completes the statement or answers the question.

1. What is an aseptic technique?

2. List two (2) reasons for washing the hands.

3. List six (6) times the hands should be washed.

4. Why is soap used as a cleansing agent?

5. How should the fingertips be pointed while washing hands?

   Why?

6. What temperature water should be used?

   Why?

7. Why are paper towels used while turning on and off the faucet?

8. List three (3) surfaces on the hands that must be cleaned.

9. Name two (2) items that can be used to clean the nails.

UNIT 13:2 Evaluation Sheet

Name _____ Date _____

Evaluated by _____

DIRECTIONS: Practice washing hands according to the criteria listed. When you are ready for your final check, give this sheet to your instructor.

PROFICIENT

Washing Hands	Points Possible	Peer Check Yes	No	Final Check* Yes	No	Points Earned**	Comments
1. Assembles supplies	5						
2. Turns faucet on with dry towel	6						
3. Regulates temperature of water	6						
4. Wets hands with fingertips pointed down	7						
5. Gets soapy lather	6						
6. Scrubs palms using friction and a circular motion for 10 to 15 seconds	7						
7. Scrubs tops of hands with opposite palm	7						
8. Interlaces fingers to wash between	7						
9. Cleans nails:							
With small brush	5						
Uses blunt edge of orange stick	5						
10. Rinses with fingertips pointed down	7						
11. Dries thoroughly	7						
12. Places towels in waste can	6						
13. Turns off faucet with dry towel	7						
14. Leaves area neat and clean	5						
15. Identifies five (5) times hands must be washed	7						
Totals	100						

* Final Check: Instructor or authorized person evaluates.
** Points Earned: Points possible times each "yes" check.

ASSIGNMENT SHEET

Grade _____ Name _____

INTRODUCTION: Observing standard precautions is one way the chain of infection can be broken. This assignment will allow you to review the main principles of standard precautions.

INSTRUCTIONS: Read the information on Observing Standard Precautions. In the space provided, print the word(s) that best completes the statement or answers the question.

1. Name two (2) pathogens spread by blood and body fluids that are a major concern to health care workers.

2. What federal agency established standards for contamination with blood or body fluids that must be followed by all health care facilities?

3. Name four (4) types of personal protective equipment (PPE) that an employer must provide.

4. Can a health care worker drink coffee in a laboratory where blood tests are performed? Why or why not?

5. What responsibilities does an employer have if an employee is splashed with blood when a tube containing blood breaks?

6. When must standard precautions be used?

7. Describe three (3) times your hands must be washed.

8. Describe four (4) situations when gloves must be worn.

9. When must gowns be worn?

10. Describe three (3) examples of situations when masks, protective eyewear, or face shields must be worn.

11. How must needles and syringes be handled after use?

12. During a blood test, some blood splashes on the laboratory counter. How must it be removed?

13. What is the purpose of mouthpieces or resuscitation devices?

14. Where must you discard a dressing contaminated with blood and pus?

15. What must you do if you stick yourself with a contaminated needle?

UNIT 13:3 Evaluation Sheet

Name _____ Date _____

Evaluated by _____

DIRECTIONS: Practice observing standard precautions according to the criteria listed. When you are ready for your final check, give this sheet to your instructor.

Observing Standard Precautions	Points Possible	Peer Check Yes	No	Final Check* Yes	No	Points Earned**	Comments
1. Assembles equipment and supplies	3						
2. Washes hands correctly	4						
3. Puts on gloves if:							
Contacting blood, body fluid, secretions, mucous membranes, or nonintact skin	3						
Handling contaminated items/surfaces	3						
Performing invasive procedures	3						
Performing blood tests	3						
4. Removes gloves correctly:							
Grasps outside of cuff of first glove	3						
Pulls glove down and turns inside out	3						
Places fingers inside cuff of second glove	3						
Pulls glove down and turns inside out	3						
Disposes of gloves correctly	3						
Washes hands immediately	3						
5. Puts on gown if splashing of blood/body fluid likely	4						
6. Removes gown correctly:							
Handles only inside while removing	2						
Folds gown inward	2						
Rolls gown	2						
Places in proper laundry bag	2						
7. Wears masks and protective eyewear if needed:							
Puts on if droplets of blood/body fluid likely	3						
Handles only ties of mask when removing	3						
Cleans and disinfects protective eyewear	3						
8. Disposes of sharps correctly	4						

PROFICIENT

Observing Standard Precautions	Points Possible	Peer Check		Final Check*		Points Earned**	Comments
		Yes	No	Yes	No		
9. Wipes up spills/splashes of blood/body fluids:							
Puts on gloves	2						
Wipes up spill with towels/gauze	2						
Discards towels/gauze in infectious waste bag	2						
Wipes area with clean towel/gauze and disinfectant	2						
Discards towel/gauze in infectious waste bag	2						
Removes gloves	2						
Washes hands immediately	2						
10. Handles infectious waste bags correctly:							
Forms cuff at top before using	2						
Discards infectious waste in bag	2						
Wears gloves to close bag	2						
Puts hands under cuff	2						
Expels excess air gently	2						
Folds top edges to seal bag	2						
Tapes or ties bag	2						
11. Uses mouthpieces or resuscitation devices correctly	4						
12. Replaces equipment	3						
13. Washes hands	3						
Totals	100						

* Final Check: Instructor or authorized person evaluates.
** Points Earned: Points possible times each "yes" check.

UNIT 13:4 STERILIZING WITH AN AUTOCLAVE

ASSIGNMENT SHEET

Grade _____   Name _____

INTRODUCTION: In order to use an autoclave correctly, you must know the following information. Read the information on Sterilizing with an Autoclave and proceed with this assignment.

INSTRUCTIONS: In the space provided, print the answer to each question.

1. The autoclave uses _____ under _____ or _____ to sterilize equipment and supplies. It will destroy all _____, both _____ and _____, including _____ and _____.

2. What must be done to any equipment or supplies before they are sterilized in the autoclave?

3. List three (3) types of wraps that can be used in the autoclave.

4. Why are autoclave indicators used?

5. List two (2) types of autoclave indicators.

6. List three (3) rules that must be followed while loading an autoclave.

7. Why is it important to separate loads before sterilizing them in an autoclave?

8. How do you determine the correct time and temperature for sterilizing different articles in the auto-clave?

9. Why do items have to be dry before being removed from an autoclave?

10. Where should sterilized items be stored?

11. How long do items remain sterile after autoclaving?

12. The wrap on a sterile bowl is wet. What should you do?

13. What is the minimum temperature required for dry heat sterilization?

What is the minimum time required for dry heat sterilization?

14. Identify two (2) items for which dry heat sterilization is more effective.

UNIT 13:4A Evaluation Sheet

Name _____ Date _____

Evaluated by _____

DIRECTIONS: Practice wrapping items for autoclaving according to the criteria listed. When you are ready for your final check, give this sheet to your instructor.

Wrapping Items for Autoclaving	Points Possible	Peer Check Yes	Peer Check No	Final Check* Yes	Final Check* No	Points Earned**	Comments
1. Assembles equipment and supplies	2						
2. Washes hands and puts on gloves	3						
3. Sanitizes item to be sterilized:							
Cleans with soapy water	2						
Rinses in cool water	2						
Rinses in hot water	2						
Dries item thoroughly	2						
Wears gloves if item contaminated with blood/body fluids	3						
Brushes serrated instruments	3						
4. Prepares linen for wrapping:							
Checks that linen is clean and dry	3						
Folds in half lengthwise	3						
Fanfolds into even sections	3						
Turns back corner tab	3						
5. Selects correct wrap for item	3						
6. Places item in center of wrap	3						
Leaves hinged instruments open	3						
7. Folds bottom corner up to center	3						
Folds back corner tab	3						
8. Folds a side corner in to center	3						
Seals edges and removes air pockets	3						
Folds back corner tab	3						
9. Folds other side corner in to center	3						
Seals edges and removes air pockets	3						
Folds back corner tab	3						
10. Brings final corner up and over top	3						
Seals edges and removes air pockets	3						
Tucks under pocket of previous folds	3						
Leaves small corner exposed for tab	3						

PROFICIENT

13:4A (cont.)

Wrapping Items for Autoclaving	Points Possible	Peer Check Yes	No	Final Check* Yes	No	Points Earned**	Comments
11. Secures with tape and/or autoclave indicator	3						
12. Labels with date, contents, and size if necessary	3						
13. Wraps with plastic or paper autoclave bag:							
Selects or cuts correct size	2						
Labels wrap or bag correctly	2						
Places clean item inside	2						
Double folds open end(s)	2						
Tapes or seals with heat	2						
14. Checks wrap carefully	3						
15. Replaces all equipment	2						
16. Removes gloves and washes hands	3						
Totals	100						

* Final Check: Instructor or authorized person evaluates.
** Points Earned: Points possible times each "yes" check.

UNIT 13:4B Evaluation Sheet

Name _____ Date _____

Evaluated by _____

DIRECTIONS: Practice sterilizing with an autoclave according to the criteria listed. When you are ready for your final check, give this sheet to your instructor.

PROFICIENT

Loading and Operating an Autoclave	Points Possible	Peer Check Yes	No	Final Check* Yes	No	Points Earned**	Comments
1. Assembles equipment and supplies	3						
2. Washes hands and dries thoroughly	3						
3. Checks plug and cord	3						
4. Fills reservoir with distilled water	4						
5. Checks pressure for zero	4						
6. Opens door properly	4						
7. Loads correctly:							
Separates items for same time and temperature	2						
Positions packages on sides	2						
Places basins on sides	2						
Leaves space between items	2						
Checks that no item is in contact with chamber sides, top, or door	2						
8. Fills chamber with correct amount of water	3						
Stops water flow at correct time	3						
9. Checks load	2						
10. Closes and locks door	3						
11. Pulls on door to check	3						
12. Sets control valve to allow temperature and pressure to increase	4						
13. Checks chart to determine time and temperature	4						
14. When temperature and pressure are correct, sets controls to maintain desired temperature	4						
15. Sets timer for correct time - moves past 10 minutes first	4						
16. Checks gauges at intervals	4						
17. Puts on safety glasses	4						

13:4B (cont.)

Loading and Operating an Autoclave	Points Possible	Peer Check		Final Check*		Points Earned**	Comments
		Yes	No	Yes	No		
18. When required time complete, sets controls so autoclave vents	4						
19. Allows steam discharge	4						
20. Checks pressure for zero	4						
21. Opens door 1/2 to 1 inch for drying	4						
22. Removes contents when dry and cool	3						
23. Leaves on vent for reuse	3						
24. Turns off if last load	3						
25. Replaces equipment	3						
26. Washes hands	3						
Totals	100						

* Final Check: Instructor or authorized person evaluates.
** Points Earned: Points possible times each "yes" check.

UNIT 13:5 USING CHEMICALS FOR DISINFECTION

ASSIGNMENT SHEET

Grade _____   Name _____

INTRODUCTION: You may be required to use chemicals for aseptic control in many health fields. This assignment will help you review the main facts.

INSTRUCTIONS: In the space provided, print the word(s) that best completes the statement or answers the question.

1. Most chemicals do not kill _____ and _____. The appropriate term is _____ because _____ does not occur.

2. List three (3) items usually disinfected with chemicals.

3. List two (2) reasons why it is important to thoroughly wash, rinse, and dry all items before placing them in a chemical solution.

4. List five (5) examples of chemical solutions.

5. List two (2) reasons why the manufacturer's directions should be read completely before using any solution.

6. What is the purpose of anti-rust tablets or solutions?

   Can they be added to all chemical solutions? Why or why not?

7. Why should the chemical solution cover the item completely?

8. While the articles are in the solution, a/an _____ should be placed on the container.

9. Where should instruments be stored after being removed from the solution?

10. When should the chemical solutions be changed or discarded?

UNIT 13:5 Evaluation Sheet

Name _____ Date _____

Evaluated by _____

DIRECTIONS: Practice using chemicals for disinfection according to the criteria listed. When you are ready for your final check, give this sheet to your instructor.

PROFICIENT

Using Chemicals for Disinfection	Points Possible	Peer Check Yes	No	Final Check* Yes	No	Points Earned**	Comments
1. Assembles equipment and supplies	4						
2. Washes hands and puts on gloves	4						
3. Washes articles thoroughly	4						
Brushes serrated edges	4						
Rinses articles	4						
Dries thoroughly	4						
4. Checks container for tight-fitting lid	5						
5. Loads properly:							
Leaves space between items	5						
Leaves hinged instruments open	5						
6. Reads manufacturer's instructions for directions on use of chemical solution	5						
Adds anti-rust substance if needed	3						
7. Pours solution over items to correct depth	5						
Reads label three times: before, during, and after pouring	5						
8. Puts lid on container	5						
9. Removes gloves and washes hands	5						
10. Checks bottle label to determine time required for disinfecting action	5						
11. Leaves instruments in solution for recommended time	5						
12. Washes hands before removing items	5						
13. Uses sterile transfer forceps to place items on sterile towel to dry	5						
14. Stores in dust-free drawer or cabinet	5						
15. Replaces equipment	4						
16. Washes hands	4						
Totals	100						

* Final Check: Instructor or authorized person evaluates.
** Points Earned: Points possible times each "yes" check.

UNIT 13:6 CLEANING WITH AN ULTRASONIC UNIT

ASSIGNMENT SHEET

Grade _____ Name _____

INTRODUCTION: Many health facilities use ultrasonic cleaning for instruments and equipment that do not penetrate body tissues. This assignment will help you review the main facts.

INSTRUCTIONS: Read the information on Cleaning with an Ultrasonic Unit. In the space provided, print the word(s) that best completes the statement or answers the question.

1. The ultrasonic unit cleans with _____ waves.

2. Explain *cavitation.*

3. Does ultrasonic cleaning remove all organisms and pathogens? Why or why not?

4. List two (2) reasons why it is important to read the labels carefully before using any cleaning solution.

5. Why should you avoid getting the solutions on the skin?

6. What solution is usually used in the permanent tank?

7. How should the beakers or pans be positioned in the permanent tank?

8. What must be done to all articles before cleaning them in the ultrasonic unit?

9. List two (2) types of jewelry that should not be cleaned in an ultrasonic unit.

10. When a white opaque coating appears on the bottom of the glass beakers, what do you do with the beakers?

11. How is the main tank cleaned?

12. How do you determine the length of time required for cleaning?

UNIT 13:6 Evaluation Sheet

Name _____ Date _____

Evaluated by _____

DIRECTIONS: Practice cleaning with an ultrasonic unit according to the criteria listed. When you are ready for your final check, give this sheet to your instructor.

PROFICIENT

Cleaning with an Ultrasonic Unit	Points Possible	Peer Check Yes	No	Final Check* Yes	No	Points Earned**	Comments
1. Assembles equipment and supplies	4						
2. Washes hands and puts on gloves if indicated	4						
3. Cleans articles with brush	4						
4. Rinses articles thoroughly	4						
5. Checks amount of solution in main tank	5						
6. Selects proper solution	5						
7. Places beaker in tank	4						
8. Adjusts beaker band	4						
9. Checks bottom of beaker to be sure it is below level of solution in permanent tank	4						
10. Checks that articles are covered with solution	4						
11. Uses auxiliary pan correctly	5						
12. Checks chart for time	5						
13. Sets timer properly (after turning it past 5)	5						
14. Checks that unit is working	5						
15. When timer signals, removes articles with transfer forceps	4						
16. Places articles on towel	4						
17. Rinses articles thoroughly	4						
18. Checks cleanliness	4						
19. Cleans unit properly:							
Sets container in place	2						
Opens drain valve	2						
Wipes tank with damp cloth or a disinfectant	2						

13:6 (cont.)

Cleaning with an Ultrasonic Unit	Points Possible	Peer Check Yes	No	Final Check* Yes	No	Points Earned**	Comments
20. Cleans beakers and pans:							
Empties solution	2						
Washes thoroughly	2						
Rinses completely	2						
Discards etched beakers	2						
21. Replaces equipment	4						
22. Removes gloves if worn and washes hands	4						
Totals	100						

* Final Check: Instructor or authorized person evaluates.
** Points Earned: Points possible times each "yes" check.

UNIT 13:7 USING STERILE TECHNIQUES

ASSIGNMENT SHEET

Grade _____ Name _____

INTRODUCTION: Following correct sterile technique is essential in many different procedures. This sheet will help stress the main facts.

INSTRUCTIONS: Read the information on Using Sterile Techniques. In the space provided, print the word(s) that best completes the statement or answers the question.

1. Define *sterile*.

   Define *contaminated*.

2. How can you avoid allowing sterile articles to touch the skin or clothing?

3. What part of a sterile field or tray is considered to be contaminated?

4. List three (3) methods for removing sterile articles from wraps and placing them on a sterile field or tray. Briefly describe each method.

5. Why must a sterile field be kept dry?

6. What should you do if you spill solution on a sterile field?

7. What part of sterile gloves are considered contaminated?

8. Before applying the sterile gloves, you must make sure what has been done in relation to the sterile tray?

9. Once gloves have been applied, where should you hold your hands to avoid contamination?

10. What should you do if you suspect an article is contaminated?

141

Name _____ Date _____

Evaluated by _____

DIRECTIONS: Practice opening sterile packages according to the criteria listed. When you are ready for your final check, give this sheet to your instructor.

PROFICIENT

Opening Sterile Packages	Points Possible	Peer Check Yes	No	Final Check* Yes	No	Points Earned**	Comments
1. Assembles equipment and supplies	4						
2. Washes hands	4						
3. Checks date and autoclave indicator on package	6						
4. Keeps work area free of all articles	5						
5. Holds package with point of top flap directed toward body	3						
Loosens fastener	3						
Grasps distal flap	3						
Pulls back and away	3						
Reaches in from side	3						
Allows no contamination	4						
6. Opens first side flap:							
Reaches in from side	3						
Pulls laterally	3						
Allows no contamination	4						
7. Opens second side flap:							
Reaches in from side	3						
Pulls laterally	3						
Allows no contamination	4						
8. Opens proximal edge:							
Pulls toward body	3						
Puts over hand/table	3						
Allows no contamination	4						
9. Transfers item with correct mitten technique	8						
10. Transfers item with correct drop technique	8						
11. Transfers item with correct transfer forcep technique	8						
12. Cleans and replaces all equipment	4						
13. Washes hands	4						
Totals	100						

* Final Check: Instructor or authorized person evaluates.
** Points Earned: Points possible times each "yes" check.

Name _____ Date _____

Evaluated by _____

DIRECTIONS: Practice preparing a sterile dressing tray according to the criteria listed. When you are ready for your final check, give this sheet to your instructor.

PROFICIENT

Preparing a Sterile Dressing Tray	Points Possible	Peer Check Yes	No	Final Check* Yes	No	Points Earned**	Comments
1. Assembles equipment and supplies	3						
2. Washes hands	3						
3. Checks date and autoclave indicator on supplies	4						
4. Opens sterile towel package:							
Unwraps correctly	3						
Picks up by outside	3						
Places on tray correctly	3						
Allows no contamination	4						
Fanfolds back edge	3						
5. Unwraps basin correctly	3						
Places on towel	3						
Allows no contamination	4						
6. Unwraps cotton balls or gauze sponges	3						
Drops into basin	3						
Allows no contamination	4						
7. Unwraps outer dressing	3						
Places on tray correctly	3						
Allows no contamnination	3						
8. Unwraps inner dressing	3						
Places on top of outer dressing correctly	3						
Allows no contamination	3						
9. Adds antiseptic solution:							
Places lid open –side up	3						
Pours off initial flow	3						
Pours into basin without splashing	3						
Allows no contamination	3						
10. Checks tray to make sure all supplies present	3						

Preparing a Sterile Dressing Tray	Points Possible	Peer Check		Final Check*		Points Earned**	Comments
		Yes	No	Yes	No		
11. Covers with towel:							
Handles outside only	3						
Keeps hands to sides of tray	3						
Unfolds fanfold on towel and covers tray	3						
Allows no contamination	3						
12. Remains with tray at all times	3						
13. Replaces equipment	3						
14. Washes hands	3						
Totals	100						

* Final Check: Instructor or authorized person evaluates.
** Points Earned: Points possible times each "yes" check.

Name _____ Date _____

Evaluated by _____

DIRECTIONS: Practice donning and removing sterile gloves according to the criteria listed. When you are ready for your final check, give this sheet to your instructor.

PROFICIENT

Donning and Removing Sterile Gloves	Points Possible	Peer Check Yes	No	Final Check* Yes	No	Points Earned**	Comments
1. Assembles equipment and supplies	4						
2. Checks date and autoclave indicator	4						
3. Washes and dries hands and removes rings	4						
4. Opens outer wrap without contamination	4						
5. Opens inner wrap:							
Handles only outside of wrap	3						
Maintains sterility of wrap and gloves	3						
Positions with cuffs close to body	3						
6. Powders hands over trash can/sink if powder packet present	4						
7. Dons first glove correctly:							
Grasps inside of cuff with thumb and forefinger	3						
Lifts out	3						
Inserts hand	3						
Holds away from body	3						
Avoids counters, etc.	3						
Maintains sterility of glove	4						
8. Dons second glove correctly:							
Puts gloved hand under cuff	3						
Lifts out	3						
Inserts hand	3						
Maintains sterility of gloves	4						
9. Straightens cuffs:							
Puts gloved hand under cuff, pulls out and up	3						
Maintains sterility of both gloves	4						
10. Handles only sterile items with gloved hands	4						

13:7C (cont.)

Donning and Removing Sterile Gloves	Points Possible	Peer Check Yes	No	Final Check* Yes	No	Points Earned**	Comments
11. Removes gloves correctly:							
Removes first glove by grasping outside with the other gloved hand	4						
Pulls glove down over hand	4						
Removes second glove by placing the ungloved hand inside the cuff	4						
Pulls glove down over hand	4						
Pulls gloves inside out while removing	4						
Puts contaminated gloves in infectious waste container	4						
12. Washes hands immediately	4						
Totals	100						

* Final Check: Instructor or authorized person evaluates.
** Points Earned: Points possible times each "yes" check.

Name _____ Date _____

Evaluated by _____

DIRECTIONS: Practice changing a sterile dressing according to criteria listed. When you are ready for your final check, give this sheet to your instructor.

PROFICIENT

Changing a Sterile Dressing	Points Possible	Peer Check Yes	No	Final Check* Yes	No	Points Earned**	Comments
1. Checks order or obtains proper authorization	3						
2. Assembles equipment and supplies	3						
3. Washes hands	3						
4. Prepares sterile tray or obtains commercially prepared kit	3						
5. Introduces self, identifies patient, and explains procedure	3						
6. Provides privacy for patient	3						
7. Prepares tape	3						
8. Positions infectious waste bag correctly	3						
9. Puts on disposable nonsterile gloves	3						
10. Removes dressing:							
Removes tape	3						
Removes dressing carefully	3						
Places tape and dressing in infectious waste bag	3						
11. Checks incision for type, amount, and color drainage	4						
12. Removes gloves and washes hands	3						
13. Opens sterile tray without contamination	4						
14. Dons sterile gloves correctly	4						
15. Cleanses wound:							
Uses circular motion	3						
Starts at center and moves out	3						
Discards cotton ball or gauze sponge	3						
Does not clean wound without specific order	3						
Goes top to bottom if cleans wound	3						
16. Applies inner dressing	3						

Changing a Sterile Dressing	Points Possible	Peer Check		Final Check*		Points Earned**	Comments
		Yes	No	Yes	No		
17. Applies outer dressing	3						
18. Removes sterile gloves correctly and discards in infectious waste bag	4						
19. Washes hands immediately	3						
20. Applies tape correctly:							
Uses proper length and width	3						
Applies in direction opposite of body movement	3						
21. Checks patient before leaving area	3						
22. Tapes/ties infectious waste bag securely	3						
23. Replaces equipment	3						
24. Washes hands immediately	3						
25. Records or reports required information	3						
Totals	100						

* Final Check: Instructor or authorized person evaluates.
** Points Earned: Points possible times each "yes" check.

UNIT 13:8 MAINTAINING ISOLATION

ASSIGNMENT SHEET

Grade _____   Name _____

INTRODUCTION: Isolation techniques will vary from area to area but the same principles are observed in all types. This sheet will help you review these main principles.

INSTRUCTIONS: Read the text information Maintaining Isolation. In the space provided, print the word(s) that best completes the statement or answers the question.

1. Define *isolation.*

2. What is the difference between standard precautions and isolation techniques?

3. What is a communicable disease?

4. List three (3) ways communicable diseases are spread.

5. Identify three (3) factors that help determine what type of isolation is used.

6. Define *contaminated.*

   Define *clean.*

7. Using the guidelines established by the Center for Disease Control and Prevention (CDC), place the letter or letters for the type of isolation used in Column B by any statement in Column A that pertains to this type of isolation.

Column A

_____ 1. Used for measles and tuberculosis

_____ 2. Used for pneumonia, pertussis, and severe viral infections

_____ 3. Used for all patients

_____ 4. Gloves should be worn when entering room

_____ 5. Uses standard precautions

_____ 6. Used for wound infections caused by multidrug-resistant organisms

_____ 7. Anyone entering room must wear high-efficiency particulate air (HEPA) mask

_____ 8. Masks must be worn when working within three feet of patient

_____ 9. Used for pathogens transmitted by airborne droplet nuclei

_____ 10. Room and items in it should receive daily cleaning and disinfection

_____ 11. Patient should be placed in a private room

_____ 12. Used for pathogens transmitted by large particle droplets

_____ 13. Room air should be discharged to outdoor air or filtered

_____ 14. Patient should wear a surgical mask if transport from room is necessary

Column B

A. Airborne

B. Contact

C. Droplet

D. Standard

8. What is protective or reverse isolation?

9. List two (2) types of patients who may require protective or reverse isolation.

10. List four (4) precautions that may be required for protective or reverse isolation.

150

Name _____ Date _____

Evaluated by _____

DIRECTIONS: Practice donning and removing isolation garments according to the criteria listed. When you are ready for your final check, give this sheet to your instructor.

PROFICIENT

Donning and Removing Isolation Garments	Points Possible	Peer Check Yes	No	Final Check* Yes	No	Points Earned**	Comments
1. Assembles equipment and supplies	4						
2. Washes hands	4						
3. Removes rings	4						
4. Places watch in plastic bag or on paper towel	4						
5. Applies mask correctly:							
Handles very little	2						
Covers mouth and nose	2						
Ties in back securely	2						
Changes mask every 30 minutes or anytime it gets wet	2						
6. Rolls up uniform sleeves	3						
7. Puts on gown correctly:							
Keeps hands inside shoulders	2						
Works arms in gently	2						
Adjusts neck with hands inside neck band	2						
Ties at neck first	2						
Ties at waist	2						
Handles only inside of gown	3						
8. Applies gloves correctly	3						
Covers cuffs of gown with gloves	3						
Removal of Garments:							
9. Unties waist ties of gown first	3						
10. Removes gloves:							
Uses gloved hand to grasp outside of opposite glove	2						
Pulls glove off inside out	2						
Places hand under cuff to remove second glove	2						

Donning and Removing Isolation Garments	Points Possible	Peer Check Yes	No	Final Check* Yes	No	Points Earned**	Comments
Pulls glove off inside out	2						
Places gloves in infectious waste container	2						
11. Washes hands thoroughly	3						
Operates faucet with towel	3						
12. Removes mask after gloves	2						
Handles ties only	2						
Places in infectious waste container	2						
13. Removes gown last	2						
Unties neck ties	2						
Places one hand inside cuff and pulls sleeve over hand	2						
Places covered hand on outside of gown to pull gown sleeve over second hand	2						
Eases out of gown gently	2						
Folds gown so inside of gown is on outside	2						
Rolls gown	2						
Places gown in linen hamper (or waste can if gown disposable)	2						
Touches only inside of gown	3						
14. Washes hands thoroughly	3						
15. Removes watch by touching only inside of plastic bag or top part of towel	2						
16. Opens door with towel, discards towel in waste can	2						
17. Washes hands immediately	3						
Totals	100						

* Final Check: Instructor or authorized person evaluates.
** Points Earned: Points possible times each "yes" check.

UNIT 13:8B Evaluation Sheet

Name _____ Date _____

Evaluated by _____

DIRECTIONS: Practice working in an isolation unit according to the criteria listed. When you are ready for your final check give this sheet to your instructor.

PROFICIENT

Working in a Hospital Isolation Unit	Points Possible	Peer Check Yes	No	Final Check* Yes	No	Points Earned**	Comments
1. Assembles equipment and supplies	2						
2. Washes hands	2						
3. Dons isolation garment	2						
4. Records vital signs:							
Tapes paper to door	3						
Keeps watch in plastic bag/paper towel	3						
Writes information on paper without touching paper on door	3						
5. Transfers food correctly:							
Obtains tray inside unit	3						
Receives glasses by bottom	3						
Receives plates from opposite side	3						
Allows no contamination	3						
6. Disposes of food:							
Pours liquids into sink	3						
Flushes soft liquids in toilet	3						
Places hard solids in waste container	3						
Places disposable utensils/dishes in trash	3						
Cleans metal utensils	3						
7. Handles linens:							
Folds and rolls	3						
Places in linen bag	3						
Folds down top edge	3						
Tells clean person to cuff outside bag	3						
Places linens in outside bag	3						
Allows no contamination	3						
Tells clean person how to label and tie final bag	3						
8. Disposes of trash:							
Ties plastic bag shut	3						
Places in cuffed outer bag	3						
Allows no contamination during transfer	3						
Tells clean person how to tape or tie and label outer bag	3						

13:8B (cont.)

Working in a Hospital Isolation Unit	Points Possible	Peer Check Yes	No	Final Check* Yes	No	Points Earned**	Comments
9. Transfers equipment:							
Cleans thoroughly inside unit	3						
Places in bag	3						
Seals top of bag	3						
Places in cuffed outer bag without contamination	3						
Tells clean person how to seal, tape, and label outer bag	3						
10. Checks patient before leaving unit	3						
Offers bedpan/urinal	3						
11. Removes isolation garments correctly	2						
12. Washes hands	2						
Totals	100						

* Final Check: Instructor or authorized person evaluates.
** Points Earned: Points possible times each "yes" check.

UNIT 14:1 MEASURING AND RECORDING VITAL SIGNS

ASSIGNMENT SHEET

Grade _____ Name _____

INTRODUCTION: Vital signs are important indicators of health states of the body. This assignment will help you review the main facts about vital signs.

INSTRUCTIONS: Read the information on Measuring and Recording Vital Signs. In the space provided, print the word(s) that best completes the statements or answers the questions.

1. Use the Key Terms to complete the crossword puzzle.

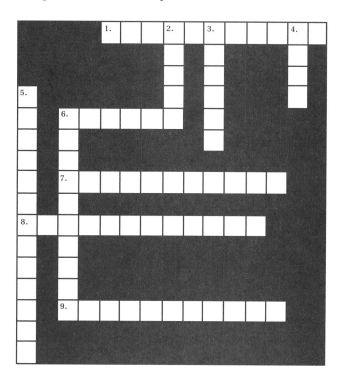

ACROSS

1. Measurement of the balance between heat lost and heat produced

6. Strength of the pulse

7. Pulse taken at the apex of the heart with a stethoscope

8. Measurement of breaths taken by a patient

9. Instrument used to take apical pulse

DOWN

2. Pressure of the blood felt against the wall of an artery

3. Regularity of the pulse or respirations

4. Number of beats per minute

5. Measurement of the force exerted by the heart against arterial walls

6. Various determinations that provide information about body conditions

---

2. List the four (4) main vital signs.

3. Why is it essential that vital signs are measured accurately?

4. Identify four (4) common sites in the body where temperature can be measured.

5. Define *pulse.*

   List three (3) factors recorded about a pulse.

6. What three (3) factors are noted about respirations?

7. Identify the two (2) readings noted on a blood pressure.

8. List three (3) times you may have to take an apical pulse.

9. What should you do if you note any abnormality or change in any vital sign?

10. What should you do if you are not able to obtain a correct reading for a vital sign?

11. Convert the following Fahrenheit (F) temperatures to Celsius (C) temperatures. Use the formula: C = (F − 32) × 5/9 or 0.5556.

For example: F is equal to 120°. What is Celsius?

Subtract 32 from F: 120 − 32 = 88

Multiply answer by 5/9 or 0.5556: 88 × 0.5556 = 48.8928 or 48.9

Celsius temperature is 48.9°.

Note: Round off answers to nearest tenth or one decimal point.

a. 140° F

b. 70° F

c. 50° F

d. 38° F

e. 86° F

f. 105° F

g. 138° F

h. 204° F

i. 99.6° F

j. 25° F

12. Convert the following Celsius (C) temperatures to Fahrenheit (F) temperatures. Use the formula: F = (C × 9/5 or 1.8) + 32

For example: C is equal to 22°. What is Fahrenheit (F)?

Multiply C by 9/5 or 1.8: 22 × 1.8 = 39.6

Add 32 to the answer: 39.6 + 32 = 71.6

Fahrenheit temperature is 71.6°.

Note: Round off answers to nearest tenth or one decimal point.

a. 32° C

b. 54° C

c. 8° C

d. 91° C

e. 0° C

f. 72° C

g. 26° C

h. 81° C

i. 99.8° C

j. 46.1° C

UNIT 14:2 MEASURING AND RECORDING TEMPERATURE

ASSIGNMENT SHEET

Grade _____   Name _____

INTRODUCTION: In addition to being able to take temperatures, it will be important for you to know the main facts about body temperature. This assignment will help you review these facts.

INSTRUCTIONS: Read the information on Measuring and Recording Temperature. In the space provided, print the word(s) that best completes the statements or answers the questions.

1. Define *temperature*.

2. List three main reasons why temperature may vary.

3. The normal range for body temperature is _____ to _____ degrees.

4. A normal oral temperature is _____ degrees. The clinical thermometer is left in place for _____ minutes.

5. A normal rectal temperature is _____ degrees. The clinical thermometer is left in place for _____ minutes.

6. A normal axillary temperature is _____ degrees. The clinical thermometer is left in place for _____ minutes.

7. What is the most accurate method for taking a temperature? Why?

8. What is the least accurate method for taking a temperature? Why?

9. What is an aural temperature?

   How does an aural thermometer measure temperature?

10. What is the difference between hyperthermia and hypothermia?

11. List two (2) ways you can tell a rectal thermometer from an oral thermometer.

12. Briefly describe the proper procedure for cleanup and disposal of a broken clinical thermometer.

13. How can you prevent cross-contamination while using the probe of an electronic thermometer?

14. How do plastic or paper thermometers register body temperature?

15. Why is it important to ask patients if they have had anything to eat or drink or if they have smoked before taking an oral temperature?

16. How long should a thermometer soak in a disinfectant (after cleaning) before it is safe to rinse in cold water and use on a patient?

READING A THERMOMETER

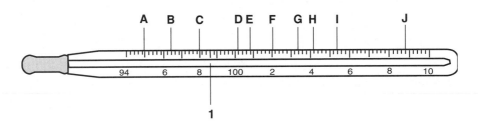

17. After the following steps is a list of temperatures that are to be recorded along the bottom of the illustrated thermometer:

    * Each temperature reading is preceded by a listed number (1, 2, 3, etc.).

    * Locate the line on the sketch that reflects the temperature reading.

    * Draw an arrow to the correct line on the thermometer.

    * Place the listed number below the arrow (1, 2, 3, etc.).

    * See Example 1.

    1. 98^6 (Example)

    2. 100^4

    3. 99

    4. 99^8

    5. 102^6

    6. 104^4

    7. 97^6

    8. 95^4

    9. 101^2

    10. 106^8

18. Note that in the previous sketch, letters appear along the top of the thermometer. Each letter has an arrow pointing to a line on the thermometer. This is the temperature reading. Record each reading beside the corresponding letter that follows. (Note Example A.)

    A. 95 (Example)

    B.

    C.

    D.

    E.

    F.

    G.

    H.

    I.

    J.

Name _____ Date _____

Evaluated by _____

DIRECTIONS: Practice cleaning a thermometer according to the criteria listed. When you are ready for your final check, give this sheet to your instructor.

PROFICIENT

Cleaning the Thermometer	Points Possible	Peer Check Yes	No	Final Check* Yes	No	Points Earned**	Comments
1. Assembles equipment and supplies	5						
2. Washes hands and puts on gloves if indicated	5						
3. Wipes thermometer from top to bulb with soapy cotton ball	7						
4. Rinses in cool water	7						
5. Shakes down correctly:							
Holds securely	5						
Uses snapping motion of wrist	5						
Shakes down to 96° F (35.6° C)	5						
6. Places in container of disinfectant	7						
7. Removes gloves and washes hands	6						
8. Soaks thermometer at least 30 minutes	7						
9. Wipes with alcohol cotton ball after soaking	6						
10. Rinses in cool water	6						
11. Checks for signs of breakage	7						
12. Reads to be sure it is 96° F (35.6°C) or less	7						
13. Places clean thermometer in clean gauze-lined container	5						
14. Replaces all equipment used	5						
15. Washes hands	5						
Totals	100						

* Final Check: Instructor or authorized person evaluates.
** Points Earned: Points possible times each "yes" check.

161

Name _____   Date _____

Evaluated by _____

DIRECTIONS: Practice measuring and recording an oral temperature according to the criteria listed. When you are ready for your final check, give this sheet to your instructor.

PROFICIENT

Measuring and Recording Oral Temperature	Points Possible	Peer Check Yes	No	Final Check* Yes	No	Points Earned**	Comments
1. Assembles equipment and supplies	4						
2. Washes hands and puts on gloves	5						
3. Introduces self and identifies patient	4						
4. Explains procedure	4						
5. Questions patient on eating, drinking, or smoking	6						
6. Wipes thermometer	4						
7. Checks and reads thermometer and applies sheath if used	6						
8. Instructs patient on holding it in mouth	6						
9. Cautions against biting thermometer	6						
10. Leaves in place 3 to 5 minutes	6						
11. Removes, wipes or removes sheath, and holds at stem end for reading	6						
12. Reads to nearest two-tenths of a degree	8						
13. Records correctly	8						
14. Cleans correctly:							
Wipes with soapy cotton ball	3						
Rinses in cool water	3						
Shakes down correctly	3						
Soaks proper time	3						
15. Replaces all equipment	4						
16. Removes gloves and washes hands	5						
17. Recognizes an abnormal reading and reports it immediately	6						
Totals	100						

* Final Check: Instructor or authorized person evaluates.
** Points Earned: Points possible times each "yes" check.

UNIT 14:2C Evaluation Sheet

Name _____ Date _____

Evaluated by _____

DIRECTIONS: Practice measuring and recording a rectal temperature according to the criteria listed. When you are ready for your final check, give this sheet to your instructor.

Measuring and Recording Rectal Temperature	Points Possible	Peer Check Yes	Peer Check No	Final Check* Yes	Final Check* No	Points Earned**	Comments
1. Assembles equipment and supplies	4						
2. Washes hands and puts on gloves	4						
3. Introduces self, identifies patient, and explains procedure	4						
4. Provides privacy for the patient	4						
5. Checks and reads thermometer	5						
6. Places lubricant on tissue to lubricate thermometer	5						
7. Positions patient on side	4						
8. Folds back covers to expose anal area	5						
9. Explains procedure to patient while inserting thermometer	4						
10. Inserts thermometer 1 to 1 ½ inches in rectum (1 inch for infant)	5						
11. Replaces bed covers while holding thermometer in place	4						
12. Leaves in place 3 to 5 minutes	5						
13. Removes thermometer and explains action to patient	4						
14. Wipes off excess lubricant with tissue or removes sheath if used	5						
15. Reads to nearest two-tenths of a degree	8						
16. Records; correctly places (R) by reading	8						
17. Repositions patient	4						
18. Cleans thermometer correctly	4						
19. Replaces equipment	4						
20. Removes gloves and washes hands	4						
21. Recognizes an abnormal reading and reports it immediately	6						
Totals	100						

* Final Check: Instructor or authorized person evaluates.
** Points Earned: Points possible times each "yes" check.

UNIT 14:2D Evaluation Sheet

Name _____ Date _____

Evaluated by _____

DIRECTIONS: Practice measuring and recording an axillary temperature according to the criteria listed. When you are ready for your final check, give this sheet to your instructor.

Measuring and Recording Axillary Temperature	Points Possible	Peer Check Yes	Peer Check No	Final Check* Yes	Final Check* No	Points Earned**	Comments
1. Assembles equipment and supplies	5						
2. Washes hands	5						
3. Introduces self and identifies patient	5						
4. Explains procedure	5						
5. Wipes thermometer	5						
6. Checks and reads thermometer	6						
7. Dries axillary area	6						
8. Positions thermometer correctly with arm over chest	6						
9. Leaves in place 10 minutes	7						
10. Removes, wipes, and holds thermometer correctly	6						
11. Reads to nearest two-tenths of a degree	8						
12. Records; correctly places (Ax) by reading	8						
13. Repositions patient for comfort and safety	6						
14. Cleans thermometer correctly	6						
15. Replaces equipment	5						
16. Washes hands	5						
17. Recognizes an abnormal reading and reports it immediately	6						
Totals	100						

* Final Check: Instructor or authorized person evaluates.
** Points Earned: Points possible times each "yes" check.

Name _____ Date _____

Evaluated by _____

DIRECTIONS: Practice measuring and recording a tympanic (aural) temperature according to the criteria listed. When you are ready for your final check, give this sheet to your instructor.

PROFICIENT

Measuring and Recording a Tympanic (Aural) Temperature	Points Possible	Peer Check		Final Check*		Points Earned**	Comments
		Yes	No	Yes	No		
1. Assembles equipment and supplies	3						
2. Washes hands	4						
3. Introduces self and identifies patient	4						
4. Explains procedure	4						
5. Removes thermometer from base and selects proper mode	5						
6. Installs probe cover correctly	5						
7. Checks that thermometer indicates "ready" with correct mode	5						
8. Positions patient correctly with easy access to ear	4						
9. Pulls ear pinna back:							
Pulls straight back for infant under 1 year	4						
Pulls up and back for children and adults	4						
10. Inserts probe into ear canal and seals canal	5						
11. Presses scan or activator button	5						
12. Holds thermometer steady for 1 or 2 seconds or time required	5						
13. Removes probe from ear	5						
14. Reads temperature correctly	7						
15. Records correctly and places (T) by reading	7						
16. Removes and discards probe cover correctly	4						
17. Returns thermometer to base unit	4						
18. Repositions patient for comfort and safety	4						
19. Replaces all equipment	3						
20. Washes hands	4						
21. Recognizes an abnormal reading and reports it immediately	5						
Totals	100						

* Final Check: Instructor or authorized person evaluates.
** Points Earned: Points possible times each "yes" check.

UNIT 14:2F Evaluation Sheet

Name _____ Date _____

Evaluated by _____

DIRECTIONS: Practice measuring and recording temperature with an electronic thermometer according to the criteria listed. When you are ready for your final check, give this sheet to your instructor.

Measuring Temperature with an Electronic Thermometer	Points Possible	Peer Check Yes	No	Final Check* Yes	No	Points Earned**	Comments
1. Assembles equipment and supplies	4						
2. Washes hands and puts on gloves if indicated	5						
3. Introduces self and identifies patient	4						
4. Explains procedure	4						
5. Positions patient correctly and questions patient on eating, drinking, or smoking for oral temperature	7						
6. If necessary, inserts probe into thermometer unit and turns unit on	6						
7. Covers probe with sheath or probe cover	6						
8. Inserts probe into desired location and holds probe in position	7						
9. Removes probe when thermometer signals that temperature has been recorded	7						
10. Reads thermometer correctly	8						
11. Records correctly	8						
12. Removes and discards sheath or probe cover correctly	6						
13. Repositions patient for comfort and safety	6						
14. If necessary, positions probe in correct storage position in thermometer unit and turns unit off	6						
15. Replaces all equipment	4						
16. Removes gloves if worn and washes hands	5						
17. Recognizes an abnormal reading and reports it immediately	7						
Totals	100						

PROFICIENT

* Final Check: Instructor or authorized person evaluates.

** Points Earned: Points possible times each "yes" check.

UNIT 14:3 MEASURING AND RECORDING PULSE

ASSIGNMENT SHEET

Grade _____ Name _____

INTRODUCTION: One of the vital signs you will be required to record is pulse. This assignment sheet will assist you in learning the sites for taking pulse and the important aspects about pulse.

INSTRUCTIONS: Read the information about Measuring and Recording Pulse. In the space provided, print the word(s) that best completes the statement or answers the question.

1. Define *pulse.*

2. (a) Study the outlined figure. As you identify each pulse site, enter the name beside the corresponding letter on the following list.

   A.

   B.

   C.

   D.

   E.

   F.

   G.

   (b) Circle the site (on the sketch) that is used most frequently for taking pulse.

3. The three (3) factors that must be noted about each and every pulse are:

4. What is the normal pulse range for each of the following?

   a. Adults:

   b. Children over 7 years old:

   c. Children from 1 to 7 years old:

   d. Infants:

5. List three (3) factors that could cause an increase in a pulse rate.

6. List three (3) factors that could cause a decrease in a pulse rate.

7. In an adult, a pulse rate under 60 beats per minute is called _____. A pulse rate above 100 beats per minute is called _____. An irregular or abnormal rhythm is a/an _____ .

167

Name _____ Date _____

Evaluated by _____

DIRECTIONS: Practice measuring and recording pulse according to the criteria listed. When you are ready for your final check, give this sheet to your instructor.

PROFICIENT

Measuring and Recording Pulse	Points Possible	Peer Check Yes	No	Final Check* Yes	No	Points Earned**	Comments
1. Assembles equipment and supplies	5						
2. Washes hands	5						
3. Introduces self, identifies patient, and explains procedure	6						
4. Positions patient with arm supported and palm down	8						
5. Places fingers correctly over selected pulse site	8						
6. Counts one minute	8						
7. Obtains correct count to ± 2 beats per minute	15						
8. Records accurately	10						
9. Notes rhythm and volume	10						
10. Checks patient before leaving	6						
11. Replaces equipment	5						
12. Washes hands	5						
13. Recognizes an abnormal measurement and reports it immediately	9						
Totals	100						

* Final Check: Instructor or authorized person evaluates.
** Points Earned: Points possible times each "yes" check.

UNIT 14:4 MEASURING AND RECORDING RESPIRATIONS

ASSIGNMENT SHEET

Grade _____   Name _____

INTRODUCTION: This assignment will help you review the main facts regarding respirations.

INSTRUCTIONS: Read the information about Measuring and Recording Respirations. In the space provided, print the word(s) that best completes the statement or answers the question.

1. Define *respiration.*

2. One respiration consists of one _____ and one _____.

3. What is the normal rate for respirations in adults?

   What is the normal rate for children?

   What is the normal rate for infants?

4. List four (4) words to describe the character or volume of respirations.

5. List two (2) words to describe the rhythm of respirations.

6. Briefly define the following words.

   dyspnea:

   apnea:

   Cheyne-Stokes:

   rales:

   tachypnea:

   bradypnea:

7. Why is it important that the patient is not aware that you are counting respirations?

8. If you are taking a TPR, how can you count respirations without letting the patient know that you are doing it?

Name _____   Date _____

Evaluated by _____

DIRECTIONS: Practice measuring and recording respirations according to the criteria listed. When you are ready for your final check, give this sheet to your instructor.

Measuring and Recording Respirations	Points Possible	Peer Check Yes	Peer Check No	Final Check* Yes	Final Check* No	Points Earned**	Comments
1. Assembles equipment and supplies	5						
2. Washes hands	5						
3. Introduces self and identifies patient	5						
4. Positions patient correctly	5						
5. Leaves hand on pulse site	7						
6. Counts 1 minute	7						
7. Keeps patient unaware of counting activity	8						
8. Obtains correct count to ± 1 breath per minute	15						
9. Records correctly	10						
10. Notes rhythm and character	10						
11. Checks patient before leaving	5						
12. Replaces equipment	5						
13. Washes hands	5						
14. Recognizes an abnormal measurement and reports it immediately	8						
Totals	100						

* Final Check: Instructor or authorized person evaluates.
** Points Earned: Points possible times each "yes" check.

UNIT 14:5 GRAPHING TPR

ASSIGNMENT SHEET #1

Grade _____   Name _____

INTRODUCTION: This assignment will provide you with practice in graphing TPRs.

INSTRUCTIONS: Use the blank graphic chart to record the following information. Be sure to include the entries that are shown under Notes in this sample case history.

Patient: Louise Simmers   Physician: Dr. James Webber
Room 238   Hospital No.: 534–23
Admitted: 11/1/ ——

Date	Time	T	P	R	Notes
11/1/—	12 Noon	98^6	88	20	BP 120/80
	4 PM	98^8	80	22	
11/2/—	8 AM	97^4	68	16	BP 124/78
	12 Noon	98^2	74	18	
	4 PM	98^8	86	22	
	8 PM	99	110	28	
11/3/—	8 AM	97^2	64	14	BP 116/78
	12 Noon	Sleeping-not disturbed			
	4 PM	96^8	88	22	
	8 PM	97^4	80	20	
	12 MN	98^2	84	18	
11/4/—	4 AM	98^8	90	22	BP 110/74
	8 AM	99^2	94	24	
	12 Noon	100^4	96	24	
	4 PM	102^6 R	92	24	
	8 PM	102^4 R	90	20	
	12 MN	103^8 R	98	22	
11/5/—	4 AM	104^6 R	110	26	Antibiotics
	8 AM	103^6 R	120	28	BP 124/86
	12 Noon	99^8 R	90	20	
	4 PM	99^6 R	82	18	
	8 PM	99	86	20	
	12 MN	98	84	18	
11/6/—	8 AM	97^6	68	14	BP 108/68
	12 Noon	98^2	72	16	
	4 PM	98^6	76	16	
	8 PM	98^6	110	24	
	12 MN	In OR-Emergency surgery			
11/7/—	8 AM	98	68	20	
	4 PM	98^6	76	18	Discharged to another hospital

GRAPHIC CHART

Family Name		First Name		Attending Physician			Room No.		Hosp. No.	

Date								
Day in Hospital								
Day P O or P P								

	Hour	A M	P M	A M	P M	A M	P M	A M	P M	A M	P M	A M	P M	A M	P M	A M	P M
		4 8 12	4 8 12	4 8 12	4 8 12	4 8 12	4 8 12	4 8 12	4 8 12	4 8 12	4 8 12	4 8 12	4 8 12	4 8 12	4 8 12	4 8 12	4 8 12

TEMPERATURE

106
105
104
103
102
101
100
99 Normal
98
97
96

PULSE

150
140
130
120
110
100
90
80
70
60

RESPIRATION

50
40
30
20
10

Blood Pressure								
Fluid Intake								
Urine								
Defecation								
Weight								

(Courtesy of Physicians Record Company)

GRAPHIC CHART

UNIT 14:5 GRAPHING TPR

ASSIGNMENT SHEET #2

Grade _____   Name _____

INTRODUCTION: Tamika Petro was admitted to Ram Hospital with an elevated temperature and abdominal pain. This assignment will provide practice in graphing her TPRs.

INSTRUCTIONS: Chart the following information on a TPR graphic chart.

Patient: Tamika Petro   Room: 238

Physician: Dr. John Vaughn   Hospital No.: 36-26-38

Date	Time	T	P	R	Notes
11/8/—	4 PM	104^6 R	128	36	Admission
	8 PM	104^4 R	126	34	BP 134/86
	12 MN	103 R	116	30	
11/9/—	4 AM	99^8 R	86	26	
	8 AM	99 R	88	20	BP 124/76
	12 Noon	103^4 R	108	28	
	4 PM	102^4 R	100	22	
	8 PM	In OR-Appendectomy by Dr. Vaughn			
	12 MN	100^6 Ax	124	28	
11/10/—	4 AM	100^4 Ax	132	24	
	8 AM	97^8 Ax	82	18	BP 110/68
	12 Noon	98	90	16	
	4 PM	99	86	18	
	8 PM	99^6	94	18	
	12 MN	98^8	80	14	
11/11/—	8 AM	98	82	12	BP 106/68
	12 Noon	98^6	90	18	
	4 PM	101^6	106	24	
	8 PM	102^8 R	110	28	
	12 MN	103^3 R	120	34	Antibiotics
11/12/—	4 AM	101^2 R	118	26	
	8 AM	99^6 R	98	18	BP 108/78
	12 Noon	98	86	12	
	4 PM	98^6	80	16	
	8 PM	98	82	20	
11/13/—	8 AM	97	64	12	BP 122/82
	4 PM	96^8	68	16	
11/14/—	8 AM	97^6	60	12	BP 120/78
	4 PM	98^6	86	18	Discharged

GRAPHIC CHART

Family Name		First Name	Attending Physician		Room No.	Hosp. No.

Date								
Day in Hospital								
Day P O or P P								

	Hour	A M / P M	A M / P M	A M / P M	A M / P M	A M / P M	A M / P M	A M / P M	A M / P M
		4 8 12 4 8 12	4 8 12 4 8 12	4 8 12 4 8 12	4 8 12 4 8 12	4 8 12 4 8 12	4 8 12 4 8 12	4 8 12 4 8 12	4 8 12 4 8 12

TEMPERATURE

106
105
104
103
102
101
100
99 Normal
98
97
96

PULSE

150
140
130
120
110
100
90
80
70
60

RESPIRATION

50
40
30
20
10

Blood Pressure								
Fluid Intake								
Urine								
Defecation								
Weight								

form D-703

(Courtesy of Physicians Record Company)

GRAPHIC CHART

174

UNIT 14:5 GRAPHING TPR

ASSIGNMENT SHEET #3

Grade _____ Name _____

INTRODUCTION: This assignment will allow you to improve your skills on graphing TPRs.

INSTRUCTIONS: Chart the following information on a blank graphic chart.

Patient: Ralph Brown   Room: 238

Physician: Dr. Jacoby   Hospital No.:   589-2112

Date	Time	T	P	R	Notes
11/14/—	8PM	103^4 R	136	38	BP 180/90
	12 MN	103^6 R	130	36	
11/15/—	4 AM	102^4 R	118	28	
	8 AM	104^8 R	120	18	BP 178/88
	12 Noon	106 R	138	28	Antibiotics
	4 PM	105^6 R	140	36	
	8 PM	99^8 R	138	20	
	12 MN	101	110	24	
11/16/—	4 AM	101^8	102	20	
	8 AM	102^6	108	24	BP 172/86
	12 Noon	101^4	102	26	
	4 PM	103 R	120	34	
	8 PM	98^6 R	102	24	
	12 MN	98^8	80	20	
11/17/—	4 AM	97^8	86	18	
	8 AM	98^2	64	12	BP 134/72
	12 Noon	99	74	18	
	4 PM	98^6	110	26	
	8 PM	99^2	86	16	
11/18/—	8 AM	97^2	66	12	
	12 Noon	98^2	78	18	
	4 PM	98^6	86	20	BP 126/88
	8 PM	99^4	82	16	
11/19/—	8 AM	97^2	68	14	BP 124/82
	12 Noon	98^4	86	20	
	4 PM	98^8	80	18	
11/20/—	8 AM	97^8	64	12	BP 120/84
	4 PM	98^4	82	18	
11/21/—	8 AM	98	72	14	Discharged

GRAPHIC CHART

Family Name		First Name		Attending Physician					Room No.		Hosp. No.	

Date								
Day in Hospital								
Day P O or P P								

	Hour	A M	P M	A M	P M	A M	P M	A M	P M	A M	P M	A M	P M	A M	P M	A M	P M
		4 8 12	4 8 12	4 8 12	4 8 12	4 8 12	4 8 12	4 8 12	4 8 12	4 8 12	4 8 12	4 8 12	4 8 12	4 8 12	4 8 12	4 8 12	4 8 12
TEMPERATURE	106																
	105																
	104																
	103																
	102																
	101																
	100																
	99 Normal																
	98																
	97																
	96																
PULSE	150																
	140																
	130																
	120																
	110																
	100																
	90																
	80																
	70																
	60																
RESPIRATION	50																
	40																
	30																
	20																
	10																

Blood Pressure								
Fluid Intake								
Urine								
Defecation								
Weight								

form D-703

(Courtesy of Physicians Record Company)

GRAPHIC CHART

UNIT 14:5 GRAPHING TPR

ASSIGNMENT SHEET #4

Grade _____   Name _____

INTRODUCTION: The following patient was admitted to Ram Hospital on 11/28/—. Admitted by Dr. Yoder, the diagnosis was mononucleosis. This assignment will give you practice in graphing TPRs.

INSTRUCTIONS: Chart the following information on a blank graphic chart. If you get this graphic 100% correct, you will not have to do graphic #5.

Patient: Roger Daugherty   Room: 238
Weight :   200 lbs   Hospital No.:   555-44

Date	Time	T	P	R	Notes
11/28/—	4 PM	103^6 R	108	30	BP 128/80
	8 PM	104^2 R	100	26	
	12 MN	103^2 R	118	28	Aspirin Gr X
11/29/—	4 AM	101^6 R	100	24	
	8 AM	100^4 R	86	20	BP 124/84
	12 Noon	103^6 R	122	28	Aspirin Gr X
	4 PM	100^2 R	106	22	
	8 PM	104^8 R	110	32	
	12 MN	105^8 R	148	38	
11/30/—	4 AM	99^4 R	88	20	
	8 AM	98^6 R	86	18	BP 118/76
	12 Noon	98^8	80	20	
	4 PM	99^8	94	18	
	8 PM	98^2	84	16	
12/1/—	8 AM	97^6	60	12	BP 130/78
	12 Noon	98^2	66	14	
	4 PM	99^2	82	20	
	8 PM	101	98	28	
	12 MN	99^8	88	22	
12/2/—	8 AM	97^2	64	12	BP 126/76
	4 PM	98^4	86	14	
12/3/—	8 AM	100	96	24	BP 114/76
	12 Noon	99^2	86	18	
	4 PM	99^8	88	22	
	8 PM	98^8	80	18	
12/4/—	8 AM	97^8	88	16	BP 118/78
	4 PM	98^6	80	18	
12/5/—	8 AM	97^2	68	14	BP 118/76
	4 PM	98^4	80	18	Discharged

177

GRAPHIC CHART

Family Name		First Name		Attending Physician			Room No.		Hosp. No.	

Date								
Day in Hospital								
Day P O or P P								

	Hour	AM / PM	AM / PM	AM / PM	AM / PM	AM / PM	AM / PM	AM / PM	AM / PM
		4 8 12 4 8 12	4 8 12 4 8 12	4 8 12 4 8 12	4 8 12 4 8 12	4 8 12 4 8 12	4 8 12 4 8 12	4 8 12 4 8 12	4 8 12 4 8 12

TEMPERATURE: 106, 105, 104, 103, 102, 101, 100, 99 Normal, 98, 97, 96

PULSE: 150, 140, 130, 120, 110, 100, 90, 80, 70, 60

RESPIRATION: 50, 40, 30, 20, 10

Blood Pressure								
Fluid Intake								
Urine								
Defecation								
Weight								

form D-703

(Courtesy of Physicians Record Company)

GRAPHIC CHART

UNIT 14:5 GRAPHING TPR

ASSIGNMENT SHEET #5

Grade _____ Name _____

INTRODUCTION: On January 1, 20— Jim Johnson was admitted to Ram Hospital by Dr. Imhoff. The diagnosis was hepatitis and exhaustion from too much holiday celebration. Dr. Imhoff placed the patient in isolation. This assignment will allow you to perfect your skills on graphing TPRs.

INSTRUCTIONS: Record all of the following information on a blank graphic chart.

ROOM: 238   HOSPITAL NO.: 54-56-54   WEIGHT: 206 lb

Date	Time	T	P	R	Notes
1/1/——	12 Noon	103^4 R	136	38	BP 138/84
	4 PM	104^6 R	136	46	Aspirin Gr X
	8 PM	102^4 R	120	30	
	12 MN	103^2 R	130	36	Aspirin Gr XX
1/2/——	4 AM	100^4 R	116	24	
	8 AM	99^6 R	98	18	BP 124/78
	12 Noon	98^4	76	18	
	4 PM	99^6	94	24	
	8 PM	101^2	108	34	
	12 MN	103^8 R	120	42	Aspirin Gr X
1/3/——	4 AM	100^4 R	96	24	
	8 AM	99^6 R	84	18	BP 128/76
	12 Noon	99^8	88	22	
	4 PM	98^4	80	16	
	8 PM	98^8	86	18	
1/4/——	8 AM	97^2 Ax	68	12	BP 118/78
	12 Noon	98^4	76	18	
	4 PM	98^6	122	28	
	8 PM	99^4	86	18	
1/5/——	8 AM	97^6 Ax	62	14	BP 120/80
	4 PM	99^8	88	20	
	8 PM	102^6 R	94	28	Aspirin Gr XX
	12 PM	99^4 R	86	20	
1/6/——	8 AM	98^2	74	16	BP 124/72
	12 Noon	98^8	86	18	
	4 PM	98^8	90	18	
1/7/——	8 AM	97^4	64	12	BP 128/74
	8 PM	98^6	62	18	
1/8/——	8 AM	97^6	66	14	BP 120/68
	4 PM	98^4	82	12	

GRAPHIC CHART

Family Name		First Name	Attending Physician		Room No.	Hosp. No.

Date								
Day in Hospital								
Day P O or P P								

	Hour	A M 4 8 12	P M 4 8 12	A M 4 8 12	P M 4 8 12	A M 4 8 12	P M 4 8 12	A M 4 8 12	P M 4 8 12	A M 4 8 12	P M 4 8 12	A M 4 8 12	P M 4 8 12	A M 4 8 12	P M 4 8 12	A M 4 8 12	P M 4 8 12
TEMPERATURE	106																
	105																
	104																
	103																
	102																
	101																
	100																
	99 Normal																
	98																
	97																
	96																
PULSE	150																
	140																
	130																
	120																
	110																
	100																
	90																
	80																
	70																
	60																
RESPIRATION	50																
	40																
	30																
	20																
	10																

Blood Pressure								
Fluid Intake								
Urine								
Defecation								
Weight								

FORM D-703

(Courtesy of Physicians Record Company)

GRAPHIC CHART

UNIT 14:6 MEASURING AND RECORDING APICAL PULSE

ASSIGNMENT SHEET

Grade _____ Name _____

INTRODUCTION: The following assignment will help you review the main facts regarding apical pulse.

INSTRUCTIONS: Read the information about Measuring and Recording an Apical Pulse. In the space provided, print the word(s) that best answers the question.

1. Define *apical pulse*.

2. List two (2) diseases or conditions a patient may have that would require that an apical pulse be taken.

3. Why are apical pulses usually taken on infants and children?

4. What causes the lubb-dupp heart sounds that are heard while taking an apical pulse?

5. What should you do if you hear any abnormal sounds or beats while taking an apical pulse?

6. What causes a pulse deficit or a higher rate for an apical pulse than a radial pulse?

7. Calculate the pulse deficit for the following readings.

   Apical pulse 104, radial pulse 80:

   Apical pulse 142, radial pulse 96:

   Apical pulse 86, radial pulse 86:

8. How is the stethoscope cleaned before and after an apical pulse is taken?

Name _____ Date _____

Evaluated by _____

DIRECTIONS: Practice measuring and recording an apical pulse according to the criteria listed. When you are ready for your final check, give this sheet to your instructor.

		PROFICIENT					
Measuring and Recording Apical Pulse	**Points Possible**	**Peer Check** Yes	No	**Final Check*** Yes	No	**Points Earned****	**Comments**
1. Assembles equipment and supplies. Cleans earpieces and bell/diaphragm with disinfectant	5						
2. Washes hands	5						
3. Introduces self, identifies patient, and explains procedure	5						
4. Avoids unnecessary exposure of patient	6						
5. Places stethoscope in ears properly	7						
6. Places stethoscope on apical area	7						
7. Counts 1 full minute	7						
8. Obtains pulse count accurate to ± 2 beats per minute	15						
9. Notes rhythm and volume of pulse	10						
10. Records apical pulse information correctly	10						
11. Checks patient before leaving	6						
12. Cleans and replaces equipment	5						
13. Washes hands	5						
14. Recognizes an abnormal measurement and reports it immediately	7						
Totals	100						

* Final Check: Instructor or authorized person evaluates.
** Points Earned: Points possible times each "yes" check.

ASSIGNMENT SHEET #1

Grade _____   Name _____

INTRODUCTION: The following assignment will help you review the main facts regarding blood pressure.

INSTRUCTIONS: Read the information about Measuring and Recording Blood Pressure. Then answer the following questions in the spaces provided.

1. Define *blood pressure.*

2. Define *systolic.*

3. Define *diastolic.*

4. The average reading for systolic pressure is _____ with a range of _____.

5. The average reading for diastolic pressure is _____ with a range of _____.

6. What is the pulse pressure if the blood pressure is 136/72?

7. Hypertension is indicated when pressures are greater than _____ systolic and _____ diastolic.

8. List three (3) causes of hypotension.

9. List three (3) factors that can increase blood pressure.

10. List three (3) factors that can decrease or lower blood pressure.

11. a. Record the following blood pressure readings correctly.

Systolic	128	Diastolic	92
Diastolic	84	Systolic	188
Systolic	136	Diastolic	76
Diastolic	118	Systolic	210

b. Name all of the above readings that fall within normal range.

c. Name the above readings that do not fall within normal range.

12. Why is it important to use the correct size cuff?

UNIT 14:7 READING A MERCURY SPHYGMOMANOMETER

ASSIGNMENT SHEET #2

Grade _____ Name _____

INTRODUCTION: The mercury gauge is a long column. Each mark represents 2 mm Hg. Complete this assignment sheet to learn how to record readings from this mercury gauge.

INSTRUCTIONS: In the space provided, place the reading to which the arrow is pointing.

1. _____
2. _____
3. _____
4. _____
5. _____
6. _____
7. _____
8. _____
9. _____
10. _____
11. _____
12. _____
13. _____
14. _____
15. _____
16. _____
17. _____
18. _____
19. _____
20. _____
21. _____
22. _____
23. _____
24. _____
25. _____
26. _____
27. _____
28. _____
29. _____
30. _____
31. _____
32. _____
33. _____
34. _____
35. _____

ASSIGNMENT SHEET #3

Grade _____ Name _____

INTRODUCTION: The aneroid gauge is a common gauge on many sphygmomanometers. Each line represents 2 mm Hg pressure. Complete this sheet to practice reading the gauge.

INSTRUCTIONS: In the spaces provided, place the reading to which the arrow is pointing.

1. _____

2. _____

3. _____

4. _____

5. _____

6. _____

7. _____

8. _____

9. _____

10. _____

11. _____

12. _____

13. _____

14. _____

15. _____

16. _____

17. _____

18. _____

19. _____

20. _____

21. _____

22. _____

23. _____

24. _____

25. _____

26. _____

Name _____ Date _____

Evaluated by _____

DIRECTIONS: Practice measuring and recording blood pressure according to the criteria listed. When you are ready for your final check, give this sheet to your instructor.

PROFICIENT

Measuring and Recording Blood Pressure	Points Possible	Peer Check Yes	No	Final Check* Yes	No	Points Earned**	Comments
1. Assembles equipment and supplies. Cleans stethoscope earpieces and bell/disk with a disinfectant	3						
2. Washes hands	3						
3. Introduces self and identifies patient	3						
4. Explains procedure	3						
5. Applies cuff correctly	4						
6. Determines palpatory systolic pressure	4						
7. Deflates cuff and waits 30-60 seconds	4						
8. Places stethoscope in ears correctly	4						
9. Locates brachial artery	4						
10. Inflates cuff 30 mm Hg above palpatory systolic pressure	4						
11. Uses aneroid sphygmomanometer:							
Places gauge correctly	4						
Untangles tubing	4						
Reads pressure to ± 2 mm Hg	8						
Records correctly	4						
12. Uses mercury sphygmomanometer:							
Sets on flat surface	4						
Reads to ± 2 mm Hg	8						
Records correctly	4						
13. Reads adult diastolic as cessation of sound	5						
14. Reads child diastolic as change in sound	5						
15. Checks patient for comfort and safety	4						
16. Cleans stethoscope earpieces and bell/disk with a disinfectant	4						
17. Replaces equipment	3						
18. Washes hands	3						
19. Recognizes an abnormal measurement and reports it immediately	4						
Totals	100						

* Final Check: Instructor or authorized person evaluates.
** Points Earned: Points possible times each "yes" check.

UNIT 15:1 PROVIDING FIRST AID

ASSIGNMENT SHEET

Grade _____ Name _____

INTRODUCTION: The following assignment will help you review the main facts on general guidelines for first aid.

INSTRUCTIONS: Study the information on Providing First Aid. In the space provided, print the word(s) that best answers the question or completes the statement.

1. Define first aid.

2. Using the correct first aid methods can mean the difference between _____ and _____, or _____ versus _____.

3. The type of first aid treatment you provide will vary depending on several factors. List three (3) factors that may affect any action taken.

4. Identify three (3) senses that can alert you to an emergency.

5. What action should you take if you notice that it is not safe to approach the scene of an accident?

6. What is the first thing you should determine when you get to the victim?

7. Why is it important to avoid moving a victim whenever possible?

8. List four (4) kinds of information that should be reported while calling emergency medical services (EMS).

9. What is triage?

10. Identify six (6) life-threatening emergencies that must be cared for first.

11. List three (3) sources of information you can use to find out the details regarding an accident, injury, or illness.

12. How can you reassure the victim?

13. Why shouldn't you discuss the victim's condition with observers at the scene?

14. While providing first aid to the victim, make every attempt to avoid further _____. Provide only the treatment you are _____ to provide.

UNIT 15:2 PERFORMING CARDIOPULMONARY RESUSCITATION (CPR)

ASSIGNMENT SHEET

Grade _____ Name _____

INTRODUCTION: This assignment will help you review the main facts regarding CPR.

INSTRUCTIONS: Review the information on Performing Cardiopulmonary Resuscitation (CPR). In the space provided, print the word(s) that best completes the statement or answers the question.

1. CPR stands for _____.

2. What do the ABCs of CPR represent?

3. How does biological death differ from clinical death?

4. When does biological death occur?

5. What method should be used to open the airway?

6. What should you determine first before starting CPR?

7. What is the three point evaluation that is used to check for breathing?

8. What pulse site is checked to determine if compression is necessary?

9. Why is it important to place the heel of the hand one finger width above the substernal notch before giving chest compressions?

10. To perform a one-person rescue on an adult victim, give _____ compressions followed by _____ respirations. Compressions are given at the rate of _____ per minute. _____ 15:2 cycles should be completed every minute. Pressure should be applied straight down to compress the sternum about _____ inches or _____ centimeters.

11. What is the ratio of compressions to ventilations when two people are giving CPR to an adult victim?

12. To rescue an infant, both the _____ and the _____ are covered for ventilations. Two fingers are placed _____ below a line drawn between the nipples, and the sternum is compressed _____ inches or _____ centimeters. Compressions are given at the rate of _____ per minute. After each _____ compressions, give one ventilation for a ratio of _____:_____ compressions to ventilations.

13. CPR for a child is similar to an infant. Compressions are given at the rate of _____ per minute. The heel of one hand is placed on the sternum _____ above the _____. The sternum is compressed _____ inches or _____ centimeters. The ratio of compressions to ventilations is _____:_____.

14. What should you do for a choking victim who is conscious, coughing , and able to breathe?

15. Briefly list the sequence of steps used to remove an obstruction in an unconscious adult victim who has an obstructed airway.

16. Briefly list the sequence of steps used to remove an obstruction in an infant with an obstructed airway.

17. You have tried to remove an obstruction from an airway for several minutes, but the airway is still blocked. Should you check the pulse and start chest compressions at this point? Why or why not?

18. List five (5) reasons for stopping CPR once it is started.

UNIT 15:2A Evaluation Sheet

Name _____   Date _____

Evaluated by _____

DIRECTIONS: Practice performing CPR with a one-person rescue according to the criteria listed. When you are ready for your final check, give this sheet to your instructor.

PROFICIENT

Performing Cardiopulmonary Resuscitation: One-Person Rescue	Points Possible	Peer Check Yes	No	Final Check* Yes	No	Points Earned**	Comments
1. Assembles equipment and supplies–places manikin on firm surface	1						
2. Checks consciousness:							
Shakes victim by tapping shoulder	3						
Asks "Are you OK?"	3						
3. If the victim is unconscious, activates EMS	5						
4. Opens airway with head tilt/chin lift method	6						
5. Looks, listens, and feels for respirations for 5 seconds	5						
6. Gives 2 slow full breaths	6						
7. Palpates carotid pulse for 5–10 seconds	5						
8. Administers chest compressions as follows:							
Locates correct hand position on sternum	5						
Places heel of hands on chest with fingers off of chest	5						
Positions shoulders above sternum to apply vertical force	5						
Keeps elbows straight	5						
Compresses $1\frac{1}{2}$ to 2 inches	5						
Gives 15 compressions at rate of 80–100 per minute	5						
Counts "one and, two and . . ."	5						
9. Gives two ventilations	5						
10. Repeats cycle of 15 compressions and 2 ventilations giving 4 cycles every minute	5						
11. Checks pulse and breathing for 5 seconds after 4 cycles	5						
12. Resumes CPR by giving 2 breaths and then continues 15:2 cycle	5						
13. Continues CPR unless:							
Victim recovers	2						
Qualified help takes over	2						
Physician orders you to discontinue attempt	2						
Too physically exhausted	2						
Scene suddenly becomes unsafe	2						
14. Cleans and replaces all equipment used	1						
Totals	100						

* Final Check: Instructor or authorized person evaluates.
** Points Earned: Points possible times each "yes" check.

Name _____ Date _____

Evaluated by _____

DIRECTIONS: Practice performing CPR with a two-person rescue according to the criteria listed. When you are ready for your final check, give this sheet to your instructor.

Performing Cardiopulmonary Resuscitation: Two-Person Rescue	Points Possible	PROFICIENT Peer Check Yes	No	Final Check* Yes	No	Points Earned**	Comments
1. Assembles equipment and supplies and places manikin on firm surface	2						
2. First rescuer begins CPR:							
Shakes victim	3						
Asks "Are you OK?"	3						
Opens airway	3						
Looks, listens, and feels for breathing for 5 seconds	3						
Gives 2 slow full breaths	3						
Checks carotid pulse for 5–10 seconds	3						
If no pulse, locates correct position for hands	3						
Administers chest compressions at the rate of 80–100 per minute	3						
Gives 2 ventilations after each 15 compressions	3						
3. Second rescuer goes to obtain help	4						
4. When second rescuer returns, the first rescuer indicates "take over compressions"	4						
5. First rescuer completes 15:2 cycle	4						
6. First rescuer does 5 second pulse and breathingcheck, states "No pulse. Continue CPR," and gives one breath	4						
7. If second rescuer takes over compressions:							
Second rescuer finds correct hand placement during pulse and breathing check	4						
Second rescuer gives compressions at rate of 80–100 per minute	3						
Counts "one and, two and, etc."	3						
Pauses slightly after 5 compressions	3						
First rescuer gives one breath after each 5 compressions	3						
Rescuers continue with 5:1 cycle with slight pause for ventilation	4						

Name _____

15:2B (cont.)

Performing Cardiopulmonary Resuscitation: Two-Person Rescue	Points Possible	Peer Check Yes	Peer Check No	Final Check* Yes	Final Check* No	Points Earned**	Comments
8. Rescuers switch positions as follows:							
Compressor gives clear signal to change positions	3						
Compressor completes cycle of 5 compressions	3						
Ventilator gives ventilation after fifth compression	3						
Compressor moves to head							
Checks pulse and breathing for 5 seconds	3						
Ventilates once	3						
Says "No pulse"	3						
Ventilator moves to chest							
Locates correct hand placement for compressions	4						
After new ventilator gives breath, begins compressions at rate of 80–100 per minute	3						
Rescuers continue with 5:1 cycle with slight pause for ventilation	4						
9. Rescuers continue CPR until help arrives, victim recovers, doctor orders attempt discontinued, or scene suddenly becomes unsafe	4						
10. Cleans and replaces all equipment used	2						
Totals	100						

* Final Check: Instructor or authorized person evaluates.
** Points Earned: Points possible times each "yes" check.

UNIT 15:2C Evaluation Sheet

Name _____ Date _____

Evaluated by _____

DIRECTIONS: Practice performing CPR on infants according to the criteria listed. When you are ready for your final check, give this sheet to your instructor.

Performing Cardiopulmonary Resuscitation: Infants	Points Possible	Peer Check		Final Check*		Points Earned**	Comments
		Yes	No	Yes	No		
1. Assembles equipment and supplies and places manikin on firm surface	2						
2. Shakes gently and calls to infant	5						
3. Calls aloud for help	5						
4. Opens airway but does not tilt head as far back as an adult	6						
5. Looks, listens, and feels for breathing for 5 seconds	6						
6. Gives 2 slow full breaths	5						
Covers mouth and nose	5						
Watches for chest to rise	5						
7. Checks brachial pulse on infants for 5–10 seconds	6						
8. Administers compressions:							
Places 2–3 fingers one finger's width below an imaginary line drawn between the nipples	6						
Gives compressions at rate of 100 per minute	6						
Counts 1, 2, 3, 4, 5, breathe	6						
Compresses $\frac{1}{2}$ to 1 inch or 1.4 to 2.5 centimeters	6						
Supports back or places victim on firm surface	6						
9. Gives one ventilation after every five compressions	6						
10. Repeats cycle of 5:1 with slight pause for ventilation	6						
11. Checks breathing and pulse after 1 minute – checks for 5 seconds	6						
12. Continues CPR if no breathing or pulse by starting with one breath	5						
13. Cleans and replaces all equipment	2						
Totals	100						

PROFICIENT

* Final Check: Instructor or authorized person evaluates.
** Points Earned: Points possible times each "yes" check.

UNIT 15:2D Evaluation Sheet

Name _____ Date _____

Evaluated by _____

DIRECTIONS: Practice performing CPR on children according to the criteria listed. When you are ready for your final check, give this sheet to your instructor.

PROFICIENT

Performing Cardiopulmonary Resuscitation: Children	Points Possible	Peer Check		Final Check*		Points Earned**	Comments
		Yes	No	Yes	No		
1. Assembles equipment and supplies and places manikin on firm surface	2						
2. Shakes gently and calls to child	5						
3. Obtains medical help as soon as possible	5						
4. Opens airway correctly	6						
5. Looks, listens, and feels for breathing for 5 seconds	6						
6. Gives 2 slow full breaths	5						
Covers nose and mouth or just mouth	5						
Watches for chest to rise	5						
7. Checks carotid pulse for 5–10 seconds	6						
8. Administers compressions if no pulse:							
Places heel of one hand one finger's width above substernal notch	6						
Gives compressions at rate of 80–100 per minute	6						
Counts 1 and 2 and 3 and 4 and 5	6						
Compresses 1–1½ inches or 2.5 to 3.8 centimeters	6						
Supports back or places child on flat surface	6						
9. Gives 1 ventilation after every 5 compressions	6						
10. Repeats cycle of 5:1 with slight pause for ventilations	6						
11. Checks breathing and pulse for 5 seconds after 1 minute	6						
12. Continues CPR if no breathing or pulse by starting with 1 breath	5						
13. Cleans and replaces all equipment	2						
Totals	100						

* Final Check: Instructor or authorized person evaluates.
** Points Earned: Points possible times each "yes" check.

UNIT 15:2 E Evaluation Sheet

Name _____ Date _____

Evaluated by _____

DIRECTIONS: Practice performing CPR on a conscious victim with an obstructed airway according to the criteria listed. When you are ready for your final check, give this sheet to your instructor. NOTE: Use only a manikin to perform thrusts.

PROFICIENT

Performing Cardiopulmonary Resuscitation: Obstructed Airway on Conscious Victim	Points Possible	Peer Check Yes	No	Final Check* Yes	No	Points Earned**	Comments
1. Assembles equipment and supplies and places manikin in upright position	5						
2. Determines if victim has an airway obstruction:							
Asks " Are you choking?"	5						
Checks if victim can cough, talk, or breathe	5						
3. Calls out for help	6						
4. Performs abdominal thrusts:							
Stands behind victim	8						
Wraps arms around victim's waist	8						
Places thumb side of fist above umbilicus but below xiphoid	8						
Grasps fist with other hand	8						
Uses quick upward thrusts	8						
5. Demonstrates chest thrusts for very obese or pregnant victim:							
Stands behind victim	4						
Wraps arms under victim's axillae	4						
Places thumb side of fist against center of sternum but well above xiphoid	4						
Grasps fist with other hand	4						
Thrusts inward	4						
6. Repeats thrusts until object expelled or victim loses consciousness	8						
7. Obtains medical help as soon as possible	6						
8. Replaces all equipment	5						
Totals	100						

* Final Check: Instructor or authorized person evaluates.
** Points Earned: Points possible times each "yes" check.

Name _____ Date _____

Evaluated by _____

DIRECTIONS: Practice performing CPR on an unconscious victim with an obstructed airway according to the criteria listed. When you are ready for your final check, give this sheet to your instructor.

PROFICIENT

Performing Cardiopulmonary Resuscitation: Obstructed Airway on Unconscious Victim	Points Possible	Peer Check Yes	No	Final Check* Yes	No	Points Earned**	Comments
1. Assembles equipment and supplies and places manikin on firm surface	1						
2. Shakes victim and asks "Are you OK?"	4						
3. If the victim is unconscious, activates EMS	4						
4. Opens airway with head tilt/chin lift method	4						
5. Looks, listens, and feels for breathing for 5 seconds	4						
6. Attempts to give breaths	4						
7. When chest does not rise, repositions head and attempts to ventilate	4						
8. Gives abdominal thrusts as follows:							
Positions victim on back	4						
Straddles victim's thighs	4						
Places heel of one hand on abdomen above umbilicus but below xiphoid	4						
Places other hand on top of first hand	4						
Gives quick upward thrusts into the abdomen	5						
Gives 5 thrusts	5						
9. Checks for object in mouth as follows:							
Opens mouth by lifting lower jaw with thumb and fingers	4						
Uses index finger to sweep mouth with c-shape or hooking motion	4						
Removes object if visible	4						
10. Opens airway and attempts to ventilate	4						
11. If chest rises, continues with steps of CPR by checking carotid pulse	4						
12. If the chest does not rise, repositions head and attempts to ventilate	4						
13. If chest still does not rise, repeats cycle of 5 thrusts, mouth check, attempt to ventilate	4						

15:2F (cont.)

Performing Cardiopulmonary Resuscitation: Obstructed Airway on Unconscious Victim	Points Possible	Peer Check		Final Check*		Points Earned**	Comments
		Yes	No	Yes	No		
14. Continues repeating cycle until object removed and airway open or help comes	4						
15. Follows same sequence for infants but observes following variations:							
Gives 4 back blows by positioning infant face down with head lower than chest	4						
Gives 4 chest thrusts using 2–3 fingers one finger's width below an imaginary line drawn between nipples with infant positioned face up and head lower than chest	4						
Looks in mouth for object but sweeps mouth with finger only if object is seen	4						
Attempts to ventilate	4						
16. Cleans and replaces all equipment	1						
Totals	100						

* Final Check: Instructor or authorized person evaluates.
** Points Earned: Points possible times each "yes" check.

UNIT 15:3 PROVIDING FIRST AID FOR BLEEDING AND WOUNDS

ASSIGNMENT SHEET

Grade _____ Name _____

INTRODUCTION: This assignment will help you review the main facts about providing first aid for bleeding and wounds.

INSTRUCTIONS: Read the information on Providing First Aid for Bleeding and Wounds. In the space provided, print the word(s) that best completes the statement or answers the question.

1. What is the difference between a closed wound and an open wound?

2. First aid care for wounds must be directed at controlling _____ and preventing _____.

3. List the correct name for each of the following types of open wounds.

   a. Scrape on the skin:

   b. Cut or injury by sharp object:

   c. Jagged irregular injury with tearing:

   d. Wound caused by sharp pointed object:

   e. Tissue torn or separated from body:

   f. Body part cut off:

4. Briefly describe the characteristics or signs and symptoms for each of the following types of bleeding.

   a. Arterial blood:

   b. Venous blood:

   c. Capillary blood:

5. List the four (4) methods for controlling bleeding in the order in which they should be used.

6. Name two (2) items that can be used to form a protective barrier while controlling bleeding.

7. The main pressure point for the arm is the _____.

   The main pressure point in the leg is the _____.

201

8. List four (4) ways to prevent infection while caring for minor wounds without severe bleeding.

9. List five (5) signs of infection.

10. If a tetanus infection is a possibility, what first aid is necessary?

11. How should objects embedded deep in the tissues be removed?

12. List six (6) signs and symptoms of a closed wound.

13. List four (4) first aid treatments for a victim of a closed wound.

14. What other condition must you be prepared to treat while caring for wounds?

15. At all times, remain _____ while providing first aid. Obtain _____ care as soon as possible.

UNIT 15:3 Evaluation Sheet

Name _____ Date _____

Evaluated by _____

DIRECTIONS: Practice providing first aid for bleeding and wounds according to the criteria listed. When you are ready for your final check, give this sheet to your instructor.

PROFICIENT

Providing First Aid for Bleeding and Wounds	Points Possible	Peer Check Yes	No	Final Check* Yes	No	Points Earned**	Comments
1. Follows priority of care:							
Checks the scene	3						
Checks consciousness and breathing	3						
Calls emergency medical services	3						
Cares for victim	3						
2. Controls severe bleeding with direct pressure:							
Put on gloves or uses protective barrier	3						
Uses dressing over wound	3						
Applies pressure directly to wound	3						
Avoids releasing pressure to check bleeding	3						
Applies second dressing if first soaks through	3						
3. Elevates injured part while applying pressure if no fracture is present	5						
4. Applies pressure bandage when bleeding under control:							
Maintains direct pressure and elevation	3						
Applies additional dressings over dressings on wound	3						
Secures dressings by wrapping with roller bandage in overlapping turns	3						
Ties off bandage with tie over dressings	3						
Checks pulse site below bandage	3						
Loosens and replaces bandage if signs of impaired circulation are present	3						
5. Applies pressure to pressure point if bleeding does not stop:							
Continues with direct pressure and elevation	4						
Applies pressure correctly to brachial artery in arm	4						
Applies pressure correctly to femoral artery in leg	4						
Releases pressure slowly when bleeding stops but continues with direct pressure and elevation	4						

15:3 (cont).

Providing First Aid for Bleeding and Wounds	Points Possible	Peer Check		Final Check*		Points Earned**	Comments
		Yes	No	Yes	No		
6. Removes gloves and washes hands thoroughly	4						
7. Observes for signs of shock and treats as necessary	4						
8. Reassures victim during care and remains calm	3						
9. Treats minor wounds without severe bleeding:							
Washes hands	2						
Puts on gloves	2						
Washes wound with soap, water and sterile gauze in outward motion	2						
Discards gauze after each use	2						
Rinses wound with cool water	2						
Blots dry with sterile gauze	2						
Applies sterile dressing	2						
Cautions victim to watch for signs of infection and get medical help	2						
Refers to doctor if danger of tetanus present	2						
Removes gloves and washes hands thoroughly	2						
10. Obtains medical help as soon as possible when needed for victim	3						
Totals	100						

* Final Check: Instructor or authorized person evaluates.
** Points Earned: Points possible times each "yes" check.

UNIT 15:4 PROVIDING FIRST AID FOR SHOCK

ASSIGNMENT SHEET

Grade _____   Name _____

INTRODUCTION: This assignment will help you review the main facts regarding shock.

INSTRUCTIONS: Review the information on Providing First Aid for Shock. In the space provided, print the word(s) that best completes the statement or answers the question.

1. Define *shock*.

2. Name the two (2) main body organs affected by an inadequate supply of blood.

3. List six (6) causes of shock.

4. List ten (10) signs or symptoms of shock.

5. Treatment for shock is directed at eliminating the _____, improving _____, providing _____, and maintaining _____.

6. The position for treating shock is based on the victim's injuries. Briefly list the best position for each of the following cases:

   a. Victim with neck or spine injuries:

   b. Victim vomiting or bleeding from the mouth:

   c. Victim with respiratory distress:

   d. Position if none of the previous conditions is present:

7. If medical help will not be available for at least an hour or more and dehydration is evident, what solution can you give to a conscious victim who has no vomiting, convulsions, brain, or abdominal injuries?

Name _____ Date _____

Evaluated by _____

DIRECTIONS: Practice providing first aid for shock according to the criteria listed. When you are ready for your final check, give this sheet to your instructor.

PROFICIENT

Providing First Aid for Shock	Points Possible	Peer Check Yes	Peer Check No	Final Check* Yes	Final Check* No	Points Earned**	Comments
1. Follows priorities:							
Checks the scene	4						
Checks consciousness and breathing	4						
Calls emergency medical services	4						
Cares for victim	4						
Controls bleeding	4						
2. Observes victim for signs of shock:							
Pale or bluish color to skin	2						
Cool, moist or clammy skin	2						
Diaphoresis	2						
Rapid, weak, irregular pulse	2						
Rapid, weak, irregular, shallow or labored respirations	2						
Low blood pressure	2						
Signs of weakness, apathy and/or confusion	2						
Nausea and/or vomiting	2						
Excessive thirst	2						
Restless or anxious	2						
Blurred vision	2						
Eyes sunken; vacant, dilated pupils	2						
3. Attempts to reduce shock by treating bleeding, providing oxygen, easing pain, and giving emotional support	6						
4. Positions victim according to injuries or illness:							
Avoids movement if neck or spine injury present	5						
Positions on side if vomiting or has a jaw/mouth injury	4						
Positions lying flat with head raised if victim having difficulty breathing	4						
Positions lying flat or with head raised slightly if head injury present	4						
Positions lying flat with feet raised 12 inches if none of the above conditions present	5						

15:4 (cont.)

Providing First Aid for Shock	Points Possible	Peer Check		Final Check*		Points Earned**	Comments
		Yes	No	Yes	No		
5. Places enough blankets on/under victim to prevent chilling but avoids overheating	6						
6. Avoids giving fluids by mouth if medical help is available, victim unconscious or convulsing, brain or abdominal injury, surgery possible, or nausea and vomiting noted	6						
7. If medical help delayed at least one hour or more and none of the above conditions noted, gives small sips of salt-soda solution	6						
8. Observes and cares for victim until medical help obtained	6						
9. Replaces all equipment used	2						
10. Washes hands	2						
Totals	100						

* Final Check: Instructor or authorized person evaluates.
** Points Earned: Points possible times each "yes" check.

UNIT 15:5 PROVIDING FIRST AID FOR POISONING

ASSIGNMENT SHEET

Grade _____   Name _____

INTRODUCTION: This assignment will help you review the main facts on providing first aid for poisoning.

INSTRUCTIONS: Read the information on Providing First Aid for Poisoning. In the space provided, print the word(s) that best completes the statement or answers the question.

1. List four (4) ways that poisoning can be caused.

2. Treatment for poisoning will vary depending on the _____ poison, the _____ involved, and the method of _____.

3. What is the first thing to do when a victim swallows a poison?

4. List three (3) types of information that should be given to a poison control center or physician.

5. What should you do if a conscious poison victim vomits?

6. How should you position an unconscious poisoning victim who is breathing? Why?

7. List two (2) ways to induce vomiting.

8. Why is activated charcoal used after a poisoning victim vomits?

9. List four (4) types of poison victims in whom vomiting should not be induced.

10. What is the first step of treatment for a victim who has been poisoned by inhaling gas?

11. How do you treat victims poisoned by chemicals splashing on the skin?

12. List five (5) signs of an allergic reaction to an injected poison.

UNIT 15:5 Evaluation Sheet

Name _____ Date _____

Evaluated by _____

DIRECTIONS: Practice providing first aid for poisoning according to the criteria listed. When you are ready for your final check, give this sheet to your instructor.

PROFICIENT

Providing First Aid for Poisoning	Points Possible	Peer Check Yes	No	Final Check* Yes	No	Points Earned**	Comments
1. Follows steps of priority care:							
Checks the scene	2						
Checks consciousness and breathing	2						
Calls emergency medical services	2						
Cares for victim	2						
Controls bleeding	2						
2. Checks victim for signs of poisoning by noting the following points:							
Burns on lips or mouth	2						
Odor	2						
Presence of poison container	2						
Presence of substance on victim or in mouth	2						
Information obtained from victim or observers	2						
3. Provides first aid for conscious victim who has swallowed poison:							
Determines type poison, how much taken, and when	2						
Calls poison control center or physician	2						
Follows instructions from poison control center	2						
Saves sample of any vomited material	2						
4. Induces vomiting only if told to do so, no medical help available, and *none* of the following present:							
Victim unconscious	2						
Victim convulsing	2						
Burns on lips or mouth	2						
Victim ingested acid, alkali, or petroleum product	2						
5. Provides first aid for unconscious victim:							
Checks breathing and gives artificial respiration if needed	3						
Positions breathing victim on side	3						
Calls poison control center and obtains medical help	3						

Providing First Aid for Poisoning	Points Possible	Peer Check		Final Check*		Points Earned**	Comments
		Yes	No	Yes	No		
Saves any vomitus and container with poison	3						
6. Provides first aid for a victim with chemicals or poisons splashed on the skin as follows:							
Washes area with large amounts of water	2						
Removes clothing containing substance	2						
Obtains medical help for burns/injuries	2						
7. Provides first aid for a victim who has come in contact with poisonous plants as follows:							
Washes area with soap and water	2						
Removes contaminated clothing	2						
Applies lotions or baking soda paste	2						
Obtains medical help if condition severe	2						
8. Provides first aid for victim who has inhaled poisonous gas as follows:							
Takes deep breath before entering area	2						
Holds breath while removing victim from area	2						
Checks breathing and gives artificial respiration as needed	2						
Obtains medical help	2						
9. Provides first aid for victim with insect bite/sting or snakebite:							
Positions affected area below level of heart	2						
Treats insect bite/sting:							
Removes embedded stinger correctly	2						
Washes area with soap and water	2						
Applies sterile dressing	2						
Applies cold pack	2						
Treats snakebite:							
Washes wound	2						
Immobilizes injured area	2						
Monitors breathing and gives artificial respiration if necessary	2						
Obtains medical help	2						
Watches for signs/symptoms of allergic reaction	3						
10. Observes all victims for signs of shock and treats as necessary	3						
11. Reassures victim while providing care	3						
12. Obtains medical help for any victim as soon as possible	3						
Totals	100						

* Final Check: Instructor or authorized person evaluates.
** Points Earned: Points possible times each "yes" check.

UNIT 15:6 PROVIDING FIRST AID FOR BURNS

ASSIGNMENT SHEET

Grade _____ Name _____

INTRODUCTION: This sheet will help you review the main facts on burns and first aid treatment for burns.

INSTRUCTIONS: Review the information on Providing First Aid for Burns. In the space provided, print the word(s) that best completes the statement or answers the question.

1. Define *burn.*

2. Briefly list the characteristics or signs and symptoms for each of the following types of burns:

   First degree or   Second degree or   Third degree or
   superficial   partial-thickness   full-thickness

3. First aid treatment for burns is directed at removing _____, cooling _____, covering _____, relieving _____, observing and treating _____, and preventing _____.

4. Identify four (4) times when medical care should be obtained for burn victims.

5. What is the main treatment for superficial and mild, partial-thickness burns?

6. Why is a sterile dressing applied to a burn?

7. If blisters appear on a burn, how should you treat these?

8. How should third degree burns be treated?

9. If chemicals or irritating gases burn the eyes, how should the eyes be treated?

10. Why is shock frequently noted in victims with severe burns?

UNIT 15:6 Evaluation Sheet

Name _____ Date _____

Evaluated by _____

DIRECTIONS: Practice providing first aid for burns according to the criteria listed. When you are ready for your final check, give this sheet to your instructor.

PROFICIENT

Providing First Aid for Burns	Points Possible	Peer Check Yes	No	Final Check* Yes	No	Points Earned**	Comments
1. Follows priorities:							
Checks the scene	2						
Checks consciousness and breathing	2						
Calls emergency medical services	2						
Cares for victim	2						
Controls bleeding	2						
2. Identifies type of burn present as follows:							
1st degree or superficial: reddened	3						
2nd degree or partial thickness: red, wet, painful, swollen, blister	3						
3rd degree or full thickness: white or charred with destruction of tissue	3						
3. Provides first aid for superficial or mild partial thickness burns:							
Cools burn by flushing it with large amounts of cool water	3						
Blots dry gently with sterile gauze	3						
Applies dry sterile dressing	3						
Avoids breaking blisters	3						
Elevates burned area if possible	3						
Obtains medical help if necessary	3						
4. Provides first aid for full-thickness or 3rd-degree burns:							
Obtains medical help immediately	3						
Applies dry sterile dressing	3						
Avoids removing charred clothing from area	3						
Elevates hands and arms or legs and feet if affected	3						
Elevates head if victim in respiratory distress	3						
5. Provides first aid for chemical burns as follows:							
Flushes area with large amounts of water	3						
Removes contaminated clothing	3						
Continues flushing with large amounts of cool water	3						
Obtains medical help	3						

15:6 (cont.)

Providing First Aid for Burns	Points Possible	Peer Check		Final Check*		Points Earned**	Comments
		Yes	No	Yes	No		
6. Provides first aid for burns of the eye as follows:							
Positions victim with head to side and injured eye down	3						
Pours water from inner to outer part of eye	3						
Irrigates for 15–30 minutes or until medical help arrives	3						
Obtains medical help	3						
7. Observes for signs of shock in all victims and treats as necessary	5						
8. Reassures victim and remains calm	5						
9. Obtains medical help for any of the following:							
Burns extensive (Over 15% of surface of adult body, 10% in child)	2						
Third-degree or full thickness burns	2						
Burns of the face	2						
Signs of shock	2						
Respiratory distress	2						
Burns of the eye/eyes	2						
Chemical burns on the skin	2						
Totals	100						

* Final Check: Instructor or authorized person evaluates.
** Points Earned: Points possible times each "yes" check.

UNIT 15:7 PROVIDING FIRST AID FOR HEAT EXPOSURE

ASSIGNMENT SHEET

Grade _____   Name _____

INTRODUCTION: This assignment will help you review the main facts regarding conditions caused by exposure to heat.

INSTRUCTIONS: Review the information on Providing First Aid for Heat Exposure. In the space provided, print the word(s) that best completes the statement or answers the question.

1. What occurs when the body is over exposed to heat?

2. What are heat cramps?

3. List three (3) first aid treatments for heat cramps.

4. List six (6) signs or symptoms of heat exhaustion.

5. List three (3) first aid treatments for heat exhaustion.

6. How does internal body temperature differ in heat exhaustion and heat stroke?

7. List three (3) signs and symptoms of heat stroke.

8. High body temperatures (such as 105° F or 41°C) can cause _____ and/or
   _____.

9. List three (3) first aid treatments for heat stroke.

10. Identify two (2) precautions a victim should take after recovering from any condition caused by exposure to heat.

Name _____ Date _____

Evaluated by _____

DIRECTIONS: Practice providing first aid for heat exposure according to the criteria listed. When you are ready for your final check, give this sheet to your instructor.

PROFICIENT

Providing First Aid for Heat Exposure	Points Possible	Peer Check Yes	No	Final Check* Yes	No	Points Earned**	Comments
1. Follows priorities:							
Checks the scene	2						
Checks consciousness and breathing	2						
Calls emergency medical services	2						
Cares for victim	2						
Controls bleeding	2						
2. Observes signs to determine condition as follows:							
Heat cramps: muscle pain	3						
Heat exhaustion: normal body temperature, skin pale and clammy, diaphoresis, nausea, headache, weakness, dizziness	4						
Heat stroke: high body temperature; skin hot, red and dry; weak or unconscious	4						
3. Provides first aid for heat cramps:							
Applies firm pressure to muscle with hand	4						
Lies victim down in cool area	4						
Gives victim small sips of water to total 4 ounces in 15 minutes	4						
Obtains medical help if cramps continue	4						
4. Provides first aid for heat exhaustion:							
Moves to cool area	3						
Positions lying down with feet elevated 12 inches	3						
Loosens tight clothing	3						
Applies cool wet cloths	3						
Gives victim small sips of water to total 4 ounces in 15 minutes	3						
Discontinues water if victim complains of nausea and/or vomits	3						
Obtains medical help if necessary	3						

15:7 (cont.)

Providing First Aid for Heat Exposure	Points Possible	Peer Check Yes	No	Final Check* Yes	No	Points Earned**	Comments
5. Provides first aid for heat stroke as follows:							
Moves to cool area	4						
Removes excess clothing	4						
Sponges skin with cool water or puts victim in tub of cool water	4						
Positions victim on side if vomiting occurs	4						
Obtains medical help immediately	4						
6. Observes for sign of shock and treats for shock in all victims	5						
7. Reassures victim while providing care, remains calm	5						
8. Obtains medical help for any of the following victims:							
Heat cramps do not subside	4						
Heat exhaustion victim with vomiting or shock	4						
All heat stroke victims	4						
Totals	100						

* Final Check: Instructor or authorized person evaluates.
** Points Earned: Points possible times each "yes" check.

UNIT 15:8 PROVIDING FIRST AID FOR COLD EXPOSURE

ASSIGNMENT SHEET

Grade _____ Name _____

INTRODUCTION: This assignment will help you review the main facts on first aid for cold exposure.

INSTRUCTIONS: Read the information on Providing First Aid for Cold Exposure. In the space provided, print the word(s) that best completes the statement or answers the question.

1. List three (3) factors that affect the degree of injury caused by exposure to the cold.

2. List five (5) symptoms that can result from prolonged exposure to the cold.

3. List three (3) first aid treatments for hypothermia.

4. What is frostbite?

5. List four (4) symptoms of frostbite.

6. Name four (4) common sites for frostbite.

7. What temperature water should be used to warm a body part injured by frostbite?

8. Why is it important not to rub or massage a body part affected by frostbite?

9. How should you treat blisters that form on frost-damaged skin?

10. Why do you place sterile gauze between fingers or toes that have been injured by frostbite?

UNIT 15:8 Evaluation Sheet

Name _____ Date _____

Evaluated by _____

DIRECTIONS: Practice providing first aid for cold exposure according to the criteria listed. When you are ready for your final check, give this sheet to your instructor.

	Points Possible	Peer Check		Final Check*		Points Earned**	Comments
Providing First Aid for Cold Exposure		Yes	No	Yes	No		
1. Follows priorities:							
Checks the scene	3						
Checks consciousness and breathing	3						
Calls emergency medical services	3						
Cares for victim	3						
Controls severe bleeding	3						
2. Observes for signs of exposure to cold	6						
3. Checks skin for signs of frostbite	6						
4. Moves victim to warm area	6						
5. Removes wet or frozen clothing and loosens constrictive clothing	6						
6. Warms victim slowly by wrapping in blankets or putting on dry clothing	6						
7. Immerses frostbitten part in water at 100°–105° F (37.8°–40.6° C)	6						
8. Discontinues warming when skin flushed	6						
9. Dries area or body by blotting gently	6						
10. Places sterile gauze between fingers and toes affected by frostbite	6						
11. Positions victim lying down with affected parts elevated	6						
12. Observes and treats for shock	6						
13. Gives warm liquids to victim if victim conscious and not nauseated or vomiting	6						
14. Reassures victim while providing care	6						
15. Obtains medical help as soon as possible	6						
Totals	100						

* Final Check: Instructor or authorized person evaluates.
** Points Earned: Points possible times each "yes" check.

UNIT 15:9 PROVIDING FIRST AID FOR BONE AND JOINT INJURIES

ASSIGNMENT SHEET

Grade _____ Name _____

INTRODUCTION: This assignment will help you review the main facts regarding bone and joint injuries.

INSTRUCTIONS: Read the information on Providing First Aid for Bone and Joint Injuries. In the space provided, print the word(s) that best completes the statement or answers the question.

1. Define each of the following:

   fracture:

   dislocation:

   sprain:

   strain:

2. What is the difference between a closed or simple fracture and an open or compound fracture?

3. List six (6) signs and symptoms of a fracture.

4. Treatment for fractures is directed at maintaining _____, treating _____, keeping the broken bone from _____, and preventing further _____.

5. List four (4) signs and symptoms of a dislocation.

6. Why is movement of the injured part dangerous when a dislocation has occurred?

7. List four (4) signs and symptoms of a sprain.

8. List three (3) first aid treatments for a sprain.

9. Why are cold applications used to treat a sprain or strain?

Why are warm applications used to treat a strain?

10. List six (6) different types of materials that can be used for splints.

11. List three (3) basic principles that should be followed when splints are applied.

12. How can you test that an air splint is inflated properly?

13. Why should the hand be positioned higher than the elbow when a sling is applied?

14. List four (4) points you can check to make sure that circulation is not impaired after a splint or sling has been applied.

15. What should you do if you notice signs of impaired circulation after applying a splint?

16. Why is it best to avoid moving any victim who has a neck or spinal injury?

Name _____ Date _____

Evaluated by _____

DIRECTIONS: Practice providing first aid for bone and joint injuries according to the criteria listed. When you are ready for your final check, give this sheet to your instructor.

PROFICIENT

Providing First Aid for Bone and Joint Injuries	Points Possible	Peer Check Yes	No	Final Check* Yes	No	Points Earned**	Comments
1. Follows priorities of care:							
Checks the scene	2						
Checks consciousness and breathing	2						
Calls emergency medical services	2						
Cares for victim	2						
Controls bleeding	2						
2. Observes victim for signs of bone or joint injury	3						
3. Immobilizes any injured area or suspected fracture and/or dislocation	3						
4. Applies splints:							
Selects appropriate splint material	3						
Uses splints that will immobilize joint above and below injured area	3						
Positions splints correctly to avoid pressure on injury	3						
Pads splints especially at bony areas	3						
Ties splints in place	3						
Avoids any unnecessary movement during application	3						
5. Applies air/inflatable splints as follows:							
Obtains correct splint	3						
Supports injured area while positioning splint	3						
Inflates splint correctly	3						
Checks inflation by pressing on splint with thumb	3						
6. Applies sling with triangular bandage:							
Provides support for arm while applying	3						
Positions bandage with long edge on uninjured side	3						
Brings lower end up over injured arm and over shoulder on injured side	3						
Ties bandage ends with square knot avoiding bony area of neck and places padding between knot and skin	3						

Providing First Aid for Bone and Joint Injuries	Points Possible	Peer Check		Final Check*		Points Earned**	Comments
		Yes	No	Yes	No		
Secures area by elbow with pin or by tying in knot	3						
Checks to be sure fingers exposed and hand elevated 5 to 6 inches above elbow	3						
7. Checks for signs of impaired circulation by noting the following:							
Pale or bluish color	2						
Cold to touch	2						
Swelling/edema	2						
Pain or pressure from splint/sling	2						
Numbness or tingling	2						
Poor return of pink color after blanching nails	2						
8. Loosens splint/sling if impaired circulation noted	4						
9. Observes for signs of shock and treats as needed	4						
10. Applies cold applications to reduce swelling and pain	4						
11. Positions victim in a comfortable position but avoids unnecessary movement and avoids all movement if neck or spine injury suspected	4						
12. Reassures victim while providing first aid care	4						
13. Obtains medical help as soon as possible	4						
Totals	100						

* Final Check: Instructor or authorized person evaluates.
** Points Earned: Points possible times each "yes" check.

UNIT 15:10 PROVIDING FIRST AID FOR SPECIFIC INJURIES

ASSIGNMENT SHEET

Grade _____   Name _____

INTRODUCTION: This assignment will help you review the specific care given to victims with injuries to the eye, ear, nose, brain, chest, abdomen, and genital organs.

INSTRUCTIONS: Read the information on Providing First Aid for Specific Injuries. In the space provided, print the word(s) that best completes the statement or answers the question.

1. Injuries to the eye always involve the danger of _____. A top priority of first aid care is to obtain the assistance of _____, preferably a/an _____.

2. Briefly describe two (2) techniques that can be used to remove a foreign object that is floating free in the eye.

3. If an object is embedded in the eye, what first aid care should be given?

4. List the steps of first aid treatment that should be followed when an object is protruding from the eye.

5. How should you care for tissue torn from the ear?

6. How should you position a victim with cerebrospinal fluid draining from the ear?

7. List six (6) signs and symptoms of injuries to the brain.

8. List four (4) aspects of first aid care for victims with brain injuries.

9. List three (3) causes of nosebleeds.

10. How should you position a victim with a nosebleed?

11. What type of dressing should be applied to a sucking chest wound? Why?

12. How should you position a victim with a sucking chest wound?

13. List four (4) signs and symptoms of abdominal injuries.

14. How should you position a victim with an abdominal injury?

15. How should you care for abdominal organs protruding from a wound?

16. List four (4) principles of first aid for injuries to genital organs.

Name _____ Date _____

Evaluated by _____

DIRECTIONS: Practice providing first aid for specific injuries according to the criteria listed. When you are ready for your final check, give this sheet to your instructor.

PROFICIENT

Providing First Aid for Specific Injuries	Points Possible	Peer Check Yes	No	Final Check* Yes	No	Points Earned**	Comments
1. Follows priorities of care:							
Checks the scene	1						
Checks consciousness and breathing	1						
Calls emergency medical services	1						
Cares for victim	1						
Controls bleeding	1						
2. Observes victim for signs and symptoms of specific injuries	2						
3. Provides first aid for eye injuries:							
Washes hands thoroughly	2						
Removes free floating foreign object:							
Draws upper lid down over lower lid	2						
Raises upper lid and removes object with sterile gauze or gently flushes eye with water	2						
Applies sterile dressing if object embedded or above techniques do not work on free floating object	2						
If an object is protruding from the eye, immobilizes with dressings and makes no attempt to remove	2						
Covers both eyes with dressings to prevent movement of injured eye	2						
Positions victim lying flat	2						
Obtains medical help	2						
4. Provides first aid for ear injuries as follows:							
Applies light pressure with sterile dressing to control bleeding	2						
Preserves torn tissue by putting in sterile cool water or gauze moistened with sterile cool water	2						
Places sterile gauze loosely in outer ear canal for perforation of eardrum	2						
If cerebrospinal fluid is draining from ear:							
Avoids any attempt to stop flow	2						

Providing First Aid for Specific Injuries	Points Possible	Peer Check		Final Check*		Points Earned**	Comments
		Yes	No	Yes	No		
Positions victim on injured side with head and shoulders elevated slightly	2						
Positions dressing to absorb flow	2						
Obtains medical help	2						
5. Provides first aid for brain injuries as follows:							
Positions victim lying flat	2						
Elevates head and shoulders if no neck/spine injury	2						
Watches closely for respiratory distress	2						
Allows cerebrospinal fluid to drain and absorbs with dressings	2						
Avoids fluids – moistens lips, tongue and mouth with cool wet cloth if necessary	2						
Notes length of time the victim is unconscious	2						
Obtains medical help	2						
6. Provides first aid for nosebleed:							
Positions victim sitting with head leaning slightly forward	2						
Presses bleeding nostril(s) to midline	2						
If bleeding does not stop, inserts gauze in nostril(s) and applies pressure	2						
Applies cold wet compress or covered ice bag	2						
Obtains medical help if bleeding does not stop, fracture suspected, or victim has repeated nosebleeds	2						
7. Provides first aid for chest injuries as follows:							
For sucking chest wound:							
Applies airtight dressing using aluminum foil or plastic	3						
Positions victim on injured side and elevates head and chest slightly	2						
For penetrating object:							
If object protruding, immobilizes in place and makes no attempt to remove it	3						
Positions victim in comfortable position but avoids unnecessary movement	2						
Watches closely for respiratory distress	2						
Obtains medical help immediately	2						

15:10 (cont.)

Providing First Aid for Specific Injuries	Points Possible	Peer Check		Final Check*		Points Earned**	Comments
		Yes	No	Yes	No		
8. Provides first aid for abdominal injuries:							
Positions victim lying flat with knees flexed	2						
Elevates head and shoulders slightly to aid breathing	2						
If organs protruding, covers organs with sterile dressing moistened with sterile water or normal saline	3						
Avoids giving oral fluids	2						
Obtains medical help immediately	2						
9. Provides first aid for injuries to genital organs as follows:							
Controls bleeding with direct pressure	2						
Positions victim lying flat with legs separated	2						
Preserves any torn tissue by placing it in sterile cool water or in gauze moistened with sterile cool water	2						
Applies cold compresses or covered ice bag	2						
Obtains medical help	2						
10. Observes all victims for signs of shock and treats for shock immediately	2						
11. Reassures victim while providing care; encourages victim to relax as much as possible	2						
Totals	100						

* Final Check: Instructor or authorized person evaluates.
** Points Earned: Points possible times each "yes" check.

UNIT 15:11 PROVIDING FIRST AID FOR SUDDEN ILLNESS

ASSIGNMENT SHEET

Grade _____   Name _____

INTRODUCTION: Sudden illness can occur in any individual, and you should know the major facts regarding first aid. This assignment will help you review these facts.

INSTRUCTIONS: Review the information on Providing First Aid for Sudden Illness. In the space provided, print the word(s) that best completes the statement or answers the question.

1. Identify three (3) sources of information you can use to help determine what illness a victim has.

2. List four (4) signs and symptoms of a heart attack.

3. List three (3) first aid treatments for a heart attack victim.

4. List six (6) signs and symptoms of a stroke.

5. List three (3) first aid treatments for a stroke.

6. If early symptoms of fainting are noted, how should you position the victim?

7. List three (3) points of first aid care for a victim who has fainted.

8. What is a convulsion?

9. First aid care for the victim with a convulsion is directed at preventing _____.

10. Should a padded tongue blade or soft object be placed between the victim's teeth during a convulsion? Why or why not?

11. Why is it important not to use force or restrain the muscle movements during a convulsion?

12. In a victim with diabetes, an increase in the level of glucose or sugar in the blood can lead to a condition called _____, and an excess amount of insulin can lead to a condition called _____.

13. List six (6) signs and symptoms of diabetic coma.

14. What is the main treatment for diabetic coma?

15. List six (6) signs and symptoms of insulin shock.

16. What is the main treatment for insulin shock?

Name _____ Date _____

Evaluated by _____

DIRECTIONS: Practice providing first aid for sudden illness according to the criteria listed. When you are ready for your final check, give this sheet to your instructor.

Providing First Aid for Sudden Illness	Points Possible	Peer Check Yes	No	Final Check* Yes	No	Points Earned**	Comments
1. Follows priorities of care:							
Checks the scene	2						
Checks consciousness and breathing	2						
Calls emergency medical services	2						
Cares for victim	2						
Controls bleeding	2						
2. Observes victim for specific signs and symptoms of sudden illnesses	3						
3. Obtains information from victim regarding illness	3						
4. Checks for medical bracelet, necklace or card if victim unconscious	3						
5. Provides first aid for **heart attack** as follows:							
Positions in most comfortable position for victim	3						
Encourages relaxation	2						
Watches for signs of shock and treats as needed	2						
Moistens lips and mouth with wet cloth or gives small sips of water but avoids ice or cold water	2						
Obtains medical help as quickly as possible	2						
6. Provides first aid for **stroke** as follows:							
Positions in comfortable position	2						
Elevates head and shoulders to aid breathing	2						
Positions on side if victim having difficulty swallowing or unconscious	2						
Reassures victim and encourages relaxation	2						
Avoids fluids-moistens lips and mouth if necessary	2						
Obtains medical help immediately	2						

PROFICIENT

Providing First Aid for Sudden Illness	Points Possible	Peer Check		Final Check*		Points Earned**	Comments
		Yes	No	Yes	No		
7. Provides first aid for **fainting:**							
Keeps victim lying flat	3						
Loosens tight clothing	2						
Bathes face with cool water	2						
Checks for other injuries	2						
Encourages victim to lie flat until color improves	2						
After recovery, allows victim to get up slowly	3						
Obtains medical help if recovery delayed, other injuries noted, or other instances of fainting	2						
8. Provides first aid for **convulsions** as follows:							
Removes dangerous objects or moves victim if objects too heavy to move	3						
Places pillow, blanket, or soft object under head	3						
Checks respirations	2						
Avoids restraining muscle movements	2						
Notes length of convulsion and parts of body involved	2						
Watches closely after convulsion ends	2						
Obtains medical assistance if necessary	2						
9. Provides first aid for **diabetic coma** as follows:							
Positions in comfortable position or on side if unconscious	3						
Checks respirations closely	3						
Obtains medical help immediately	3						
10. Provides first aid for **insulin shock** as follows:							
Gives conscious victim drink with sugar	3						
Places sugar under tongue of unconscious victim	3						
Positions in comfortable position or on side if unconscious	3						
Obtains medical help if recovery not prompt	2						
11. Observes for signs of shock and treats as needed	3						
12. Reassures victim while providing care	3						
Totals	100						

* Final Check: Instructor or authorized person evaluates.
** Points Earned: Points possible times each "yes" check.

UNIT 15:12 APPLYING DRESSINGS AND BANDAGES

ASSIGNMENT SHEET

Grade _____ Name _____

INTRODUCTION: This assignment will help you review the main facts on dressings and bandages.

INSTRUCTIONS: Review the information on Applying Dressings and Bandages. In the space provided, print the word(s) that best completes the statement or answers the question.

1. What is a dressing?

2. List three (3) purposes or functions of dressings.

3. Why should you avoid using fluff cotton as a dressing?

4. What are bandages?

5. Bandages should be applied snugly enough to control _____ and prevent _____, but not so tightly that they interfere with _____.

6. List three (3) types or examples of bandages.

7. List three (3) uses for triangular bandages.

8. Why are elastic bandages hazardous?

9. List four (4) signs that indicate poor circulation.

10. If any signs of impaired or poor circulation are noted after a bandage has been applied, what should you do?

UNIT 15:12 Evaluation Sheet

Name _____ Date _____

Evaluated by _____

DIRECTIONS: Practice applying dressings and bandages according to the criteria listed. When you are ready for your final check, give this sheet to your instructor.

Applying Dressings and Bandages	Points Possible	Peer Check Yes	No	Final Check* Yes	No	Points Earned**	Comments
1. Assembles supplies	1						
2. Washes hands and puts on gloves	1						
3. Applies dressing as follows:							
Obtains correct size dressing	2						
Opens package without touching dressing	2						
Uses pinching action to pick up dressing	2						
Touches only one part of outside	2						
Holds dressing over wound and lowers onto wound	2						
Secures dressing with tape or bandage	2						
4. Applies triangular bandage to head or scalp:							
Folds two-inch hem in base	2						
Places sterile dressing on wound	2						
Positions middle of base on forehead with hem on outside	2						
Brings ends around head, above ears, crosses in back, and returns to forehead	2						
Ties ends in center of forehead with square knot	2						
Supports head while pulling point down in back to make bandage snug	2						
Tucks point into area where bandage crosses in back	2						
5. Folds a cravat with a triangular bandage:							
Brings point down to base	2						
Folds lengthwise until desired width obtained	2						
6. Applies circular bandage with cravat as follows:							
Places sterile dressing on wound	2						
Places center of cravat over dressing	2						
Carries ends around area and crosses when they meet	2						
Brings ends back to starting point	2						
Ties ends with square knot	2						

PROFICIENT

Applying Dressings and Bandages	Points Possible	Peer Check Yes	No	Final Check* Yes	No	Points Earned**	Comments
7. Applies spiral wrap with roller gauze:							
Places sterile dressing on wound	2						
Holds bandage with loose end coming off bottom	2						
Starts at bottom of limb and moves upward	2						
Anchors bandage correctly	2						
Circles area with spiral motion	2						
Overlaps each turn ½ width of bandage	2						
Ends with 1 or 2 circular turns around limb	2						
Secures with tape, pins, or by tying	2						
8. Applies figure-eight wrap as follows:							
Places sterile dressing on wound	2						
Anchors bandage on instep	2						
Circles foot once or twice	2						
Angles over top of foot	2						
Goes behind ankle	2						
Circles down over top of foot and under instep	2						
Repeats pattern overlapping each turn ½ to ⅔ width of bandage	2						
Ends with 1 or 2 circular wraps around ankle	2						
Secures with tape, pins, or by tying	2						
9. Applies bandage to finger as follows:							
Places dressing on wound	2						
Holds gauze with loose end coming off bottom of roll	2						
Overlaps bandage on finger with 3–4 recurrent folds	2						
Uses spiral wrap to hold folds in position	2						
Uses figure-eight wrap around wrist to secure	2						
Ends by circling wrist	2						
Ties at wrist	2						
10. Checks circulation in area below bandage by noting following points:							
Pale or bluish	1						
Swelling	1						
Coldness	1						
Numbness or tingling	1						
Poor return of color after nailbeds pressed lightly	1						
11. Loosens bandage immediately if any signs of impaired circulation noted	2						
12. Obtains medical help for victim as soon as possible	2						
13. Removes gloves and washes hands	1						
Totals	100						

* Final Check: Instructor or authorized person evaluates.
** Points Earned: Points possible times each "yes" check.

UNIT 16:1 DEVELOPING JOB-KEEPING SKILLS

ASSIGNMENT SHEET

Grade _____   Name _____

INTRODUCTION: To keep a job, it will be essential for you to learn job-keeping skills. This assignment will help you evaluate your job-keeping skills.

INSTRUCTIONS: Read the information on Developing Job-Keeping Skills. In the space provided, print the word(s) that best completes the statement or answers the question.

1. Identify ten (10) deficiencies that employers feel are common in high school students.

2. Choose at least three (3) job-keeping skills for which you feel you are proficient. Give at least two (2) reasons why you feel you are competent in each of the skills.

3. Choose at least three (3) job-keeping skills for which you feel you need improvement. Explain why you are not competent in these skills. Then identify at least two (2) ways you can improve your competency in each of these skills.

UNIT 16:2 WRITING A LETTER OF APPLICATION AND PREPARING A RESUMÉ

ASSIGNMENT SHEET

Grade _____ Name _____

INTRODUCTION: A letter of application and a resumé are two important parts of obtaining employment. This assignment will help you review the main facts regarding the letter and resumé.

INSTRUCTIONS: Read the information on Writing a Letter of Application and Resumé. In the space provided, print the word(s) that best completes the statement or answers the question.

1. What is the main purpose of the letter of application?

2. The letter should be _____ on good quality paper. It must be _____, _____, and done according to correct _____ for letters. Care must be taken to ensure that _____ and _____ are correct.

3. Briefly state the contents for each of the paragraphs in a letter of application.

   a. paragraph 1:

   b. paragraph 2:

   c. paragraph 3:

   d. paragraph 4:

4. What is a resumé?

5. Briefly list the type of information found in each of the following parts of a resumé.

   a. personal identification:

   b. employment objective:

   c. educational background:

   d. work or employment experience:

   e. skills:

   f. other activities:

   g. references:

6. Why is honesty always the best policy when completing resumés?

7. What type of envelope should you use to mail the letter of application and resumé?

8. What is the purpose of a career passport or portfolio?

List five (5) items that might be included in a career passport or portfolio.

237

UNIT 16:2 INVENTORY SHEET FOR RESUMÉS

Grade _____ Name _____

INTRODUCTION: The following information is required for resumés.

INSTRUCTIONS: Use a telephone book, address books, school records, and other sources to complete the following information about yourself.

Name _____

Address _____
    Number & Street   City   State   Zip

Telephone ( ) _____ Social Security _____

Name of School _____

School Address _____
        No. & Street   City   State   Zip

Dates of Attendance _____

Degree Earned _____ Major _____

Special Skills Learned _____

Computer Skills/Courses _____

Grade Average _____ Awards Earned _____

_____

_____

Other Schools Attended: Name _____

    Address _____

Previous Employers: Most recent first

Names	Address City, State, Zip	Dates of Employment	Duties Job Titles

References: Names (at least 3)   Full Address and Telephone   Title

_____

_____

_____

Other Activities: Include clubs, offices, volunteer work, hobbies

_____

_____

_____

Name _____ Date _____

Evaluated by _____

DIRECTIONS: Practice writing a letter of application according to the criteria listed. When you are ready for your final check, give this sheet to your instructor along with the letter of application.

PROFICIENT

Writing a Letter of Application	Points Possible	Peer Check Yes	Peer Check No	Final Check* Yes	Final Check* No	Points Earned**	Comments
1. Uses good quality paper	6						
2. Computer prints or types all information neatly and accurately	6						
3. Follows correct form for either block or modified block style letters	6						
4. Completes contents of letter as follows:							
Addresses to correct individual	8						
States purpose for writing	8						
States position applying for	8						
Lists source of advertisement or referring person	8						
States why qualified	8						
States resumé enclosed or furnished on request	8						
Includes information on how employer can contact	8						
Thanks employer for considering application	8						
5. Spells all words correctly	6						
6. Punctuates all information and sentences correctly	6						
7. Uses complete sentences and correct grammar	6						
Totals	100						

* Final Check: Instructor or authorized person evaluates.
** Points Earned: Points possible times each "yes" check.

UNIT 16:2B Evaluation Sheet

Name _____ Date _____

Evaluated by _____

DIRECTIONS: Practice writing a resumé according to the criteria listed. When you are ready for your final check, give this sheet to your instructor along with the resumé.

Writing a Resumé	Points Possible	Peer Check Yes	No	Final Check* Yes	No	Points Earned**	Comments
1. Uses good quality paper	6						
2. Computer prints or types all information neatly and accurately	6						
3. Follows consistent format and spacing throughout resumé	6						
4. Includes all of the following information:							
Personal identification: name, address, telephone	10						
Employment objective	10						
Educational background: name and address of school, special courses, or training	10						
Work or employment experience: name and address of employers, dates employed, job title, description of duties, in order from most recent backward	10						
Skills and specific knowledge	10						
Other activities: organizations, offices held, awards, volunteer work, hobbies, interests	10						
References: full name, title, and address or states "References will be furnished on request"	10						
5. Spells all words correctly	6						
6. Punctuates all information correctly	6						
Totals	100						

* Final Check: Instructor or authorized person evaluates.
** Points Earned: Points possible times each "yes" check.

UNIT 16:3 COMPLETING JOB APPLICATION FORMS

ASSIGNMENT SHEET #1

Grade _____   Name _____

INTRODUCTION: This assignment will help you review the main facts about completing job application forms.

INSTRUCTIONS: Read the information about Completing Job Application Forms. In the space provided, print the word(s) that best completes the statement or answers the question.

1. Why do employers use job application forms?

2. List three (3) reasons why you should read the application form completely before you fill in the information.

3. If questions do not apply to you, what should you put in the space provided for the answer to the question?

4. Why is it important to watch spelling and punctuation?

5. If the application does not state otherwise, it is best to type or _____. Use _____ if printing.

6. Why must all information be correct and truthful?

7. If a space is labeled "office use only," how do you complete this section? Why?

8. What should you do before using anyone's name as a reference?

9. What is the purpose of the wallet card?

10. Identify three (3) things you should look for when you proofread your completed application.

UNIT 16:3 COMPLETING JOB APPLICATION FORMS: WALLET CARD

ASSIGNMENT SHEET #2

Grade _____   Name _____

INTRODUCTION: When you are looking for a job, you must be prepared. To be sure that you always have the needed information, it is wise to carry a "wallet card" with you. A sample form is given.

INSTRUCTIONS: Complete the information listed. This is information that can be used during job interviews, but most of the time it is required for application forms. The sheet can then be glued to an index card and kept in your wallet for easy reference. The information itself may also be written on a small index card.

Registration/License number _____   Social Security _____

Grade School Name _____

     Address _____   Zip _____

     Date Attended _____

Junior High Name _____

     Address _____   Zip _____

     Date Attended _____

High School Name _____

     Address _____   Zip _____

     Date Attended _____

Special Training–Major _____

Computer Skills/ Courses _____

Activities _____

Special Skills _____

_____

Employment:

Dates	Name	Position	Full Address and Telephone	Salary

References: Include name, title, full address, telephone (Include at least 3)

_____

_____

_____

Other Facts _____

_____

ASSIGNMENT SHEET #3

Grade _____ Name _____

INTRODUCTION: To obtain a job, you will probably have to complete an application form. The sample form that follows will help prepare you for this task.

INSTRUCTIONS: Review the information about Completing Job Application Forms. Complete the information on your "wallet card." Then use this information to complete the following form.

Health Careers Unlimited Application

Please type or print all information required. Be sure all information is accurate and complete.

Name in Full _____

Full Address _____

City _____ State _____ Zip _____

Social Security _____ Telephone _____

Position Desired _____

What prompted you to apply here? _____

When will you be available to start work? _____

Will you work (check if yes) any shift? _____ Holidays? _____

      Weekends? _____ Part time? _____ Full Time? _____

Salary Expected _____ Registration Number _____

Education: (Circle last grade completed)

High School   1   2   3   4   Name _____

      From _____ Address in Full _____

      To _____ _____

College   1   2   3   4   Name _____

      From _____ Address in Full _____

      To_____ _____

Military Record: Branch of Service _____

      Date Entered _____ Date Discharged _____

      Discharge Status _____ Rank _____

Activities/Organizations/Special Skills _____

Computer Skills/Courses _____

    243

Employment Record (list most recent position first)

Name of Employer _____

Full Address _____

Telephone _____ Dates: From _____ To _____

Supervisor's Name _____

Average Salary _____ Job Title _____

Reason for Leaving _____

Name of Employer _____

Full Address _____

Telephone _____ Dates: From _____ To _____

Supervisor's Name _____

Average Salary _____ Job Title _____

Reason for Leaving _____

Name of Employer _____

Full Address _____

Telephone _____ Dates: From _____ To _____

Supervisor's Name _____

Average Salary _____ Job Title _____

Reason for Leaving _____

References: List names, titles, full address, and telephone

1. _____

   _____

2. _____

   _____

3. _____

   _____

I affirm that all of these statements are true and correct. I grant permission for verification of any of these facts.

Date _____ Signature _____

Do not write below this line:

Date Interviewed _____ Position _____

Salary _____ Starting Date _____ Initials _____

UNIT 16:3 Evaluation Sheet

Name _____   Date _____

Evaluated by _____

DIRECTIONS: Practice completing job application forms according to the criteria listed. When you are ready for your final check, give this sheet to your instructor.

PROFICIENT

Completing Job Application Forms	Points Possible	Peer Check Yes	Peer Check No	Final Check* Yes	Final Check* No	Points Earned**	Comments
1. Completes wallet card correctly:							
Prints or types neatly	8						
Inserts accurate information	8						
Lists full addresses, zip codes, names, etc.	8						
2. Types or prints in ink on application form unless writing requested on form	7						
3. Follows all directions provided on form completely	8						
4. Completes all of the following information on form:							
Personal information	8						
Education	8						
Work experience	8						
References	8						
Signature in correct area	8						
5. Spells all words correctly	7						
6. Leaves "office space" and similar areas blank	7						
7. Completes form neatly and thoroughly; places "none" or "NA" in spaces as necessary	7						
Totals	100						

* Final Check: Instructor or authorized person evaluates.
** Points Earned: Points possible times each "yes" check.

UNIT 16:4 PARTICIPATING IN A JOB INTERVIEW

ASSIGNMENT SHEET

Grade _____   Name _____

INTRODUCTION: A job interview is an essential part of obtaining a job. This assignment will review the main facts.

INSTRUCTIONS: Review the information on Participating in a Job Interview. In the space provided, print the word(s) that best completes the statement or answers the question.

1. List two (2) purposes of the job interview.

2. List two (2) things containing information that you should take to the job interview with you.

3. List four (4) rules for dress or appearance that should be observed.

4. How early should you arrive for a job interview?

5. List eight (8) rules of conduct that should be observed during a job interview.

6. What should you do after the job interview to let the employer know you are still interested in the position?

7. Write a brief response to each of the following questions as though you were being asked during a job interview.

    a. "Why do you feel you are qualified for this position?"

    b. "What are your strengths or strong points?"

    c. "I see you recently got married. Do you plan to start a family soon?"

    d. "What do you feel are the three most important features of a job?"

    e. "What do you hope to accomplish during the next two years?"

UNIT 16:4 Evaluation Sheet

Name _____ Date _____

Evaluated by _____

DIRECTIONS: Practice participating in a job interview according to the criteria listed. When you are ready for your final check, give this sheet to your instructor.

PROFICIENT

Participating in a Job Interview	Points Possible	Peer Check Yes	No	Final Check* Yes	No	Points Earned**	Comments
1. Dresses appropriately for interview	6						
2. Prepares wallet card, resumé, job application	5						
3. Arrives 5–10 minutes early for interview	5						
4. Introduces self to employer and shakes hands firmly if indicated	5						
5. Refers to employer by name	5						
6. Sits correctly with good posture	5						
7. Listens closely to employer's questions and comments	6						
8. Answers all questions thoroughly but keeps answers pertinent	6						
9. Speaks slowly and clearly without mumbling	6						
10. Smiles when appropriate but avoids excessive laughter or giggling	5						
11. Maintains eye contact with employer	6						
12. Avoids mannerisms during interview	6						
13. Uses correct English and avoids slang terms	6						
14. Uses correct manners and acts polite	6						
15. Avoids smoking, chewing gum, eating candy, etc.	5						
16. Asks questions pertaining to job responsibility and avoids questioning fringe benefits, raises, etc.	6						
17. Thanks employer for the interview at the end	6						
18. Shakes hands firmly if indicated	5						
Totals	100						

* Final Check: Instructor or authorized person evaluates.
** Points Earned: Points possible times each "yes" check.

UNIT 16:5 DETERMINING NET INCOME

ASSIGNMENT SHEET

Grade _____ Name _____

INTRODUCTION: To determine how much money you have available after deductions, you must figure out your net income. This assignment will help you do this.

INSTRUCTIONS: Follow the instructions in each of the following sections. Place your answers in the blanks on the right. Double-check all figures for accuracy. Your teacher will supply an hourly wage rate if you are not employed.

1. List your wage per hour (how much you make an hour).

   1. _____

2. Multiply your wage per hour times the number of hours you work per week. Usually a 40 hour work week is an average amount.

   Wage Per Hour × Hours Worked Per Week =

   2. _____

   This amount is your gross weekly pay.

3. Determine the average deductions that will be taken out of your gross weekly pay.

   a. Determine deduction for federal tax by multiplying the gross pay times the percentage of deduction found on federal tax tables. (An average amount is 15 percent or 0.15.)

   _____ × _____ =
   Gross Pay   Federal Tax Percentage

   a. _____

   b. Determine deduction for state tax by multiplying the gross pay times the percentage of deduction found on state tax tables. (An average amount is 2 percent or 0.02.)

   _____ × _____ =
   Gross Pay   State Tax Percentage

   b. _____

   c. Determine deduction for city/corporation tax by multiplying the gross pay times the percentage found on city tax tables. (An average amount is 1 percent or 0.01.)

   _____ × _____ =
   Gross Pay   City Tax Percentage

   c. _____

   d. Determine the deduction for FICA or Social Security by multiplying gross pay times the current deduction. (Use 7.65 percent or 0.0765 if unknown.)

   _____ × _____ =
   Gross Pay   Social Security Percentage

   d. _____

Name _____

e. List any other deductions that are subtracted from your gross pay. This can include payments for insurance, charity, union dues, etc. Add all of these deductions together to get the total for miscellaneous deductions.

e. _____

_____

_____

f. Add the answers in a., b., c., d., and e. together to get the total amount of deductions.

f. _____

4. Subtract the amount in answer f. (total amount of all deductions) from the gross weekly pay listed in question 2. This amount will be your net weekly pay or "take home" weekly pay.

_____ − _____ = _____
Gross Pay   Deductions   Net Weekly Pay

4. _____

5. To determine your net pay per month, multiply the weekly net pay times 4 for four week months. Multiply the weekly net pay times 5 for five week months.

_____ × _____ = _____
Net Weekly Pay   Weeks Per Month   Net Monthly Pay

5. _____

NOTE: The weekly net pay can be multiplied by 52 weeks to determine yearly net pay.

249

Name _____ Date _____

Evaluated by _____

DIRECTIONS: Practice determining net income according to the criteria listed. When you are ready for your final check, give this sheet to your instructor.

PROFICIENT

Determining Net Income	Points Possible	Peer Check Yes	No	Final Check* Yes	No	Points Earned**	Comments
1. Lists wage per hour	10						
2. Determines gross weekly pay by multiplying wage per hour times the number of hours worked per week	14						
3. Determines deduction for federal tax by multiplying correct percentage times gross weekly pay	10						
4. Determines deduction for state tax by multiplying correct percentage times gross weekly pay	10						
5. Determines deduction for city/corporation tax by multiplying correct percentage times gross weekly pay	10						
6. Determines deduction for social security by multiplying correct percentage times gross weekly pay	10						
7. Lists any miscellaneous deductions and obtains a total for these by adding all miscellaneous deductions together	10						
8. Adds amounts for federal tax, state tax, city/corporation tax, social security, and miscellaneous deductions together	12						
9. Subtracts total amount of deductions from gross weekly pay to get net weekly pay	14						
Totals	100						

* Final Check: Instructor or authorized person evaluates.
** Points Earned: Points possible times each "yes" check.

UNIT 16:6 CALCULATING A BUDGET

ASSIGNMENT SHEET

Grade _____   Name _____

INTRODUCTION: To avoid financial problems, planning and foresight is required. This assignment will help you prepare a budget and plan monthly expenses. Follow the instructions in each section to calculate a budget.

1. List monthly expenses for the following items:

   Rent (you may have to share an apartment)   _____

   Utilities: heat, electricity, telephone, water, garbage, etc.   _____

   Food: include all food items purchased, money for food away from home   _____

   Car Expenses:

       Gasoline   _____

       Insurance (divide yearly payment by 12)   _____

       Oil, maintenance, tires, repairs   _____

       Payment for purchase   _____

       Other: (note what)   _____

   Laundry or cleaning of clothes   _____

   Clothing purchase (include uniforms)   _____

   Payments: Furniture   _____

                     Charge accounts   _____

                     Other bills   _____

   Personal items: shampoo, toothpaste, etc.   _____

   Donations: Church, charities   _____

   Medical or Life Insurance payments (divide yearly payment by 12)   _____

   Education expenses (fees, books, etc.)   _____

   Savings (strive for 10%)   _____

   Other items: List _____   _____

              _____   _____

   Entertainment, hobbies, etc.   _____

   Miscellaneous: "Mad" money, etc.   _____

                                           TOTAL 1. $ _____

2. List your net pay per four week month.

                                           TOTAL 2. $ _____

3. If the total in number 2 is larger than the total in number 1, you may add more money to items in your budget. If number 1 is larger, you have overspent. Refigure your budget. Figure in number 1 should equal figure in number 2 for a balanced budget.

UNIT 16:6 Evaluation Sheet

Name _____ Date _____

Evaluated by _____

DIRECTIONS: Practice calculating a budget according to the criteria listed. When you are ready for your final check, give this sheet to your instructor.

PROFICIENT

Calculating a Budget	Points Possible	Peer Check Yes	No	Final Check* Yes	No	Points Earned**	Comments
1. Lists realistic monthly amounts for each of the following items:							
Rent or house payments	5						
Utilities	5						
Food	5						
Car expenses:							
Gasoline	3						
Insurance (divides yearly payment by 12)	3						
Oil, maintenance, etc.	3						
Payment for purchase	3						
Laundry or cleaning of clothes	5						
Clothing purchase	5						
Payments:							
Furniture	3						
Charge accounts	3						
Other bills	3						
Personal items	5						
Donations	5						
Medical or life insurance (divides yearly payment by 12)	5						
Education expenses	5						
Savings	5						
Entertainment, hobbies	5						
Miscellaneous expenses	5						
2. Determines net monthly income accurately	6						
3. Totals all expenses in budget for total monthly expenses accurately	6						
4. Balances budget by making monthly expenses equal net monthly income	7						
Totals	100						

* Final Check: Instructor or authorized person evaluates.
** Points Earned: Points possible times each "yes" check.

UNIT 17:1 IDENTIFYING THE STRUCTURES AND TISSUES OF A TOOTH

ASSIGNMENT SHEET

Grade _____   Name _____

INTRODUCTION: This assignment will help you learn the main structures and tissues of a tooth.

INSTRUCTIONS: Read the information on Identifying the Structures and Tissues of a Tooth. In the space provided, print the word(s) that best completes the statement or answers the question.

1. Label the following diagram of a tooth:

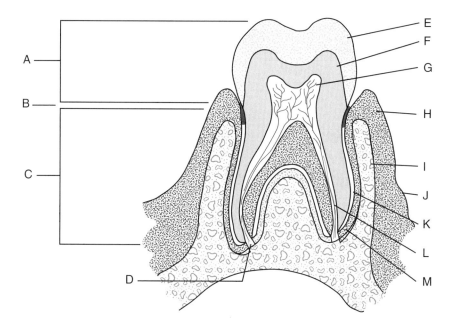

A. _____   H. _____

B. _____   I. _____

C. _____   J. _____

D. _____   K. _____

E. _____   L. _____

F. _____   M. _____

G. _____

2. How many teeth are present in primary or deciduous dentition?

3. At what age do primary teeth begin to erupt in the mouth?

4. List two (2) functions of primary or deciduous teeth.

5. When do permanent or succedaneous teeth begin to erupt into the mouth?

6. How many teeth are present in permanent or succedaneous dentition?

7. A child with both primary and permanent teeth erupted in the mouth is said to have_____dentition.

8. Name the following division or tissue of a tooth:
    a. tissue making up main bulk of a tooth:
    b. opening in tip of root of tooth:
    c. made of nerves and blood vessels:
    d. area where crown joins root:
    e. section of tooth visible in mouth:
    f. forms protective outer layer on tooth:
    g. tissue that helps hold tooth in place:
    h. section of tooth below gingiva or gums:
    i. provides sensation and nourishment for tooth:
    j. hardest tissue in the body:

9. The structures that surround and support the teeth are called the _____.

10. Place the letter(s) of the correct structure of the periodontium in column B in the space provided by the description in column A.

<u>Column A</u>   <u>Column B</u>

_____ 1. Contains nerves and blood vessels that provide nourishment   A. Alveolar process

_____ 2. Contains a series of sockets, one for each tooth in the mouth   B. Attached gingiva

_____ 3. Fibers of connective tissue that attach to the cementum and alveolus   C. Free gingiva

_____ 4. Gum tissue that surrounds cervix and fills interproximal spaces   D. Peridontal ligament

_____ 5. Bone tissues that surround the roots of the teeth

_____ 6. Acts as a shock absorber and prevents teeth from resting on bone

_____ 7. Gum tissue attached to alveolar bone

_____ 8. Produces sensation when pressure is applied to a tooth

_____ 9. Made of epithelial tissue covered with mucous membrane

_____ 10. Aids in production of cementum

UNIT 17:1 Evaluation Sheet

Name _____ Date _____

Evaluated by _____

DIRECTIONS: Practice identifying the structures and tissues of a tooth according to the criteria listed. When you are ready for your final check, give this sheet to your instructor.

PROFICIENT

Identifying Structures and Tissues of a Tooth	Points Possible	Peer Check Yes	No	Final Check* Yes	No	Points Earned**	Comments
1. Obtains model or unlabeled chart of a tooth	2						
2. Washes hands	3						
3. Identifies primary/deciduous teeth:							
States age when teeth begin to erupt	5						
States age when all teeth erupted	5						
States total number of primary teeth	5						
4. Identifies permanent/succedaneous teeth:							
States ages when teeth begin to erupt	5						
States total number of secondary teeth	5						
Defines "mixed" dentition	5						
5. Identifies sections or divisions of a tooth:							
Crown	5						
Root	5						
Cervix, neck, or cemento-enamel junction	5						
Apex	5						
Apical foramen	5						
6. Identifies and states function of tissues of a tooth:							
Enamel	5						
Cementum	5						
Dentin	5						
Pulp	5						
7. Identifies and states function of structures that surround a tooth:							
Periodontium:							
Alveolar process	5						
Periodontal ligament	5						
Gingiva	5						
8. Replaces all equipment	2						
9. Washes hands	3						
Totals	100						

* Final Check: Instructor or authorized person evaluates.
** Points Earned: Points possible times each "yes" check.

UNIT 17:2 IDENTIFYING THE TEETH

ASSIGNMENT SHEET

Grade _____ Name _____

INTRODUCTION: As an assistant, you must know the name of each tooth in the mouth. This assignment will help you learn the correct names.

INSTRUCTIONS: Review the information on Identifying the Teeth. In the space provided in the two following diagrams, label each tooth by its correct name. Be sure to put right or left, and maxillary or mandibular by each tooth.

1. PRIMARY OR DECIDUOUS TEETH

2. PERMANENT OR SUCCEDANEOUS TEETH

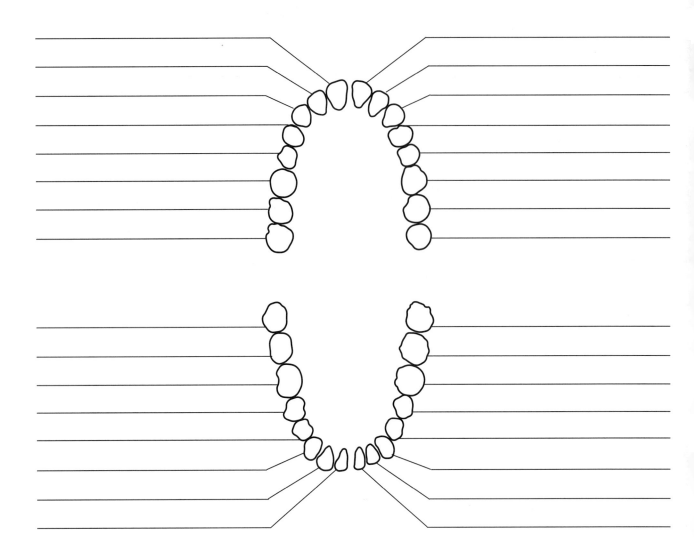

3. Place the letter(s) of the correct type of tooth in Column B in the space provided by the description in Column A.

Column A   Column B

_____ 1. Used to tear food   A. Bicuspids

_____ 2. Also called premolars   B. Cuspids

_____ 3. Broad, sharp edge   C. Incisors

_____ 4. Largest and strongest teeth   D. Molars

_____ 5. Also called canines or eyeteeth

_____ 6. Pulverize or grind food

_____ 7. Use to cut food

_____ 8. Located at angles of lips

_____ 9. Longest teeth in the mouth

_____ 10. Teeth in the back of the mouth

4. What is the name of the plane that separates the mouth into a maxillary and mandibular section?

5. What is the name of the plane that divides the mouth into a right and left half?

Name _____   Date _____

Evaluated by _____

DIRECTIONS: Practice identifying the teeth according to the criteria listed. When you are ready for your final check, give this sheet to your instructor.

Identifying the Teeth	Points Possible	Peer Check Yes	No	Final Check* Yes	No	Points Earned**	Comments
PROFICIENT							
1. Obtains model or unlabeled chart of teeth	1						
2. Washes hands	2						
3. States full name for each of the twenty primary or deciduous teeth:							
Max. rt. 2nd molar							
Max. rt. 1st molar							
Max. rt. cuspid							
Max. rt. lateral incisor							
Max. rt. central incisor							
Max. lft. central incisor							
Max. lft. lateral incisor							
Max. lft. cuspid							
Max. lft. 1st molar							
Max. lft. 2nd molar							
Mand. lft. 2nd molar							
Mand. lft. 1st molar							
Mand. lft. cuspid							
Mand. lft. lateral incisor							
Mand. lft. central incisor							
Mand. rt. central incisor							
Mand. rt. lateral incisor							
Mand. rt. cuspid							
Mand. rt. 1st molar							
Mand. rt. 2nd molar							
1½ points for each tooth	30						
4. States full name for each of the thirty-two permanent or succedaneous teeth:							
Max. rt. 3rd molar							
Max. rt. 2nd molar							
Max. rt. 1st molar							
Max. rt. 2nd bicuspid							
Max. rt. 1st bicuspid							
Max. rt. cuspid							

17:2 (cont.)

Identifying the Teeth	Points Possible	Peer Check		Final Check*		Points Earned**	Comments
		Yes	No	Yes	No		
Max. rt. lateral incisor							
Max. rt. central incisor							
Max. lft. central incisor							
Max. lft. lateral incisor							
Max. lft. cuspid							
Max. lft. 1st bicuspid							
Max. lft. 2nd bicuspid							
Max. lft. 1st molar							
Max. lft. 2nd molar							
Max. lft. 3rd molar							
Mand. lft. 3rd molar							
Mand. lft. 2nd molar							
Mand. lft. 1st molar							
Mand. lft. 2nd bicuspid							
Mand. lft. 1st bicuspid							
Mand. lft. cuspid							
Mand. lft. lateral incisor							
Mand. lft. central incisor							
Mand. rt. central incisor							
Mand. rt. lateral incisor							
Mand. rt. cuspid							
Mand. rt. 1st bicuspid							
Mand. rt. 2nd bicuspid							
Mand. rt. 1st molar							
Mand. rt. 2nd molar							
Mand. rt. 3rd molar							
2 points for each tooth	64						
5. Replaces equipment	1						
6. Washes hands	2						
Totals	100						

* Final Check: Instructor or authorized person evaluates.
** Points Earned: Points possible times each "yes" check.

UNIT 17:3 IDENTIFYING TEETH USING THE UNIVERSAL NUMBERING SYSTEM AND FEDERATION DENTAIRE INTERNATIONAL SYSTEM

ASSIGNMENT SHEET

Grade _____   Name _____

INTRODUCTION: This sheet will allow you to practice using the Universal Numbering System and Federation Dentaire International System for identifying teeth.

INSTRUCTIONS: Put your name on each paper. Read all instructions carefully.

1. Following is a diagram of primary dentition (deciduous teeth). Label each tooth using the Universal Numbering System.

2. Recheck the diagram to be sure it is correct. Refer to the previous diagram to complete the following information. Full names of the lettered teeth should be entered in column I. You may abbreviate right, left, maxillary and mandibular. The correct letter for each tooth listed should be entered in column II.

Column I	Column II
A is _____	Max. Lft. Cuspid is _____
G is _____	Mand. Rt. 1st Molar is _____
K is _____	Mand. Lft. Lateral Incisor is _____
P is _____	Max. Rt. 1st Molar is _____
T is _____	Mand. Rt. Cuspid is _____
I is _____	Mand. Lft. Central Incisor is _____
C is _____	Max. Rt. Lateral Incisor is _____
E is _____	Mand. Lft. 1st Molar is _____
M is _____	Max. Lft. Central Incisor is _____
Q is _____	Max. Lft. 2nd Molar is _____

3. Following is a diagram of the permanent or succedaneous teeth. Label each tooth using the Universal Numbering System.

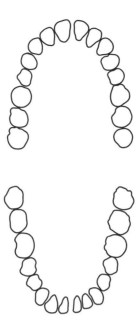

4. Check the previous diagram for accuracy. Then refer to it to complete the following information. Full names of the numbered teeth should be printed in Column I. Abbreviations may be used for right, left, maxillary and mandibular. The correct number for each tooth should be entered in Column II.

Column I	Column II
1 is _____	Max. Rt. Lateral Incisor is _____
8 is _____	Mand. Rt. 2nd Bicuspid is _____
15 is _____	Mand. Lft. 1st Molar is _____
20 is _____	Mand. Lft. Central Incisor is _____
28 is _____	Max. Lft. Cuspid is _____
32 is _____	Max. Rt. Cuspid is _____
16 is _____	Mand. Lft. 2nd Molar is _____
4 is _____	Max. Lft. 2nd Bicuspid is _____
23 is _____	Mand. Rt. Lateral Incisor is _____
17 is _____	Mand. Lft. 1st Bicuspid is _____
12 is _____	Max. Lft. Central Incisor is _____
30 is _____	Mand. Rt. 2nd Molar is _____
3 is _____	Mand. Lft. Cuspid is _____
25 is _____	Max. Rt. 2nd Molar is _____
10 is _____	Mand. Rt. Cuspid is _____
5 is _____	Max. Lft. 1st Molar is _____

263

5. Following is a diagram of primary (deciduous) teeth. Divide the diagram into four (4) quadrants and label each quadrant. Then label each tooth using the Federation Dentaire International System.

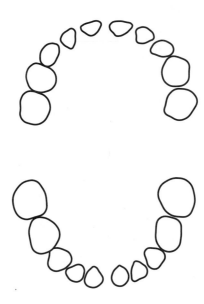

6. Check the previous diagram for accuracy. Then refer to it to complete the following information. Full names of the numbered teeth should be printed in Column I. Abbreviations may be used for right, left, maxillary, and mandibular. The correct number for each tooth listed should be entered in Column II.

Column I	Column II
51 is _____	Max. Rt. 2nd Molar is _____
74 is _____	Mand. Lft. Cuspid is _____
63 is _____	Mand. Rt. Central Incisor is _____
85 is _____	Max. Lft. Lateral Incisor is _____
82 is _____	Mand. Rt. 1st Molar is _____
53 is _____	Max. Lft. Central Incisor is _____
72 is _____	Mand. Lft. 2nd Molar is _____
65 is _____	Max. Rt. Lateral Incisor is _____
54 is _____	Mand. Rt. Cuspid is _____
71 is _____	Max. Lft. 1st Molar is _____

7. Following is a diagram of permanent (succedaneous) teeth. Divide the diagram into four (4) quadrants and label each quadrant. Then label each tooth using the Federation Dentaire International System.

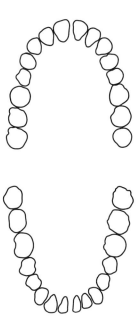

8. Check the previous diagram for accuracy. Then refer to it to complete the following information. Full names of the numbered teeth should be printed in Column I. Abbreviations may be used for right, left, maxillary, and mandibular. The correct number for each tooth listed should be entered in Column II.

Column I	Column II
11 is _____	Max. Rt. Lateral Incisor is _____
23 is _____	Mand. Rt. 2nd Bicuspid is _____
28 is _____	Mand. Lft. 2nd Molar is _____
47 is _____	Max. Lft. Central Incisor is _____
35 is _____	Mand. Rt. 1st Molar is _____
22 is _____	Mand. Lft. Lateral Incisor is _____
15 is _____	Max. Rt. Cuspid is _____
43 is _____	Max. Lft. 1st Molar is _____
18 is _____	Mand. Rt. 1st Bicuspid is _____
41 is _____	Mand. Lft. Central Incisor is _____
24 is _____	Max. Rt. 1st Molar is _____
36 is _____	Max. Lft. 2nd Bicuspid is _____
14 is _____	Mand. Lft. 1st Bicuspid is _____
33 is _____	Mand. Rt. 3rd Molar is _____
42 is _____	Max. Rt. 2nd Molar is _____
38 is _____	Max. Lft. 2nd Molar is _____

265

Name _____ Date _____

Evaluated by _____

DIRECTIONS: Practice identifying teeth using the Universal Numbering System according to the criteria listed. When you are ready for your final check, give this sheet to your instructor.

PROFICIENT

Identifying Teeth Using the Universal Numbering System	Points Possible	Peer Check Yes	No	Final Check* Yes	No	Points Earned**	Comments
1. Obtains model or chart of teeth	1						
2. Washes hands	2						
3. States universal letter for each of the twenty primary teeth (state names at random)							
Max. rt. 2nd molar - A							
Max. rt. 1st molar - B							
Max. rt. cuspid - C							
Max. rt. lateral incisor - D							
Max. rt. central incisor - E							
Max. lft. central incisor - F							
Max. lft. lateral incisor - G							
Max. lft. cuspid - H							
Max. lft. 1st molar - I							
Max. lft. 2nd molar - J							
Mand. lft. 2nd molar - K							
Mand. lft. 1st molar - L							
Mand. lft. cuspid - M							
Mand. lft. lateral incisor - N							
Mand. lft. central incisor - O							
Mand. rt. central incisor - P							
Mand. rt. lateral incisor - Q							
Mand. rt. cuspid - R							
Mand. rt. 1st molar - S							
Mand. rt. 2nd molar - T							
1½ points for each letter	30						
4. States universal number for each of the thirty-two permanent teeth (state names at random)							
Max. rt. 3rd molar - 1							
Max. rt. 2nd molar - 2							
Max. rt. 1st molar - 3							
Max. rt. 2nd bicuspid - 4							
Max. rt. 1st bicuspid - 5							

17:3A (cont.)

Identifying Teeth Using the Universal Numbering System	Points Possible	Peer Check Yes	No	Final Check* Yes	No	Points Earned**	Comments
Max. rt. cuspid - 6							
Max. rt. lateral incisor - 7							
Max. rt. central incisor - 8							
Max. lft. central incisor - 9							
Max. lft. lateral incisor - 10							
Max. lft. cuspid - 11							
Max. lft. 1st bicuspid - 12							
Max. lft. 2nd bicuspid - 13							
Max. lft. 1st molar - 14							
Max. lft. 2nd molar - 15							
Max. lft. 3rd molar - 16							
Mand. lft. 3rd molar - 17							
Mand. lft. 2nd molar - 18							
Mand. lft. 1st molar - 19							
Mand. lft. 2nd bicuspid - 20							
Mand. lft. 1st bicuspid - 21							
Mand. lft. cuspid - 22							
Mand. lft. lateral incisor - 23							
Mand. lft. central incisor - 24							
Mand. rt. central incisor - 25							
Mand. rt. lateral incisor - 26							
Mand. rt. cuspid - 27							
Mand. rt. 1st bicuspid - 28							
Mand. rt. 2nd bicuspid - 29							
Mand. rt. 1st molar - 30							
Mand. rt. 2nd molar - 31							
Mand. rt. 3rd molar - 32							
2 points for each number	64						
5. Replaces equipment	1						
6. Washes hands	2						
Totals	100						

* Final Check: Instructor or authorized person evaluates.
** Points Earned: Points possible times each "yes" check.

UNIT 17:3B Evaluation Sheet

Name _____ Date _____

Evaluated by _____

DIRECTIONS: Practice identifying teeth using the Federation Dentaire International System according to the criteria listed. When you are ready for your final check, give this sheet to your instructor.

PROFICIENT

Identifying Teeth Using the Federation Dentaire International System	Points Possible	Peer Check Yes	No	Final Check* Yes	No	Points Earned**	Comments
1. Obtains model or chart of teeth	1						
2. Washes hands	2						
3. States Federation Dentaire number for each of the twenty primary teeth (state names at random)							
Max. rt. 2nd molar - 55							
Max. rt. 1st molar - 54							
Max. rt. cuspid - 53							
Max. rt. lateral incisor - 52							
Max. rt. central incisor - 51							
Max. lft. central incisor - 61							
Max. lft. lateral incisor - 62							
Max. lft. cuspid - 63							
Max. lft. 1st molar - 64							
Max. lft. 2nd molar - 65							
Mand. lft. 2nd molar - 75							
Mand. lft. 1st molar - 74							
Mand. lft. cuspid - 73							
Mand. lft. lateral incisor - 72							
Mand. lft. central incisor - 71							
Mand. rt. central incisor - 81							
Mand. rt. lateral incisor - 82							
Mand. rt. cuspid - 83							
Mand. rt. 1st molar - 84							
Mand. rt. 2nd molar - 85							
1 1/2 points for each number	30						
4. States Federation Dentaire number for each of the thirty-two permanent teeth (state names at random)							
Max. rt. 3rd molar - 18							
Max. rt. 2nd molar - 17							
Max. rt. 1st molar - 16							
Max. rt. 2nd bicuspid - 15							
Max. rt. 1st bicuspid - 14							

17:3B (cont.)

Identifying Teeth Using the Federation Dentaire International System	Points Possible	Peer Check		Final Check*		Points Earned**	Comments
		Yes	No	Yes	No		
Max. rt. cuspid - 13							
Max. rt. lateral incisor - 12							
Max. rt. central incisor - 11							
Max. lft. central incisor - 21							
Max. lft. lateral incisor - 22							
Max. lft. cuspid - 23							
Max. lft. 1st bicuspid - 24							
Max. lft. 2nd bicuspid - 25							
Max. lft. 1st molar - 26							
Max. lft. 2nd molar - 27							
Max. lft. 3rd molar - 28							
Mand. lft. 3rd molar - 38							
Mand. lft. 2nd molar - 37							
Mand. lft. 1st molar - 36							
Mand. lft. 2nd bicuspid - 35							
Mand. lft. 1st bicuspid - 34							
Mand. lft. cuspid - 33							
Mand. lft. lateral incisor - 32							
Mand. lft. central incisor - 31							
Mand. rt. central incisor - 41							
Mand. rt. lateral incisor - 42							
Mand. rt. cuspid - 43							
Mand. rt. 1st bicuspid - 44							
Mand. rt. 2nd bicuspid - 45							
Mand. rt. 1st molar - 46							
Mand. rt. 2nd molar - 47							
Mand. rt. 3rd molar - 48							
2 points for each number	64						
5. Replaces equipment	1						
6. Washes hands	2						
Totals	100						

* Final Check: Instructor or authorized person evaluates.
** Points Earned: Points possible times each "yes" check.

UNIT 17:4 IDENTIFYING THE SURFACES OF THE TEETH

ASSIGNMENT SHEET

Grade _____   Name _____

INTRODUCTION: To chart dental conditions, you must know the crown surfaces of the teeth. This sheet will help you practice identifying the surfaces.

INSTRUCTIONS: Put your name on this paper. Read all directions carefully.

A. The following diagram represents an anterior tooth. It is a right anterior tooth and you are looking at a tongue (back) view of the tooth. Identify the surfaces, line angles, and point angles and write them in the spaces provided.

   NOTE: Make sure you understand the position of the tooth. Do not attempt to do the assignment until you can visualize the position of the tooth (Hint: Put your tongue on a right anterior tooth.)

Crown Surfaces: Name and abbreviation for each answer.

   1.

   2.

   3.

   4.

   5. The surface not seen on the other side of the tooth, facing the lips is the _____ (surface).

Line Angles: Name and Abbreviation

   6.

   7.

   8.

   9.

   10.

Point Angles: Name and Abbreviation

   11.

   12.

B. Following is a diagram of a posterior tooth. It is a right posterior tooth. You are looking at the inside or back surface of the tooth.

Label the surfaces, line angles, and point angles in the spaces provided following the sketch. List each name correctly and place the abbreviation by the name as requested.

NOTE: Make sure you understand the position of the tooth.

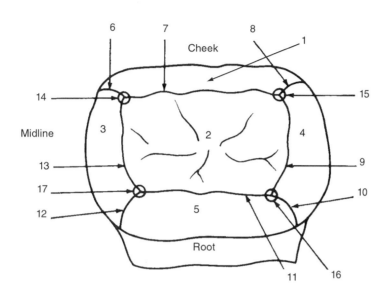

Crown Surfaces: List Name and Abbreviation

1.

2.

3.

4.

5.

Line Angles: List Name and Abbreviation

6.

7.

8.

9.

10.

11.

12.

13.

Point Angles: List Name and Abbreviation

14.

15.

16.

17.

UNIT 17:4 Evaluation Sheet

Name _____ Date _____

Evaluated by _____

DIRECTIONS: Practice identifying the surfaces of teeth according to the criteria listed. When you are ready for your final check, give this sheet to your instructor.

PROFICIENT

Identifying the Surfaces of the Teeth	Points Possible	Peer Check Yes	No	Final Check* Yes	No	Points Earned**	Comments
1. Obtains model or unlabeled chart of teeth	3						
2. Washes hands	3						
3. Identifies anterior teeth	5						
4. Identifies posterior teeth	5						
5. Identifies surfaces on anterior teeth:							
Labial	3						
Incisal	3						
Mesial	3						
Distal	3						
Lingual	3						
6. Identifies surfaces on posterior teeth:							
Buccal	3						
Occlusal	3						
Mesial	3						
Distal	3						
Lingual	3						
7. Identifies line angles on anterior teeth:							
Linguoincisal	2						
Labioincisal	2						
Mesiolabial	2						
Mesioincisal	2						
Mesiolingual	2						
Distolingual	2						
Distoincisal	2						
Distolabial	2						
8. Identifies line angles on posterior teeth:							
Mesioocclusal	2						
Mesiolingual	2						
Mesiobuccal	2						
Distoocclusal	2						
Distolingual	2						
Distobuccal	2						
Linguoocclusal	2						
Buccoocclusal	2						

Name _____

17:4 (cont.)

Identifying the Surfaces of the Teeth	Points Possible	Peer Check Yes	No	Final Check* Yes	No	Points Earned**	Comments
9. Identifies point angles on anterior teeth:							
Mesiolinguoincisal	2						
Mesiolabioincisal	2						
Distolabioincisal	2						
Distolinguoincisal	2						
10. Identifies point angles on posterior teeth:							
Mesiolinguoocclusal	2						
Mesiobuccoocclusal	2						
Distobuccoocclusal	2						
Distolinguoocclusal	2						
11. Replaces equipment	3						
12. Washes hands	3						
Totals	100						

* Final Check: Instructor or authorized person evaluates.
** Points Earned: Points possible times each "yes" check.

273

UNIT 17:5 CHARTING CONDITIONS OF THE TEETH

ASSIGNMENT SHEET #1

Grade _____   Name _____

INTRODUCTION: This assignment sheet will allow you to practice charting a variety of dental conditions.

INSTRUCTIONS: Carefully read the information on Charting Conditions of the Teeth. Refer to it as needed to complete this assignment.

Use the blank dental record chart to record the following conditions, which represent dental services performed on a series of visits. Draw the correct symbols for the listed conditions on both the anatomic and geometric diagrams.

NOTE: The information pertains to permanent teeth.

DATE	NO	DESCRIPTION	DEBIT	DATE	AMT.	BAL

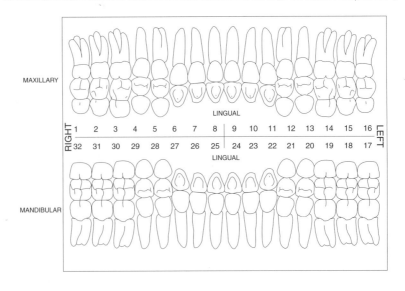

Name _____

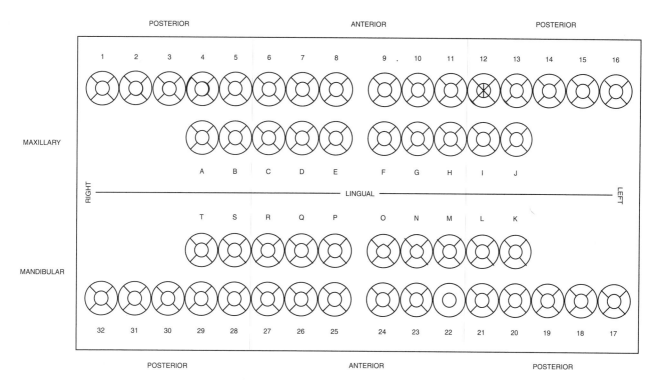

Date	Conditions noted/treatment done
1/20/—	Initial visit to office
	Clinical examination done
	Full-mouth series of X rays taken
	Prophylaxis treatment and fluoride application done
	Following conditions noted on exam:
	Maxillary right 3rd molar is impacted
	Mandibular right 3rd molar needs to be extracted
	Mandibular left 2nd bicuspid is missing
	Mandibular left 1st molar has a mesioocclusal carious lesion (decay)
	Mandibular left central incisor has a lingual carious lesion
	Maxillary right 1st bicuspid has a distoocclusal carious lesion
1/23/—	Amalgam restoration to occlusal surface of maxillary right 2nd molar
	Composite restoration to the mesiolabioincisal edge of the maxillary right central incisor
	Dycal placed under restoration
3/10/—	Bite wing X rays taken, four X rays
	Root canal treatment to maxillary left cuspid
5/3/—	Amalgam restoration to mesial occlusal distal surfaces of maxillary left 1st bicuspid
5/20/—	Mandibular left third molar extracted
6/2/—	Composite restoration to the distal lingual incisal edge of the mandibular left lateral incisor
7/12/—	Clinical examination, prophylaxis treatment
	Maxillary left lateral incisor has a lingual carious lesion
	Alginate impression taken on mandibular arch
7/30/—	Amalgam restoration to the buccal surface of the maxillary right 2nd bicuspid
8/15/—	Gold crown placed on mandibular right 1st molar

UNIT 17:5 CHARTING CONDITIONS OF THE TEETH

ASSIGNMENT SHEET #2

Grade _____ Name _____

INTRODUCTION: This assignment will provide additional practice on charting a variety of dental conditions.

INSTRUCTIONS: Put your name on this paper. Refer to the information on Charting Conditions of the Teeth.

Use the blank dental record chart to record the following dental conditions performed during a series of visits to the dental office. Draw the correct symbols for the listed conditions on both the anatomic and geometric diagrams.

NOTE: The information pertains to permanent teeth.

DATE	NO	DESCRIPTION	DEBIT	DATE	AMT.	BAL

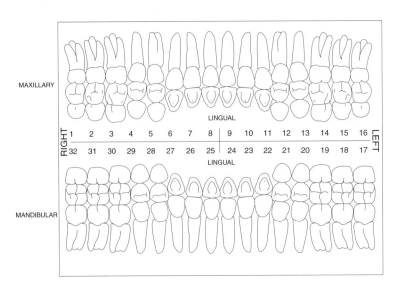

Name _____

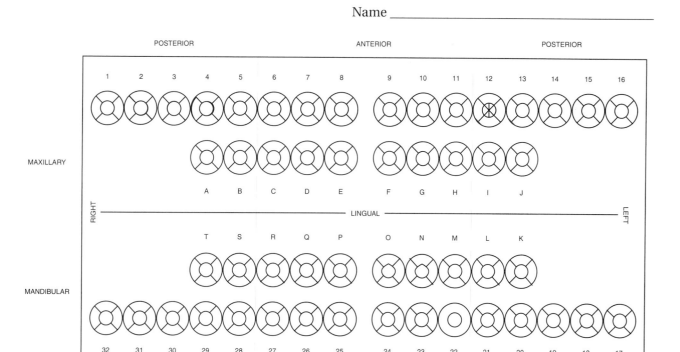

Date	Conditions noted/treatment done
1/1/—	Initial visit to office
	Clinical examination done. Conditions noted:
	Mandibular left third molar is impacted
	Maxillary right lateral incisor has mesiolabioincisal decay
	Maxillary left 3rd molar needs to be extracted
	Gold crown on maxillary left 1st molar
	Mandibular right 1st molar is missing
	Maxillary left 2nd bicuspid is missing
	Maxillary left central incisor has a composite restoration on distolabial surface
	Mandibular right cuspid has a lingual composite restoration
	Full mouth series of X rays taken
1/23/—	Amalgam restoration to mesioocclusal edge of mandibular left 2nd bicuspid
1/30/—	Amalgam restoration to mesioocclusodistal edge of maxillary right 1st molar
2/3/—	Root canal treatment done to maxillary left cuspid
6/2/—	Clinical exam, bite wing X rays, prophylaxis treatment
7/4/—	Composite restoration to mesiolinguoincisal edge of maxillary right central incisor, Dycal used
8/9/—	Rubber base impression taken of maxillary right cuspid
8/20/—	Porcelain crown placed on maxillary right cuspid
2/11/—	Clinical exam, prophylaxis, bite wing X rays (4)
3/8/—	Amalgam restoration to lingual surface of mandibular left cuspid
4/6/—	Amalgam restoration to mesioocclusal edge of mandibular right 2nd molar
4/28/—	Composite restoration to lingual surface of mandibular left central incisor

UNIT 17:5 CHARTING CONDITIONS OF THE TEETH

ASSIGNMENT SHEET #3

Grade _____ Name _____

INTRODUCTION: Use information learned on previous assignments to chart the following dental conditions. Refer to text information on charting dental conditions as needed.

INSTRUCTIONS: Use the blank dental chart to record the following dental conditions performed during a series of visits to the dental office. Draw the correct symbols for the listed conditions on both the anatomic and geometric diagrams.

DATE	NO	DESCRIPTION	DEBIT	DATE	AMT.	BAL

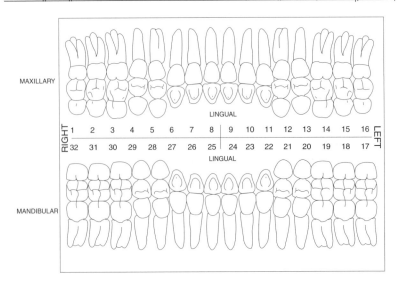

Name _____

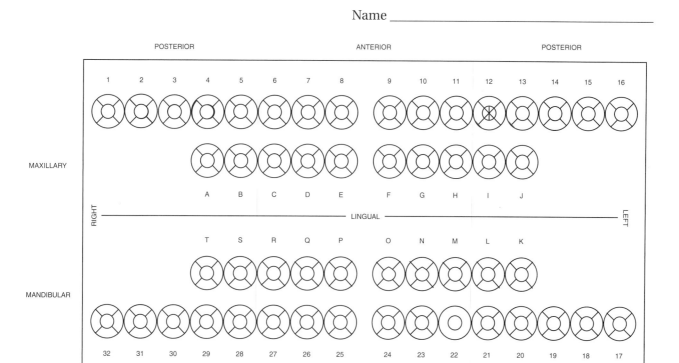

Date   *Conditions noted/treatment done*

5/7/—   Initial visit to office

Full mouth series of X rays taken, prophylaxis treatment

Clinical examination done. Following conditions noted:

Maxillary right 3rd molar is impacted

Maxillary right 1st molar has mesioocclusal decay

Mandibular right cuspid has lingual decay

Gold crown present on maxillary left 2nd molar

Mandibular right 2nd molar needs to be extracted

Maxillary left 1st molar has a mesioocclusodistal amalgam restoration

Mandibular left central incisor has a mesiolinguoincisal composite restoration

6/1/—   Amalgam restoration to distoocclusal edge of mandibular left 2nd bicuspid, I.R.M. under restoration

6/15/—   Mandibular left third molar extracted

7/2/—   Rubber base impression taken of maxillary right cuspid

7/20/—   Porcelain crown placed on maxillary right cuspid

10/1/—   Clinical examination, prophylaxis treatment, 4 bite wing X rays, maxillary right central incisor has labial decay

10/15/—   Composite restoration to labioincisal edge of maxillary left cuspid

10/22/—   Amalgam restoration to distoocclusal edge of maxillary left 2nd bicuspid

11/3/—   Amalgam restoration to distobuccal edge of maxillary right 2nd bicuspid

3/3/—   Clinical examination, full mouth X rays, prophylaxis treatment

3/20/—   Composite restoration to lingual surface of mandibular left cuspid, Dycal under restoration

4/2/—   Amalgam restoration to mesioocclusal edge of mandibular right 2nd bicuspid, I.R.M. used

4/15/—   Root canal treatment to mandibular right central incisor

5/3/—   Amalgam placed on occlusal surface of mandibular right 1st molar

279

Name _____ Date _____

Evaluated by _____

DIRECTIONS: Practice charting conditions of the teeth by completing the 3 assignments. The instructor will use the following criteria to grade the charts.

PROFICIENT

Charting Conditions of the Teeth	Points Possible	Peer Check Yes	No	Final Check* Yes	No	Points Earned**	Comments
1. Assembles supplies	2						
2. Washes hands	2						
3. Charts conditions of teeth on anatomic and geometric diagrams:							
Charts on the correct teeth	20						
Uses the correct symbols	20						
4. Charts services rendered:							
Charts all required information	20						
Uses correct abbreviations	20						
5. Charts all information in a neat legible manner	12						
6. Replaces supplies	2						
7. Washes hands	2						
Totals	100						

* Final Check: Instructor or authorized person evaluates.
** Points Earned: Points possible times each "yes" check.

UNIT 17:6 OPERATING AND MAINTAINING DENTAL EQUIPMENT

ASSIGNMENT SHEET

Grade _____ Name _____

INTRODUCTION: This assignment will help you review the main facts regarding dental equipment.

INSTRUCTIONS: Review the information on Operating and Maintaining Dental Equipment. In the space provided, print the answer that best completes the statement or answers the question.

1. During dental procedures, equipment can be contaminated with _____,
_____, and _____. _____ must be observed at all
times. _____ barriers must be placed on many parts of the equipment prior to use.
When the procedure is complete, the assistant must wear _____ to remove the
contaminated barriers. The areas should then be _____ or _____ if
possible.

2. Give the main use or function of each of the following:

   a. dental light

   b. dental chair

   c. air compressor

   d. oral evacuation system

   e. air-water syringe

   f. saliva ejector

   g. high-velocity evacuator

   h. cuspidor

   i. low speed handpiece

   j. high speed handpiece

3. How far is the light positioned from the oral cavity?

   Why is a soft cloth used to clean the light shield?

4. Why do dental chairs have thin and narrow headrests?

   Why do chairs have a foot control to lock the chair in position?

5. The air compressor units are usually set to provide _____ pounds of pressure. Notify the doctor if the pressure gauge goes above _____ pounds of presssure.

6. List two (2) types of maintenance required on the air compressor units.

7. What is the purpose for the solids collector trap on the oral evacuation system?

   How is it cleaned?

   Why is a germicide spray or liquid used?

8. What should be done with the tip of the air–water syringe after each patient?

9. How should the saliva ejector tip holder and tubing be cleaned after each patient?

10. What is the purpose of the filter screen on a high-velocity oral evacuator?

11. Why is the slide valve on the high-velocity oral evacuator lubricated after cleaning?

12. List two (2) attachments that can be placed on a low speed handpiece. What is the main use for each attachment?

13. How should the low speed and high speed handpieces be cleaned after each patient?

14. How can you learn the correct maintenance required for different types of dental equipment?

UNIT 17:6 Evaluation Sheet

Name _____ Date _____

Evaluated by _____

DIRECTIONS: Practice operating and maintaining dental equipment according to the criteria listed. When you are ready for your final check, give this sheet to your instructor.

PROFICIENT

Operating and Maintaining Dental Equipment	Points Possible	Peer Check Yes	Peer Check No	Final Check* Yes	Final Check* No	Points Earned**	Comments
1. Assembles equipment and supplies	1						
2. Washes hands and puts on gloves	1						
3. Dental Light							
Turns on and off	2						
Positions 30-42 inches from oral cavity	2						
Operates dimmer switch	2						
Applies protective barriers to handles and/or switches	2						
Cleans shield with soft cloth	2						
Lubricates moving parts	2						
4. Dental Chair							
Locks and unlocks chair	2						
Operates elevation control	2						
Operates forward-backward control	2						
Operates reset button	2						
Covers headrest with disposable cover	2						
Washes with mild detergent or upholstery cleaner	2						
5. Air Compressor							
Turns unit on and off	2						
Checks pressure gauge	2						
Notifies doctor if pressure goes above 120	2						
Checks oil reservoir if system has one	2						
Drains water from main tank with pressure at zero	2						
6. Oral Evacuation System							
Turns unit on and off	2						
Cleans solids collector trap correctly	2						
7. Air-Water Syringe							
Operates for air, water, and combination of air and water	2						
Removes and replaces syringe tip	2						
Sterilizes tip after use	2						
Wipes tip holder and tubing with disinfectant	2						

Operating and Maintaining Dental Equipment	Points Possible	Peer Check		Final Check*		Points Earned**	Comments
		Yes	No	Yes	No		
8. Saliva Ejector							
Turns on and off	2						
Inserts tip correctly	2						
Disposes of tip after use	2						
Brushes inside of tip holder	2						
Wipes tip holder and tubing with disinfectant	2						
Draws disinfecting solution into unit to sanitize tubing	2						
9. High-Velocity Oral Evacuator							
Inserts tip correctly	2						
Operates slide valve to turn on and off	2						
Cleans and lubricates slide valve	2						
Cleans filter screen on unit correctly	2						
Disposes of plastic tip or brushes, rinses and sterilizes metal tip	2						
Wipes tip holder and tubing with disinfectant	2						
Draws disinfecting solution into unit to sanitize tubing	2						
10. Cuspidor							
Cleans and disinfects after each patient	2						
11. Low Speed Handpiece							
Inserts and removes contra-angle head	2						
Inserts and removes prophylactic angle head	2						
Inserts and removes bur in contra-angle	2						
Lubricates contra-angle and prophylactic heads correctly	2						
Cleans tubing with disinfectant	2						
Sterilizes handpiece correctly	2						
Lubricates handpiece correctly and operates handpiece after lubrication	2						
12. High Speed Handpiece							
Inserts and removes F.G. bur	2						
Cleans tubing with disinfectant	2						
Sterilizes handpiece correctly	2						
Lubricates correctly and operates after lubrication to remove excess	2						
13. Replaces equipment	1						
14. Removes gloves and washes hands	1						
Totals	100						

* Final Check: Instructor or authorized person evaluates.

** Points Earned: Points possible times each "yes" check.

UNIT 17:7 IDENTIFYING DENTAL INSTRUMENTS AND PREPARING DENTAL TRAYS

ASSIGNMENT SHEET

Grade _____   Name _____

INTRODUCTION: This assignment will help you review the main facts regarding setting up basic dental trays.

INSTRUCTIONS: Read the information on Identifying Dental Instruments and Preparing Dental Trays. In the space provided, print the word(s) that best completes the statement or answers the question.

1. List two (2) methods used to set up trays for various dental procedures.

2. Items placed on the trays should be organized and in _____. Usually instruments are arranged on the tray in the _____.

3. Briefly describe the purpose of each of the following trays.

   a. prophylactic or general examination tray:

   b. amalgam restoration tray:

   c. composite restoration tray:

   d. surgical extraction tray:

4. Name the following parts of an instrument.

   a. cutting portion:

   b. working end of a condensing instrument:

   c. portion that connects shaft or handle with the blade:

   d. handle of the instrument:

5. The crossword puzzle that follows will allow you to review the use of some dental instruments. To complete the crossword, refer to the information sheet for 17:7 Identifying Dental Instruments and Preparing Dental Trays, and the abbreviations in 5:1, Using Medical Abbreviations, of the textbook.

285

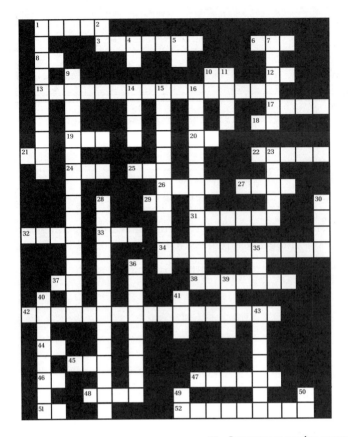

ACROSS:

1. Special string used to clean between the teeth
3. Correct name for silver filling material
6. Abbreviation for amount
8. Abbreviation for urine
10. Abbreviation for axilla or axillary
12. Abbreviation for right
13. Instrument used to carve or shape amalgam restoration
17. Another word for mouth is _____ cavity
18. Abbreviation for bedrest
19. Abbreviation for gynecology
20. Abbreviation for operating room
21. Abbreviation for Barium Enema
22. Instrument used to remove soft decay
24. Abbreviation for red blood cell
25. Abbreviation for blood urea nitrogen
26. Abbreviation for pediatrics
27. Before every procedure, a dental worker must _____ his/her hands
29. Abbreviation for blood
31. _____ material is used to put stitches in the mouth
32. A matrix _____ may be used to wall in a cavity before placing amalgam
33. A Tri-flow syringe is also called an _____ – water syringe
34. Instrument used to remove small tips of root or bone from a tooth socket
37. Abbreviation for vital signs
38. The doctor who uses all of the dental instruments
42. Instruments used to extract or remove teeth
44. Abbreviation for lumbar puncture
45. Abbreviation for temperature, pulse and respiration
46. Abbreviation for registered nurse
47. Instrument used to remove tartar or calculus from teeth
48. Abbreviation for eye, ear, nose and throat
51. Abbreviation for recovery room
52. If you study hard you may become a dental _____ and assist the dentist.

DOWN:

1. The dentist and assistant working together use the _____ method of dental assisting
2. Abbreviation for South America
4. Abbreviation for morning, before noon
5. Abbreviation for before meals
7. Instrument used to reflect light or look at the teeth
9. Instrument used to pack and condense amalgam into cavity
10. Abbreviation for "of each"
11. A picture taken of the teeth and developed in a darkroom
14. Small tips placed in handpieces to prepare cavities
15. Instruments used to carry cotton rolls and/or pellets to and from the mouth
16. Special carving instrument with one round end and one pointed end
23. To brush the teeth, use a brush and tooth _____
28. Instrument used to carry amalgam to the mouth
30. Abbreviation for blood work
35. Abbreviation for plastic filling instrument
36. A person with 2-4 years of special training who can clean teeth in a dental office is a _____
39. Abbreviation for at night, night
40. Instrument used to examine or explore the teeth
41. Abbreviation for plastic filling instrument
43. The person you help take care of is called a _____
49. Abbreviation for cancer
50. Abbreviation for occupational therapy

UNIT 17:7 Evaluation Sheet

Name _____   Date _____

Evaluated by _____

DIRECTIONS: Practice identifying dental instruments and preparing dental trays according to the criteria listed. When you are ready for your final check, give this sheet to your instructor.

Identifying Dental Instruments and Preparing Dental Trays	Points Possible	Peer Check Yes	No	Final Check* Yes	No	Points Earned**	Comments
A. Prophylactic or General Examination Tray:							
1. Assembles equipment and supplies	4						
2. Washes hands and puts on personal protective equipment	4						
3. Prepares for patient:							
Drape	5						
Clips	5						
Records and X rays	5						
4. Checks condition of handpieces to be used:							
Low speed handpiece	5						
Prophylactic attachment	5						
Air-water syringe	5						
Saliva ejector	5						
Evacuator	5						
5. Sets up tray with following instruments and supplies:							
Explorer	5						
Mouth mirror	5						
Cotton pliers	5						
Scalers	5						
Periodontal probe	5						
Prophylactic cup	4						
Prophylactic paste	4						
Fluoride Tray	4						
6. Prepares film for X rays	4						
7. Sets out equipment to demonstrate brushing and flossing	4						
8. Scrubs and sterilizes all instruments and replaces all equipment after use	4						
9. Removes personal protective equipment and washes hands	3						
Totals	100						

* Final Check: Instructor or authorized person evaluates.
** Points Earned: Points possible times each "yes" check.

Identifying Dental Instruments and Preparing Dental Trays	Points Possible	Peer Check		Final Check*		Points Earned**	Comments
		Yes	No	Yes	No		
B. *Amalgam Restoration Tray:*							
1. Assembles equipment and supplies	2						
2. Washes hands and puts on personal protective equipment	2						
3. Prepares supplies:							
Drape and clip	2						
Patient records/X rays	2						
4. Checks condition of handpieces and attachments to be used:							
Low speed handpiece and contra-angle	3						
High speed handpiece	3						
Burs and bur remover	3						
Air-water syringe	3						
Evacuator/saliva ejector	3						
5. Sets up tray with following instruments and supplies:							
Explorer	3						
Mouth mirror	3						
Cotton pliers	3						
Spoons	4						
Hatchet	4						
Gingival Margin trimmer	4						
Amalgam carrier	4						
Condenser plugger	4						
Hollenback carver	4						
Cleoid Discoid carver	4						
Burnishers	3						
Plastic filling instruments	3						
Matrix retainer and band and wooden wedges	3						
Cotton pellets/rolls	3						
Articulating paper	3						
Finishing strips	3						
6. Prepares following equipment/supplies for use:							
Amalgam alloy and mercury	3						
Amalgamator	3						
Capsule and pestle if needed	3						
Amalgam well, dappen dish, or squeeze cloth	3						
Bases and cements	3						
7. Loads anesthetic aspirating syringe	3						
8. Scrubs and sterilizes all instruments and replaces all equipment after use	2						
9. Removes personal protective equipment and washes hands	2						
Totals	100						

*   Final Check: Instructor or authorized person evaluates.
** Points Earned: Points possible times each "yes" check.

17:7 (cont.)

Identifying Dental Instruments and Preparing Dental Trays	Points Possible	Peer Check		Final Check*		Points Earned**	Comments
		Yes	No	Yes	No		
C. Composite or Aesthetic Restoration Tray:							
1. Assembles equipment and supplies	2						
2. Washes hands and puts on personal protective equipment	2						
3. Prepares supplies:							
Drape and clips	2						
Patient records/X rays	2						
4. Checks condition of handpieces and attachments to be used:							
Low speed handpiece and contra-angle	4						
High speed handpiece	4						
Burs and bur remover	4						
Air-water syringe	4						
Evacuator/saliva ejector	4						
5. Sets up tray with instruments and supplies:							
Explorer	4						
Mouth mirror	4						
Cotton pliers	4						
Spoons	4						
Hoes or hatchets	4						
Plastic filling instruments	4						
Composite instruments	4						
Matrix strip	4						
Cotton pellets/rolls	3						
Finishing strips	3						
6. Prepares following supplies for use:							
Etching liquid	4						
Resin	4						
Composite pastes/premixed syringe	4						
Mixing pads/plastic wells	3						
Mixing sticks/brushes	3						
Cements and bases	4						
7. Loads anesthetic aspirating syringe	4						
8. Prepares curing light	4						
9. Scrubs and sterilizes all instruments and replaces all equipment after use	2						
10. Removes personal protective equipment and washes hands	2						
Totals	100						

* Final Check: Instructor or authorized person evaluates.
** Points Earned: Points possible times each "yes" check.

Identifying Dental Instruments and Preparing Dental Trays	Points Possible	Peer Check		Final Check*		Points Earned**	Comments
		Yes	No	Yes	No		
D. *Surgical Extraction Tray:*							
1. Assembles equipment and supplies	2						
2. Washes hands and puts on personal protective equipment	3						
3. Prepares supplies:							
Drape and clips	3						
Patient records/X rays	3						
4. Checks condition of handpieces and attachments to be used:							
Low speed handpiece	5						
Air-water syringe	5						
Saliva ejector/evacuator	5						
5. Sets up tray with following instruments and supplies:							
Explorer	5						
Mouth mirror	5						
Cotton pliers	5						
Extracting forceps	5						
Periosteal elevator	5						
Root elevator	5						
Root tip pick	5						
Rongeur forceps	5						
Lancets as needed	5						
Bone chisels and mallet as needed	5						
Needle holder with suture material as needed	5						
Cotton pellets/rolls	4						
Gauze sponges	4						
6. Loads anesthetic aspirating syringe	5						
7. Scrubs and sterilizes all instruments and replaces all equipment after use	3						
8. Removes personal protective equipment and washes hands	3						
Totals	100						

* Final Check: Instructor or authorized person evaluates.
** Points Earned: Points possible times each "yes" check.

UNIT 17:8 POSITIONING A PATIENT IN THE DENTAL CHAIR

ASSIGNMENT SHEET

Grade _____   Name _____

INTRODUCTION: This assignment will allow you to review the main facts regarding correct positioning of a patient in a dental chair.

INSTRUCTIONS: Review the information on Positioning a Patient in a Dental Chair. In the space provided, print the word(s) that best completes the statement or answers the question.

1. In four-handed dentistry, the patient is placed in a/an _____ or
   _____ position.

2. Why is the patient's head placed at the upper narrow headrest on the chair?

3. How high should the chair be positioned from the floor?

4. List two (2) times the chair must be locked into position so it will not move.

5. Why is it important to recline the back of the chair slowly?

6. Why is it important to inform the patient before moving or changing the position of the chair?

7. Why is a drape placed on the patient during dental procedures?

   Which side of the drape should be placed against the patient's clothing? Why?

8. The dental light should be positioned _____ from the oral cavity. Care must be taken to ensure that the light _____ but does not
   _____.

UNIT 17:8 Evaluation Sheet

Name _____ Date _____

Evaluated by _____

DIRECTIONS: Practice positioning a patient in a dental chair according to the criteria listed. When you are ready for your final check, give this sheet to your instructor.

Positioning a Patient in the Dental Chair	Points Possible	Peer Check Yes	No	Final Check* Yes	No	Points Earned**	Comments
1. Assembles equipment and supplies	3						
2. Washes hands	3						
3. Covers headrest with a disposable cover	4						
4. Covers handles and/or switches of dental light with protective barriers	4						
5. Introduces self, identifies patient, and explains procedure	5						
6. Locks chair in low position	5						
7. Seats patient in chair	5						
8. Adjusts headrest to correct position	5						
9. Drapes patient correctly	5						
10. Informs patient before any movement of the chair	5						
11. Elevates chair correctly	5						
12. Reclines chair correctly	5						
13. Positions light 30-42 inches from oral cavity	5						
14. Locks chair to prevent movement after examination complete	5						
15. Cautions patient not to get out of chair until movement stops	5						
16. Operates reset button	5						
17. Removes drape	5						
18. Assists patient out of chair	5						
19. Removes protective barriers and cleans equipment:							
Puts on gloves	2						
Removes protective barriers	2						
Wipes contaminated areas with disinfectant	3						
Cleans and prepares items for sterilization	2						
20. Replaces all equipment	3						
21. Removes gloves and washes hands	4						
Totals	100						

* Final Check: Instructor or authorized person evaluates.
** Points Earned: Points possible times each "yes" check.

UNIT 17:9 DEMONSTRATING BRUSHING AND FLOSSING TECHNIQUES

ASSIGNMENT SHEET

Grade _____   Name _____

INTRODUCTION: This assignment will help you review the main facts regarding brushing and flossing of the teeth.

INSTRUCTIONS: Review the information on Demonstrating Brushing and Flossing Techniques. In the space provided, print the word(s) that best completes the statement or answers the question.

1. List three (3) purposes or reasons for using correct brushing-flossing techniques.

2. Demonstrations on brushing and flossing should be given to _____. Talk _____ and _____. _____ and _____ important parts.

3. While using the Bass technique for brushing, the brush is placed at _____ and then a _____ motion is used.

4. List the five (5) surfaces that must be cleaned on each tooth.

5. Which surfaces are not cleaned by brushing but are cleaned by flossing?

6. Which type of toothbrush is recommended in most cases? Why?

7. When should brushes be discarded?

8. What is the purpose of toothpaste or dentifrices?

9. Why is fluoride added to toothpaste?

10. List two (2) types of dental floss.

    Which type of floss should patients use?

UNIT 17:9A Evaluation Sheet

Name _____ Date _____

Evaluated by _____

DIRECTIONS: Practice demonstrating brushing techniques according to the criteria listed. When you are ready for your final check, give this sheet to your instructor.

PROFICIENT

Demonstrating Brushing Techniques	Points Possible	Peer Check Yes	No	Final Check* Yes	No	Points Earned**	Comments
1. Assembles equipment and supplies	4						
2. Washes hands	4						
3. Introduces self and identifies patient	4						
4. Stresses importance of brushing	8						
5. Uses soft textured brush	8						
6. Suggests systematic method for brushing	8						
7. Places brush at 45 degree angle at gumline	8						
8. Rotates brush gently to get bristles in place	8						
9. Vibrates with short back and forth motion to clean tooth	8						
10. Cleans facial (front) surface	5						
11. Cleans lingual (tongue) surface	5						
12. Places brush vertically to do lingual (tongue) surface of front teeth	5						
13. Cleans biting surface	5						
14. Uses very short vibrating motion on biting surface	6						
15. Ascertains that patient understands method	6						
16. Replaces equipment	4						
17. Washes hands	4						
Totals	100						

* Final Check: Instructor or authorized person evaluates.
** Points Earned: Points possible times each "yes" check.

Name _____ Date _____

Evaluated by _____

DIRECTIONS: Practice demonstrating flossing techniques according to the criteria listed. When you are ready for your final check, give this sheet to your instructor.

PROFICIENT

Demonstrating Flossing Techniques	Points Possible	Peer Check Yes	No	Final Check* Yes	No	Points Earned**	Comments
1. Assembles equipment and supplies	3						
2. Washes hands	3						
3. Introduces self and identifies patient	3						
4. Stresses importance of flossing	7						
5. Uses 12-18 inches of floss	6						
6. Anchors floss on middle fingers	6						
7. Wraps floss around index fingers and/or thumb	6						
8. Leaves 1 to 2 inches of floss between fingers	6						
9. Inserts floss gently into space between gum and tooth	7						
10. Stresses not to snap floss in place	7						
11. Forms C around side of tooth	6						
12. Holds floss firmly by tooth and uses up and down motion	7						
13. Cleans both sides of every tooth	7						
14. Warns patient about bleeding or soreness	6						
15. Tells patient to call doctor if bleeding persists	6						
16. Ascertains that patient understands procedure	8						
17. Replaces equipment	3						
18. Washes hands	3						
Totals	100						

* Final Check: Instructor or authorized person evaluates.
** Points Earned: Points possible times each "yes" check.

UNIT 17:10 TAKING IMPRESSIONS AND POURING MODELS

ASSIGNMENT SHEET

Grade _____   Name _____

INTRODUCTION: This assignment will help you review the main facts about dental impressions and models.

INSTRUCTIONS: Review the information on Taking Impressions and Pouring Models. Print the word(s) that best completes the statement or answers the question.

1. What is an impression?

2. Why is an impression taken?

3. Name three (3) materials used to take impressions.

4. List three (3) advantages and three (3) disadvantages of alginate.

   Advantages   *Disadvantages*

5. What advantage does rubber base impression material have that alginate does not have?

6. Identify three (3) advantages of polysiloxane or polyvinylsiloxane impression materials.

7. What is a model?

8. What are the purposes or uses for a model?

9. List two (2) materials that can be used for pouring models.

10. What advantage does a stone model have that a plaster model does not have?

11. Why must impression and model materials be stored in a tightly closed container in a cool, dry area?

12. List two (2) ways to prevent air bubbles in the preparation of a model.

UNIT 17:10A Evaluation Sheet

Name _____ Date _____

Evaluated by _____

DIRECTIONS: Practice preparing alginate according to the criteria listed. When you are ready for your final check, give this sheet to your instructor.

PROFICIENT

Preparing Alginate	Points Possible	Peer Check		Final Check*		Points Earned**	Comments
		Yes	No	Yes	No		
1. Assembles equipment and supplies	2						
2. Washes hands and puts on personal protective equipment	3						
3. Cleans bowl and spatula	3						
4. Measures water first	3						
Regulates temperature of water to 70° F or 21° C	3						
Measures correct amount	3						
Puts water in bowl	3						
5. Measures powder:							
Fluffs powder in can	3						
Fills scoop	3						
Taps scoop with spatula	3						
Levels scoop with spatula	3						
Places powder in bowl	3						
Measures correct amount	3						
6. Uses circular motion to mix powder and water	3						
7. Uses stropping action to produce a smooth mix	3						
8. Presses mix against side and rotates bowl	3						
9. Places alginate in tray:							
Sprays tray first	3						
Places in tray correctly	3						
Presses slightly to secure	3						
Smooths top of tray	3						
10. Takes an impression with a denture:							
Shakes excess water off denture	3						
Presses anterior teeth in place	3						
Pushes arch into place	3						
Applies gentle pressure	3						
Holds steady for 1 minute	3						
Removes when alginate set	3						

297

Preparing Alginate	Points Possible	Peer Check		Final Check*		Points Earned**	Comments
		Yes	No	Yes	No		
11. Rinses impression with room temperature water for at least 30 seconds	3						
12. Sprays impression with a disinfectant	3						
13. Wraps alginate impression in wet towel until ready to pour model	3						
14. Disposes of alginate in waste can	3						
Washes other equipment thoroughly	3						
Sterilizes tray correctly	3						
15. Replaces all equipment	2						
16. Removes personal protective equipment and washes hands	3						
Totals	100						

* Final Check: Instructor or authorized person evaluates.
** Points Earned: Points possible times each "yes" check.

UNIT 17:10 B Evaluation Sheet

Name _____ Date _____

Evaluated by _____

DIRECTIONS: Practice preparing rubber base according to the criteria listed. When you are ready for your final check, give this sheet to your instructor.

Preparing Rubber Base	Points Possible	Peer Check Yes	Peer Check No	Final Check* Yes	Final Check* No	Points Earned**	Comments
				PROFICIENT			
1. Assembles all equipment and supplies	3						
2. Washes hands and puts on personal protective equipment	3						
3. Prepares tray:							
Paints tray with adhesive	4						
Uses heavy bodied base	4						
4. Prepares syringe:							
Applies tip correctly	4						
Makes paper funnel	4						
Uses light bodied base	4						
5. Marks length of strip desired on paper	5						
6. Dispenses even line of accelerator first	5						
7. Dispenses equal length strip of base	5						
8. Coats spatula with accelerator	5						
9. Mixes until mix even with no streaks of color	6						
10. Completes mix in 45-60 seconds	6						
11. Loads syringe correctly	4						
Fills tray correctly	4						
12. Passes filled syringe first	4						
13. Passes impression tray next	4						
14. Rinses impression with room temperature water for 30 seconds	4						
15. Sprays impression with a disinfectant or soaks it in a disinfecting solution	4						
16. Cleans syringe or tray:							
Soaks 15 minutes in warm water	3						
Uses brush as needed	3						
Discards excess material in trash can	3						
Sterilizes syringe and/or tray correctly	3						
17. Replaces all equipment	3						
18. Removes personal protective equipment and washes hands	3						
Totals	100						

*Final Check: Instructor or authorized person evaluates.
** Points Earned: Points possible times each "yes" check.

Name _____ Date _____

Evaluated by _____

DIRECTIONS: Practice pouring plaster models according to the criteria listed. When you are ready for your final check, give this sheet to your instructor.

PROFICIENT

Pouring a Plaster Model	Points Possible	Peer Check Yes	No	Final Check* Yes	No	Points Earned**	Comments
1. Assembles equipment and supplies	3						
2. Washes hands and puts on personal protective equipment	3						
3. Dries impression before using	4						
4. Measures water first	4						
Uses 45-50 cc	5						
Adjusts to room temperature or cooler	5						
Puts water in bowl	3						
5. Measures plaster next	4						
Weighs out 100 grams	5						
Sifts into bowl	4						
Allows water to absorb plaster	4						
6. Uses wiping and scraping motion to mix	5						
7. Puts bowl on vibrator platform to remove air bubbles	5						
8. Pours model:							
Puts bag on vibrator platform	3						
Places impression on vibrator platform	3						
Places small amount of mix on heel	5						
Vibrates to cause flow into teeth areas	5						
Repeats process until impression filled	5						
Adds base correctly	5						
Smooths sides	5						
9. Allows model to set at least one hour	3						
10. Places waste plaster in trash container	3						
11. Cleans and replaces all equipment	3						
12. Rinses sink thoroughly	3						
13. Removes personal protective equipment and washes hands	3						
Totals	100						

* Final Check: Instructor or authorized person evaluates.
** Points Earned: Points possible times each "yes" check.

Name _____ Date _____

Evaluated by _____

DIRECTIONS: Practice pouring stone models according to the criteria listed. When you are ready for your final check, give this sheet to your instructor.

PROFICIENT

Pouring a Stone Model	Points Possible	Peer Check Yes	No	Final Check* Yes	No	Points Earned**	Comments
1. Assembles equipment and supplies	3						
2. Washes hands and puts on personal protective equipment	3						
3. Dries impression before using	4						
4. Measures water first	4						
Uses 30–35 cc	5						
Adjusts to 70°F (21°C) or cooler	5						
Puts water in bowl	3						
5. Measures stone next	4						
Weighs out 100 grams	5						
Sifts into bowl	4						
Allows water to absorb stone	4						
6. Uses wiping and scraping motion to mix	5						
7. Puts bowl on vibrator platform to remove air bubbles	5						
8. Pours model:							
Puts bag on vibrator platform	3						
Places impression on vibrator platform	3						
Places small amount of mix on heel	5						
Vibrates to cause flow into teeth areas	5						
Repeats process correctly until impression filled	5						
Adds base correctly	5						
Smooths sides	5						
9. Allows model to set at least one hour	3						
10. Places waste stone material in trash container	3						
11. Cleans and replaces all equipment	3						
12. Rinses sink thoroughly	3						
13. Removes personal protective equipment and washes hands	3						
Totals	100						

* Final Check: Instructor or authorized person evaluates.
** Points Earned: Points possible times each "yes" check.

UNIT 17:10E Evaluation Sheet

Name _____ Date _____

Evaluated by _____

DIRECTIONS: Practice trimming a model according to the criteria listed. When you are ready for your final check, give this sheet to your instructor.

Trimming a Model	Points Possible	Peer Check		Final Check*		Points Earned**	Comments
		Yes	No	Yes	No		
1. Assembles equipment and supplies	2						
2. Washes hands	2						
3. Soaks model in water	3						
4. Wears safety glasses	5						
5. Turns on trimmer water supply to moisten wheel	4						
6. Trims base to following specifications:							
Smooth and even	5						
1/2 inch thick	5						
1/3 of total height	5						
7. Trims heel to following specifications:							
Smooth and even	5						
1/4 inch from back of third molar	5						
Perpendicular to base	5						
8. Makes side cuts to following specifications:							
Correct angle of 55° on mandibular and 63° on maxillary	5						
1/4 to 3/8 inch from bicuspids	5						
Smooth and even	5						
9. Trims heel cuts to following specifications:							
Even on both sides	5						
1/2 inch long	5						
125° angle to heel	5						
10. Makes anterior cuts to:							
Arc on mandibular and even angle cuts on maxillary	5						
Starts cuts at cuspids	5						
11. Checks teeth to be sure they are correct and well formed	5						
12. Cleans model trimmer	3						
13. Replaces all equipment	2						
14. Rinses sink thoroughly	2						
15. Washes hands	2						
Totals	100						

PROFICIENT

* Final Check: Instructor or authorized person evaluates.
** Points Earned: Points possible times each "yes" check.

UNIT 17:11 MAKING CUSTOM TRAYS

ASSIGNMENT SHEET

Grade _____ Name _____

INTRODUCTION: This assignment will help you review the main facts regarding custom trays.

INSTRUCTIONS: Review the information on Making Custom Trays. In the space provided, print the word(s) that answers the question or completes the statement.

1. What are custom trays?

2. List two (2) materials that can be used to produce a custom tray.

3. Which material is more popular?

   Why?

4. What must be made first before a custom tray can be made?

5. The stone or plaster model of the patient's mouth is used as a/an _____ to form the _____. In this way, the tray is _____ for an individual patient.

6. Acrylic resins are difficult to remove from the mixing jars or containers. What can you use to mix the materials?

7. How can you prevent the acrylic materials from sticking to your hands or fingers?

Name _____ Date _____

Evaluated by _____

DIRECTIONS: Practice making a custom tray according to the criteria listed. When you are ready for your final check, give this sheet to your instructor.

PROFICIENT

Making Custom Trays	Points Possible	Peer Check Yes	No	Final Check* Yes	No	Points Earned**	Comments
1. Assembles all equipment and supplies	3						
2. Washes hands	3						
3. Applies wax to model	5						
4. Prepares mix correctly:							
Measures liquid and places in cup	6						
Measures powder and places in cup	6						
Uses tongue blade for mixing	5						
Mixes thoroughly	6						
5. Coats model and slab with petroleum jelly	5						
6. Forms wafer of even thickness with mix	5						
7. Fits tray to model:							
Adapts slowly	5						
Fits at palate first	5						
Moves to sides	5						
8. Forms handle correctly	5						
9. Removes excess with knife	5						
10. Allows tray to cure for 7 to 10 minutes	5						
11. Removes tray correctly	5						
12. Removes wax spacer	5						
13. Puts on safety glasses and uses burs-stone to smooth	5						
14. Labels tray with patient's name	5						
15. Cleans and replaces all equipment	3						
16. Washes hands	3						
Totals	100						

* Final Check: Instructor or authorized person evaluates.
** Points Earned: Points possible times each "yes" check.

UNIT 17:12 MAINTAINING AND LOADING AN ANESTHETIC ASPIRATING SYRINGE

ASSIGNMENT SHEET

Grade _____   Name _____

INTRODUCTION: As you assist the doctor with anesthesia, it will be essential for you to know the following facts.

INSTRUCTIONS: Read the information on Maintaining and Loading an Anesthetic Aspirating Syringe. In the space provided, print the word(s) that best completes the statement or answers the question.

1. Define *anesthesia:*

2. Why are topical anesthetics used?

   How are these applied?

3. List the two (2) types of injections used for local anesthesia. State the dental area where each is used.

4. What is the main anesthetic medication used in dental offices?

5. List two (2) reasons why vasoconstrictors are used with the anesthetic?

   What is the name of the most common vasoconstrictor used?

6. What are the main points to be observed about each of the following items on an anesthetic carpule?
   a. glass:
   b. solution:
   c. rubber plunger:
   d. bubbles:
   e. aluminum cap:

7. How should you clean or sterilize the carpule before use?

   Why do most manufacturers state that carpules are not to soak in a disinfectant prior to use?

8. Why does the doctor aspirate before injecting the dental anesthesia?

9. Below are two (2) diagrams of the aspirating syringe. The top sketch shows the assembled syringe. The other shows the parts. In the space provided below the diagrams, label the parts shown.

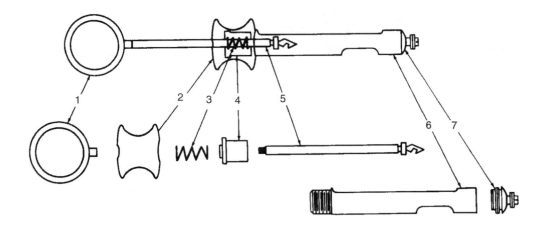

1.

2.

3.

4.

5.

6.

7.

10. What three (3) main steps of care should be given the syringe after each use?

11. After each five (5) uses, what special care should be given to the syringe?

12. After an injection has been given, the needle must be removed from the syringe and placed in a/an
_____. It must not be _____, _____, or
_____.

UNIT 17 : 12 A E v a l u a t i o n   S h e e t

Name _____ Date _____

Evaluated by _____

DIRECTIONS: Practice maintaining an anesthetic aspirating syringe according to the criteria listed. When you are ready for your final check, give this sheet to your instructor.

PROFICIENT

Maintaining an Anesthetic Aspirating Syringe	Points Possible	Peer Check Yes	No	Final Check* Yes	No	Points Earned**	Comments
1. Assembles equipment and supplies	3						
2. Washes hands and puts on personal protective equipment	3						
3. Takes syringe apart	6						
4. Identifies the parts:							
Thumb ring	5						
Finger grip	5						
Spring	5						
Guide bearing	5						
Piston with harpoon	5						
Barrel	5						
Needle adaptor	5						
5. Cleans all parts thoroughly	6						
6. Checks piston and harpoon	6						
7. Checks hole on adaptor	6						
8. Replaces defective parts	5						
9. Lubricates threaded parts	6						
10. Reassembles syringe correctly	6						
11. Washes, rinses, and autoclaves after each use	6						
12. Dismantles and lubricates after each five uses	6						
13. Replaces equipment used	3						
14. Removes personal protective equipment and washes hands	3						
Totals	100						

* Final Check: Instructor or authorized person evaluates.
** Points Earned: Points possible times each "yes" check.

Name _____ Date _____

Evaluated by _____

DIRECTIONS: Practice loading an anesthetic aspirating syringe according to the criteria listed. When you are ready for your final check, give this sheet to your instructor.

PROFICIENT

Loading an Anesthetic Aspirating Syringe	Points Possible	Peer Check Yes	No	Final Check* Yes	No	Points Earned**	Comments
1. Assembles equipment and supplies	2						
2. Washes hands and puts on personal protective equipment	2						
3. Checks carpule or cartridge for:							
Breaks in glass	4						
Abnormal size bubbles	4						
Rust on aluminum cap	4						
Color of solution	4						
Level of plunger	4						
4. Disinfects carpule correctly	6						
5. Checks syringe	6						
6. Retracts piston	6						
7. Inserts plunger end of carpule first	6						
8. Engages harpoon in plunger securely	6						
9. Attaches needle without contamination	6						
10. Expels a few drops of solution without contamination	6						
11. Removes bubbles	6						
12. Passes anesthetic syringe to doctor correctly	6						
13. After use, removes needle and places in sharps container	6						
14. Unloads syringe correctly	6						
15. Records type and amount of anesthetic used on patient's chart	5						
16. Cleans and sterilizes syringe correctly and replaces all equipment	3						
17. Removes personal protective equipment and washes hands	2						
Totals	100						

* Final Check: Instructor or authorized person evaluates.
** Points Earned: Points possible times each "yes" check.

UNIT 17:13 MIXING DENTAL CEMENTS AND BASES

ASSIGNMENT SHEET

Grade _____ Name _____

INTRODUCTION: As an assistant, you may work with a wide variety of dental cements and bases. This sheet will help you review some key points.

INSTRUCTIONS: Review the information on Mixing Dental Cements and Bases. In the space provided, print the word(s) that completes the statement or answers the question.

1. Define the following words. Give one (1) example of each.

   a. liner:

   b. base:

   c. cement:

   d. temporary:

2. Give at least three (3) brand names for each of the following.

   a. varnish:

   b. zinc oxide eugenol:

   c. calcium hydroxide:

   d. carboxylates:

3. Can zinc oxide eugenol (ZOE) be used as a base under resins or composites? Why or why not?

4. Can calcium hydroxide be used as a temporary restoration? Why or why not?

5. List two (2) uses for zinc phosphate.

6. Why is it important to use correct mixing techniques?

7. How do you determine the correct mixing technique for a dental cement or base?

8. Why is it important to use clean measuring devices and to follow precautions to prevent mixing the materials together?

Name _____ Date _____

Evaluated by _____

DIRECTIONS: Practice preparing varnish according to the criteria listed. When you are ready for your final check, give this sheet to your instructor.

PROFICIENT

Mixing Dental Cements and Bases: Preparing Varnish	Points Possible	Peer Check Yes	No	Final Check* Yes	No	Points Earned**	Comments
1. Assembles equipment and supplies	5						
2. Washes hands and puts on personal protective equipment	6						
3. Checks thickness of varnish - adds thinner as needed	7						
4. Passes air syringe to dry area	6						
5. Places cotton pellet in cotton pliers	6						
6. Saturates pellet with varnish and passes to doctor	6						
7. Passes air syringe to doctor	6						
8. Discards used pellet	6						
9. Passes second pellet with varnish applied	6						
10. Passes air syringe to doctor	6						
11. Discards used pellet	6						
12. Cleans screw threads on varnish bottle with thinner	6						
13. Uses thinner to clean instruments	6						
14. Scrubs and sterilizes cotton pliers	6						
15. Closes lids securely	6						
16. Replaces equipment	5						
17. Removes personal protective equipment and washes hands	5						
Totals	100						

* Final Check: Instructor or authorized person evaluates.
** Points Earned: Points possible times each "yes" check.

Name _____ Date _____

Evaluated by _____

DIRECTIONS: Practice preparing calcium hydroxide according to the criteria listed. When you are ready for your final check, give this sheet to your instructor.

PROFICIENT

Mixing Dental Cements and Bases: Preparing Calcium Hydroxide	Points Possible	Peer Check		Final Check*		Points Earned**	Comments
		Yes	No	Yes	No		
1. Assembles equipment and supplies	5						
2. Washes hands and puts on personal protective equipment	5						
3. Uses equal amounts of base and catalyst	10						
4. Places materials side by side on mixing pad	10						
5. Allows no contamination of the tubes	10						
6. Uses ball instrument to mix	10						
7. Mixes until material has a uniform color	10						
8. Completes mix in 10 seconds	10						
9. Places mix on mixing instrument to pass to doctor	10						
10. Cleans and sterilizes all instruments and replaces all equipment used	5						
11. Secures caps on both tubes	5						
12. Discards used sheet of mixing pad in trash container	5						
13. Removes personal protective equipment and washes hands	5						
Totals	100						

* Final Check: Instructor or authorized person evaluates.
** Points Earned: Points possible times each "yes" check.

U N I T 17 : 13 C   E v a l u a t i o n   S h e e t

Name _____ Date _____

Evaluated by _____

DIRECTIONS: Practice preparing carboxylate according to the criteria listed. When you are ready for your final check, give this sheet to your instructor.

PROFICIENT

Mixing Dental Cements and Bases: Preparing Carboxylate	Points Possible	Peer Check Yes	No	Final Check* Yes	No	Points Earned**	Comments
1. Assembles equipment and supplies	4						
2. Washes hands and puts on personal protective equipment	4						
3. Measures powder:							
Presses scoop in powder	5						
Uses spatula to remove excess	5						
Levels scoop with spatula	5						
Taps scoop with spatula to place powder on mixing pad	6						
4. Measures liquid:							
Holds bottle vertical	5						
Places drop by the side of the powder	6						
Uses correct amount of liquid for mix	6						
Closes lid immediately	6						
5. Adds all of powder to liquid	6						
6. Mixes vigorously	6						
7. Mixes until final mix is glossy	6						
8. Completes mixing in 30 seconds	6						
9. Closes lids of liquid and powder bottles immediately after use	6						
10. Cleans and sterilizes instruments right after use	5						
11. Discards used sheet of mixing pad in trash container	5						
12. Replaces all equipment	4						
13. Removes personal protective equipment and washes hands	4						
Totals	100						

* Final Check: Instructor or authorized person evaluates.
** Points Earned: Points possible times each "yes" check.

Name _____ Date _____

Evaluated by _____

DIRECTIONS: Practice preparing zinc oxide eugenol according to the criteria listed. When you are ready for your final check, give this sheet to your instructor.

PROFICIENT

Mixing Dental Cements and Bases: Preparing Zinc Oxide Eugenol	Points Possible	Peer Check Yes	No	Final Check* Yes	No	Points Earned**	Comments
1. Assembles equipment and supplies	5						
2. Washes hands and puts on personal protective equipment	5						
3. Fluffs powder	5						
4. Fills scoop	5						
5. Levels scoop with spatula	5						
6. Places powder on mixing pad	5						
7. Uses one drop of liquid per scoop of powder	5						
8. Dispenses liquid by side of powder on pad	5						
9. Closes liquid lid immediately	5						
10. Places dropper in holder	5						
11. Mixes $1/2$ of the powder with the liquid	6						
12. Adds remaining powder in 2-3 increments	6						
13. Whips vigorously for 5–10 seconds	6						
14. Mixes until smooth	6						
15. Completes mix in 1 to $1^1/2$ minutes	6						
16. Secures lid on powder and liquid containers	5						
17. Cleans and sterilizes instruments and replaces all equipment	5						
18. Discards used sheet from mixing pad in trash container	5						
19. Removes personal protective equipment and washes hands	5						
Totals	100						

* Final Check: Instructor or authorized person evaluates.
** Points Earned: Points possible times each "yes" check.

UNIT 17:14 PREPARING RESTORATIVE MATERIALS—AMALGAM AND COMPOSITE

ASSIGNMENT SHEET

Grade _____ Name _____

INTRODUCTION: Read the information about Preparing Restorative Materials. This assignment will help you review the main facts.

INSTRUCTIONS: In the space provided, print the word(s) that completes the statement or answers the question.

1. Define *restoration*.

2. The restorative material (filling material) used most frequently in anterior teeth is _____. The restorative material used most frequently in posterior teeth is _____.

3. Dental amalgam pellets or powder contain four main metals. List the four metals and their properties.

   Metal   *Properties*

4. The liquid metal that is added to dental amalgam to form a new alloy is called _____.

5. List three (3) safety rules for handling this liquid metal.

6. Where should scrap amalgam be stored?

7. What is trituration?

8. List three (3) reasons why composite is used.

9. When does polymerization of light-cured composite occur?

10. Why are etching and bonding agents applied to the cavity before composite is used?

314

UNIT 17:14A Evaluation Sheet

Name _____ Date _____

Evaluated by _____

DIRECTIONS: Practice preparing amalgam according to the criteria listed. When you are ready for your final check, give this sheet to your instructor.

PROFICIENT

Preparing Restorative Materials: Amalgam	Points Possible	Peer Check Yes	No	Final Check* Yes	No	Points Earned**	Comments
1. Washes hands and puts on personal protective equipment	4						
2. Assembles equipment and supplies and cleans capsule if needed	3						
3. Assists doctor as required for cavity preparation	3						
4. Prepares bonding agent if used	4						
5. Puts correct amount of alloy and mercury in capsule or uses premeasured capsule and twists or presses it to release mercury	6						
6. Prepares amalgamator - determines correct time	6						
7. Places capsule in amalgamator	5						
8 Triturates correctly	5						
9. Empties capsule into amalgam well, dappen dish, or squeeze cloth	5						
10. Loads amalgam carrier	5						
11. Fills carrier until it is smooth and well packed	6						
12. Hands carrier correctly	6						
13. Refills as above	5						
14. Works quickly before mix sets	5						
15. Passes following as needed:							
Condensation instruments	5						
Carving instruments	5						
Articulation paper	5						
16. Gives patient correct instructions	5						
17. Cleans and replaces all equipment used	3						
18. Discards disposables contaminated with mercury in a sealed polyethylene bag and places scrap amalgam in a tightly sealed unbreakable jar	5						
19. Removes personal protective equipment and washes hands thoroughly	4						
Totals	100						

* Final Check: Instructor or authorized person evaluates.
** Points Earned: Points possible times each "yes" check.

Copyright © 2001 Delmar Thomson Learning. All rights reserved.

315

Name _____ Date _____

Evaluated by _____

DIRECTIONS: Practice preparing composite according to the criteria listed. When you are ready for your final check, give this sheet to your instructor.

PROFICIENT

Preparing Restorative Materials: Composite	Points Possible	Peer Check Yes	No	Final Check* Yes	No	Points Earned**	Comments
1. Assembles equipment and supplies	4						
2. Washes hands and puts on personal protective equipment	4						
3. Prepares etching liquid:							
Places 1–2 drops on pad/plastic well	4						
Places pellet in cotton pliers or uses brush	4						
Saturates pellet or brush with etching liquid	4						
4. Passes air-water syringe	5						
5. Prepares resin:							
Places equal amounts of universal and catalyst on mixing pad/ plastic well	4						
Mixes thoroughly	4						
Allows no contamination of either bottle	4						
6. Prepares composite using 2 pastes:							
Removes equal amounts of catalyst and universal	5						
Allows no contamination of either jar	5						
Mixes until uniform and even color	5						
Completes mix in 20 seconds	5						
Prepares premixed light-cured composite:							
Reads instructions on syringe	5						
Dispenses correct amount from syringe	5						
7. Passes instruments for placement	6						
8. Works quickly before mix sets	5						
9. Puts on light-filtering glasses and passes curing light if needed	5						
10. Passes finishing and polishing strips	5						
11. Scrubs and sterilizes all instruments thoroughly	4						
12. Replaces all equipment; secures lids on all containers	4						
13. Removes personal protective equipment and washes hands	4						
Totals	100						

* Final Check: Instructor or authorized person evaluates.
** Points Earned: Points possible times each "yes" check.

UNIT 17:15 DEVELOPING AND MOUNTING DENTAL X RAYS

ASSIGNMENT SHEET

Grade _____　Name _____

INTRODUCTION: As a dental assistant, you may be involved with developing and mounting dental X rays. This sheet will help you review the main facts.

INSTRUCTIONS: Study the information on Developing and Mounting Dental X rays. In the space provided below, print the word(s) that best completes the statement or answers the question.

1. Areas that appear dark on X rays are called _____. Examples of these areas are _____ and _____. Areas that appear light or white on X rays are called _____. Examples include _____, and _____.

2. Identify the following types of X rays.

   a.　X rays that show only the crowns of teeth:

   b.　X rays that show the root and surrounding area:

   c.　X ray that shows the entire dental arch on one film:

3. What is the function of the lead foil in the packet of dental film?

4. Why must dental films be developed in a dark room?

5. Why is the silver halide on dental film suspended in a gelatin?

6. What is the correct temperature for the developer, fix, and water bath?

7. What is the purpose of the developing solution?

   Is it acid or alkaline?

8. What is the purpose of the fix solution?

   Is it acid or alkaline?

9. What surface are you viewing if the dimples on the X ray are mounted so they are convex (pointing out)?

10. What surface are you viewing if the dimples on the X ray are mounted so they are concave (pointing inward)?

Name _____ **Date** _____

Evaluated by _____

DIRECTIONS: Practice developing dental X rays according to the criteria listed. When you are ready for your final check, give this sheet to your instructor.

PROFICIENT

Developing Dental X rays	Points Possible	Peer Check Yes	No	Final Check* Yes	No	Points Earned**	Comments
1. Assembles equipment and supplies	3						
2. Washes hands and puts on personal protective equipment	3						
3. Stirs solutions in tank	4						
4. Turns on water supply	3						
Regulates temperature at 68°F or 20°C	4						
5. Closes door of darkroom tightly	3						
6. Turns warning light on	4						
7. Turns safe lights on	4						
8. Unwraps film:							
Pulls up tab	3						
Pulls out inner wrap	3						
Handles film by edges	4						
Places film on clip	3						
Tugs gently on film to check if secure on clip	4						
9. Labels wrap with patient's name and puts on rack	3						
10. Places film in developing solution:							
Immerses smoothly	4						
Closes lid to tank	3						
Sets timer for five minutes or per manufacturer's instructions	4						
11. Shakes off excess liquid when time complete	3						
12. Places film in rinse	3						
13. Rinses 30 seconds	3						
14. Shakes off excess water	3						
15. Places in fix solution:							
Agitates film in fix	3						
Leaves in twice as long as developing time	4						
Covers tank with lid	3						
16. Places in water bath - agitates	3						
17. Rinses at least 20 minutes	4						
18. Hangs clip on drying rack	3						
19. Cleans and replaces all equipment used	3						
20. Turns off water supply	3						
21. Removes personal protective equipment and washes hands	3						
Totals	100						

* Final Check: Instructor or authorized person evaluates.
** Points Earned: Points possible times each "yes" check.

UNIT 17:15B Evaluation Sheet

Name _____ Date _____

Evaluated by _____

DIRECTIONS: Practice mounting dental X rays according to the criteria listed. When you are ready for your final check, give this sheet to your instructor.

Mounting Dental X rays	Points Possible	Peer Check Yes	No	Final Check* Yes	No	Points Earned**	Comments
1. Assembles equipment and supplies	2						
2. Washes hands	2						
3. Mounts bite wing X rays:							
Identifies crowns on X ray	4						
Positions dimples all in same direction	4						
Mounts two sets correctly	16						
4. Mounts full mouth series:							
Identifies periapical view	4						
Places dimples all in same direction	4						
Mounts two full series correctly	32						
5. Mounts child films:							
Places all dimples in same direction	4						
Mounts one set correctly	8						
6. Identifies dimple placement							
Convex placement:							
Identifies facial surface	4						
Points out right and left teeth correctly	4						
Concave placement:							
Identifies lingual surface	4						
Points out right and left teeth correctly	4						
7. Replaces equipment	2						
8. Washes hands	2						
Totals	100						

* Final Check: Instructor or authorized person evaluates.
** Points Earned: Points possible times each "yes" check.

UNIT 18:1 OPERATING THE MICROSCOPE

ASSIGNMENT SHEET

Grade _____ Name _____

INTRODUCTION: This assignment will help you understand the parts of the microscope and basic operating principles.

INSTRUCTIONS: Review the information on Operating the Microscope. In the space provided, print the word(s) that best completes the statement or answers the question. Identify the parts of the microscope, and write their names beside the corresponding number in the column.

1.

2.

3.

4.

5.

6.

7.

8.

9.

10.

11.

12. What do electron microscopes use to view objects?

13. Why is an epifluorescence microscope used?

14. What might happen if you lower the objective with the coarse adjustment while looking through the eyepiece?

15. How do you increase the amount of light that enters the microscope through the hole in the stage?

16. Why must you use special lens paper to clean the eyepiece and the objectives?

17. What is the function (use of) the coarse adjustment knob?

18. What is the function of the fine adjustment knob?

19. What is an oil immersion objective used for?

20. If the eyepiece you are using has a magnification power of 10X, what would the total magnification be with the following objectives? (How much would you enlarge each object?)

    a. 4X

    b. 10X

    c. 40X

21. If the eyepiece you are using is 2OX, what would the total magnification be with the following objectives?

    a. 4X

    b. 10X

    c. 40X

22. How should a microscope be stored?

UNIT 18:1 Evaluation Sheet

Name _____ Date _____

Evaluated by _____

DIRECTIONS: Practice operating the microscope according to the criteria listed. When you are ready for your final check, give this sheet to your instructor.

PROFICIENT

Operating the Microscope	Points Possible	Peer Check Yes	No	Final Check* Yes	No	Points Earned**	Comments
1. Assembles equipment and supplies	2						
2. Washes hands and puts on gloves if needed	2						
3. Identifies parts:							
Arm	2						
Base	2						
Stage	2						
Eyepiece	2						
Revolving nosepiece	2						
Objectives	2						
Light	2						
Iris diaphragm	2						
Slide clips	2						
Coarse adjustment	2						
Fine adjustment	2						
Body tube	2						
4. Cleans slide and cover slip	3						
5. Places specimen on slide	3						
6. Adds drop of water or normal saline to slide	3						
7. Adds cover slip without air bubbles	3						
8. Positions low objective	3						
9. Turns on illuminating light	3						
10. Anchors slide on stage with slide clips	3						
11. Lowers objective while watching slide	3						
12. Uses coarse adjustment for rough focus	3						
13. Uses fine adjustment for precise focus	3						
14. Increases or decreases amount of light as needed by turning iris diaphragm	3						
15. Switches to high power	3						

18:1 (cont.)

Operating the Microscope	Points Possible	Peer Check Yes	No	Final Check* Yes	No	Points Earned**	Comments
16. Focuses with fine adjustment	3						
17. Uses oil immersion objective:							
Positions oil immersion objective	2						
Focuses with fine adjustment	2						
Moves objective to side	2						
Puts small drop of oil on slide	2						
Repositions objective in oil	2						
Focuses with fine adjustment	2						
Cleans objective with lens paper when done	2						
18. Cleans slide and cover slip thoroughly	3						
19. Cleans eyepiece(s) and objectives with lens paper	3						
20. Lowers low power objective to stage	3						
21. Turns off light	3						
22. Covers for storage	3						
23. Cleans and replaces all equipment	2						
24. Removes gloves if worn and washes hands	2						
Totals	100						

* Final Check: Instructor or authorized person evaluates.
** Points Earned: Points possible times each "yes" check.

UNIT 18:2 OBTAINING AND HANDLING CULTURES

ASSIGNMENT SHEET

Grade _____   Name _____

INTRODUCTION: This assignment will help you understand some basic facts about cultures and Gram's stain technique.

INSTRUCTIONS: Review the information on Obtaining and Handling Cultures. In the space provided, print the word(s) that best completes the statement or answers the question.

1. Why are culture specimens obtained?

2. Why is a sterile applicator swab used to obtain the specimen?

3. What is agar?

   What does it do?

4. Define the following words.

   resistant:

   sensitive:

5. Why is it important to know if an organism is sensitive or resistant to an antibiotic?

6. What is meant by the term *fixing* the slide?

   What is the purpose of fixing?

7. List the four (4) solutions that are used for a Gram's stain. Give the purpose for each solution and the time that it is applied to the slide.

Solution	*Purpose*	*Time*

8. In addition to coloring the organisms so they are visible, what is the purpose of the Gram's stain technique?

Name _____ Date _____

Evaluated by _____

DIRECTIONS: Practice obtaining a culture specimen according to the criteria listed. When you are ready for your final check, give this sheet to your instructor.

Obtaining a Culture Specimen	Points Possible	Peer Check Yes	Peer Check No	Final Check* Yes	Final Check* No	Points Earned**	Comments
PROFICIENT							
1. Checks order for obtaining culture specimen	4						
2. Assembles equipment and supplies	4						
3. Washes hands and puts on gloves	4						
4. Introduces self and identifies patient	4						
5. Explains procedure	4						
6. Checks site for specimen	4						
7. Removes applicator from package without contamination	7						
8. Holds applicator at wooden end only	7						
9. Rolls applicator tip over site to cover tip	8						
10. Places applicator in medium	8						
11. Avoids contamination of specimen	7						
12. Checks that tip is down in medium	7						
13. Labels specimen with:							
Patient's name	2						
Doctor's name	2						
Address/room number/patient number	2						
Date/time	2						
Type of test ordered	2						
Site of specimen	2						
14. Takes specimen to laboratory or places in safe area away from sunlight or heat	4						
15. Places contaminated disposables in infectious waste bag	4						
16. Wipes contaminated areas with a disinfectant	4						
17. Replaces equipment	4						
18. Removes gloves and washes hands	4						
Totals	100						

* Final Check: Instructor or authorized person evaluates.
** Points Earned: Points possible times each "yes" check.

Name _____ Date _____

Evaluated by _____

DIRECTIONS: Practice preparing a direct smear according to the criteria listed. When you are ready for your final check, give this sheet to your instructor.

PROFICIENT

Preparing a Direct Smear	Points Possible	Peer Check Yes	No	Final Check* Yes	No	Points Earned**	Comments
1. Assembles equipment and supplies	4						
2. Washes hands and puts on gloves	4						
3. Cleans slide thoroughly	4						
4. Removes specimen from medium without contamination	6						
5. Holds slide correctly	6						
6. Rolls applicator swab to opposite end of slide	6						
7. Uses firm, even pressure to transfer organisms to slide	6						
8. Avoids contamination of fingers, thumb, slide, and applicator swab	6						
9. Discards applicator swab in infectious waste bag	6						
10. Allows slide to air dry at room temperature	6						
11. Fixes slide:							
Places slide in hemostats or slide clamps	5						
Turns on bunsen burner/alcohol lamp	5						
Holds slide 1–2 inches above flame for 1–2 seconds 3–4 times	5						
Checks temperature of slide to avoid excess heat	5						
12. Extinguishes bunsen burner or alcohol lamp	4						
13. Places slide on staining rack	5						
14. Labels slide correctly	5						
15. Cleans and replaces all equipment:							
Places contaminated disposables in infectious waste bag	4						
Wipes contaminated areas with a disinfectant	4						
16. Removes gloves and washes hands	4						
Totals	100						

* Final Check: Instructor or authorized person evaluates.
** Points Earned: Points possible times each "yes" check.

Name _____ Date _____

Evaluated by _____

DIRECTIONS: Practice streaking an agar plate according to the criteria listed. When you are ready for your final check, give this sheet to your instructor.

PROFICIENT

Streaking an Agar Plate	Points Possible	Peer Check Yes	No	Final Check* Yes	No	Points Earned**	Comments
1. Assembles equipment and supplies	4						
2. Washes hands and puts on gloves	4						
3. Removes culture specimen from medium without contamination	7						
4. Checks moisture of applicator swab	6						
5. Opens agar plate without contamination	6						
6. Holds plate firmly or places it on flat surface	6						
7. Streaks plate correctly	8						
8. Checks agar to be sure all areas streaked	6						
9. Discards applicator swab in infectious waste bag	6						
10. Applies disks correctly for sensitivity test	7						
11. Closes agar plate without contamination	6						
12. Labels specimen with:							
Patient's name	2						
Doctor's name	2						
Date	2						
Time	2						
Address/room number/identification number	2						
Site of specimen	2						
13. Checks temperature of incubator for 36–37° C (97–99° F)	6						
14. Incubates agar plate for 24–36 hours with agar side up	6						
15. Cleans and replaces all equipment:							
Places contaminated disposables in infectious waste bag	3						
Wipes contaminated areas with a disinfectant	3						
16. Removes gloves and washes hands	4						
Totals	100						

* Final Check: Instructor or authorized person evaluates.
** Points Earned: Points possible times each "yes" check.

UNIT 18:2D Evaluation Sheet

Name _____ Date _____

Evaluated by _____

DIRECTIONS: Practice transferring culture from agar plate to slide according to the criteria listed. When you are ready for your final check, give this sheet to your instructor.

PROFICIENT

Transferring Culture from Agar Plate to Slide	Points Possible	Peer Check Yes	No	Final Check* Yes	No	Points Earned**	Comments
1. Assembles equipment and supplies	4						
2. Washes hands and puts on gloves	5						
3. Lights bunsen burner or alcohol lamp	5						
4. Heats loop until it is red hot	7						
5. Opens agar plate without contamination	7						
6. Picks up small amount of culture in cooled loop	7						
7. Closes lid on agar plate immediately	7						
8. Places drop of normal saline on slide	7						
9. Suspends organisms on loop in saline solution	7						
10. Spreads solution over entire width of slide	7						
11. Heats loop until it is red hot	7						
12. Allows slide to air dry	7						
13. Fixes slide correctly	7						
14. Labels slide correctly	5						
15. Cleans and replaces all equipment:							
Places contaminated disposables in infectious waste bag	3						
Wipes contaminated areas with a disinfectant	3						
16. Removes gloves and washes hands	5						
Totals	100						

* Final Check: Instructor or authorized person evaluates.
** Points Earned: Points possible times each "yes" check.

Name _____ Date _____

Evaluated by _____

DIRECTIONS: Practice staining with Gram's stain according to the criteria listed. When you are ready for your final check, give this sheet to your instructor.

PROFICIENT

Staining with Gram's Stain	Points Possible	Peer Check Yes	No	Final Check* Yes	No	Points Earned**	Comments
1. Assembles equipment and supplies	2						
2. Washes hands and puts on gloves	2						
3. Places fixed slide on rack with smear facing up	4						
4. Covers slide with gentian violet or crystal violet	4						
Leaves in place one minute	4						
5. Rinses slide with distilled water	3						
6. Applies iodine correctly:							
Covers slide with iodine	4						
Tilts slide to drain	4						
Reapplies iodine	4						
Leaves in place 1 minute	4						
7. Rinses slide with distilled water	3						
8. Decolorizes with ethyl alcohol/acetone-alcohol:							
Covers slide with alcohol	4						
Tilts slide to drain solution	4						
Reapplies alcohol and again tilts slide to drain	4						
Checks color of solution as it runs off of slide	4						
Stops applying alcohol when draining solution is no longer purple	4						
9. Rinses slide with distilled water	3						
10. Applies safranin:							
Covers slide with safranin	4						
Tilts slide to drain	4						
Reapplies safranin	4						
Leaves in place 30–60 seconds	4						
11. Rinses with distilled water	3						
12. Dries back of slide with paper towel	4						
13. Allows smear side of slide to air dry	4						
14. Identifies organisms:							
Gram positive as purple	4						
Gram negative organisms as red	4						
15. Cleans up and replaces all equipment	2						
16. Removes gloves and washes hands	2						
Totals	100						

* Final Check: Instructor or authorized person evaluates.
** Points Earned: Points possible times each "yes" check.

UNIT 18:3 PUNCTURING THE SKIN TO OBTAIN CAPILLARY BLOOD

ASSIGNMENT SHEET

Grade _____ Name _____

INTRODUCTION: This assignment will help you review the main facts regarding performing a skin puncture.

INSTRUCTIONS: Read the information on Puncturing the Skin to Obtain Capillary Blood. In the space provided, print the word(s) that best completes the statement or answers the question.

1. List three (3) ways blood can be obtained for blood tests.

2. Why is it important for you to determine your legal responsibility involving the obtaining of blood for blood tests?

3. List three (3) points you must observe to follow aseptic techniques while performing a finger puncture.

4. List five (5) points that must be checked before a finger is used to perform a finger puncture.

5. How deep should the skin puncture be?

6. The puncture should be made _____ the grain of lines in the finger or at _____ to the fingerprint striations.

7. Why is the first drop of blood removed? Why can't it be used for various blood tests?

8. How long should you stay with the patient after performing a finger puncture?

9. Why is it important to handle any blood sample with extreme care?

10. How should you dispose of the lancet used to puncture the skin?

UNIT 18:3 Evaluation Sheet

Name _____ Date _____

Evaluated by _____

DIRECTIONS: Practice puncturing the skin to obtain capillary blood according to the criteria listed. When you are ready for your final check, give this sheet to your instructor.

PROFICIENT

Puncturing the Skin to Obtain Capillary Blood	Points Possible	Peer Check Yes	No	Final Check* Yes	No	Points Earned**	Comments
1. Assembles equipment and supplies	4						
2. Washes hands and puts on gloves	4						
3. Introduces self, identifies patient and explains procedure	5						
4. Selects finger after checking for absence of:							
Edema	2						
Cyanosis/pale color	2						
Scars	2						
Sores	2						
Calluses	2						
5. Cleans finger with alcohol	6						
6. Lets finger dry	6						
7. Punctures finger with quick, clean stab	6						
Punctures finger at correct angle	6						
Punctures in right area	6						
8. Places lancet in sharps container	6						
9. Uses gentle pressure to start blood flow	6						
10. Wipes off first drop	6						
11. Uses second or succeeding drops of blood for tests	6						
12. When sufficient blood is obtained, instructs patient to hold sterile gauze firmly against puncture	5						
13. Checks patient for cessation of bleeding before leaving	6						
14. Cleans and replaces all equipment :							
Places contaminated disposables in infectious waste bag	4						
Wipes contaminated areas with a disinfectant	4						
15. Remove gloves and washes hands	4						
Totals	100						

* Final Check: Instructor or authorized person evaluates.
** Points Earned: Points possible times each "yes" check.

UNIT 18:4 PERFORMING A MICROHEMATOCRIT

ASSIGNMENT SHEET

Grade _____ Name _____

INTRODUCTION: This assignment will help you review the main facts regarding the microhematocrit blood test.

INSTRUCTIONS: Read the information on Performing a Microhematocrit. In the space provided, print the word(s) that best completes the statement or answers the question.

1. Define *hematocrit.*

2. Red blood cells carry _____ from the lungs to body cells and _____ from the body cells to the lungs.

3. Why is a microhematocrit a popular method for determining hematocrit?

4. The microhematocrit centrifuge separates the blood into three main layers. What are the three (3) layers?

5. Why are the microhematocrit capillary tubes lined with an anticoagulant?

6. Why is the empty end of the capillary tube sealed with special plastic sealing clay?

7. Give the normal microhematocrit value for the following.

   a. Adult women:

   b. Adult men:

   c. Newborns:

   d. Children 6 years old:

8. What does a low hematocrit reading indicate?

9. What does a high hematocrit reading indicate?

10. Why is accuracy essential when performing a microhematocrit?

11. If any results are questionable, what should you do?

12. Who should report the results of the test to the patient?

Name _____ Date _____

Evaluated by _____

DIRECTIONS: Practice performing a microhematocrit according to the criteria listed. When you are ready for your final check, give this sheet to your instructor.

Performing a Microhematocrit	Points Possible	Peer Check Yes	Peer Check No	Final Check* Yes	Final Check* No	Points Earned**	Comments
1. Assembles equipment and supplies	4						
2. Washes hands and puts on gloves	4						
3. Introduces self, identifies patient, and explains procedure	4						
4. Performs finger puncture	4						
5. Puts lancet in sharps container	4						
6. Wipes off first drop of blood	4						
7. Fills tube(s) to correct level	6						
8. Seals tube(s) properly	6						
9. When sufficient blood obtained, instructs patient to hold gauze against puncture	5						
10. Places tube(s) in centrifuge in correct area	6						
11. Closes lids on centrifuge securely	6						
12. Centrifuges proper amount of time	6						
13. Aligns tube correctly for reading	6						
14. Reads microhematocrit accurately (to ±1 percent)	7						
15. Records reading accurately	7						
16. Checks patient to be sure bleeding has stopped	5						
17. Cleans and replaces all equipment:							
Places contaminated disposables in infectious waste bag	4						
Wipes contaminated areas with a disinfectant	4						
18. Removes gloves and washes hands	4						
19. Reports abnormal readings immediately	4						
Totals	100						

PROFICIENT

* Final Check: Instructor or authorized person evaluates.
** Points Earned: Points possible times each "yes" check.

UNIT 18:5 MEASURING HEMOGLOBIN

ASSIGNMENT SHEET

Grade _____   Name _____

INTRODUCTION: This assignment will help you review the main facts on the hemoglobin test.

INSTRUCTIONS: Read the information about Measuring Hemoglobin. In the space provided, print the word(s) that best completes the statement or answers the question.

1. What is hemoglobin?

2. What is the function of hemoglobin?

3. What does a hemoglobin test determine?

4. What is a hemoglobinometer?

5. Define *hemolysis.*

   What happens to hemoglobin when hemolysis occurs?

6. How can you determine when hemolyzation of the blood has occurred?

7. State the normal hemoglobin value for the following.

   a. Males: c. Newborns:

   b. Females: d. Children from 1 to 10 years old:

8. A low hemoglobin level can be an indication of _____. A high level can be an indication of _____.

9. What should be done if the test results are questionable?

10. Why is an automated photometer test more accurate to check hemoglobin?

Name _____ Date _____

Evaluated by _____

DIRECTIONS: Practice measuring hemoglobin with a hemoglobinometer according to the criteria listed. When you are ready for your final check, give this sheet to your instructor.

PROFICIENT

Measuring Hemoglobin with a Hemoglobinometer	Points Possible	Peer Check		Final Check*		Points Earned**	Comments
		Yes	No	Yes	No		
1. Assembles equipment and supplies	3						
2. Washes hands and puts on gloves	3						
3. Cleans chamber with lens paper	4						
4. Introduces self, identifies patient, and explains procedure	4						
5. Performs finger puncture	5						
6. Puts lancet in sharps container	5						
7. Wipes off first drop of blood	5						
8. Places blood on chamber correctly	5						
9. When sufficient blood is obtained, instructs patient to hold gauze against puncture	5						
10. Hemolyzes blood with agitating action	5						
11. Stops hemolyzation when blood is clear and transparent	5						
12. Covers chamber with cover slip and inserts in clip	5						
13. Checks color match on hemoglobinometer	5						
14. Loads chamber into hemoglobinometer	5						
15. Sets color match correctly	6						
16. Reads scale within ± 0.5 gram/100 mL of blood	6						
17. Records reading accurately	6						
18. Checks patient to be sure finger puncture has stopped bleeding	5						
19. Cleans and replaces all equipment :							
Cleans chamber and glass with disinfectant	2						
Places contaminated disposables in infectious waste bag	2						
Wipes contaminated areas with a disinfectant	2						
20. Removes gloves and washes hands	3						
21. Reports abnormal readings immediately	4						
Totals	100						

* Final Check: Instructor or authorized person evaluates.
** Points Earned: Points possible times each "yes" check.

UNIT 18:5B Evaluation Sheet

Name _____ Date _____

Evaluated by _____

DIRECTIONS: Practice measuring hemoglobin with a photometer according to the criteria listed. When you are ready for your final check, give this sheet to your instructor.

Measuring Hemoglobin with a Photometer	Points Possible	Peer Check Yes	No	Final Check* Yes	No	Points Earned**	Comments
1. Assembles equipment and supplies	3						
2. Washes hands and puts on gloves	3						
3. Uses control cuvette to calibrate photometer correctly	5						
4. Introduces self, identifies patient, and explains procedure	4						
5. Performs finger puncture	5						
6. Puts lancet in sharps container	5						
7. Wipes off first drop of blood	5						
8. Fills cuvette correctly:							
Holds cuvette at square rear end	4						
Places angled tip of cuvette in middle of drop of blood	4						
Holds cuvette steady while it fills with blood	4						
Checks to make sure no air bubbles are present	4						
9. When sufficient blood is obtained, instructs patient to hold gauze against puncture	5						
10. Wipes off excess blood on outside of cuvette	5						
11. Activates photometer to "ready" display	5						
12. Places filled cuvette in holder	5						
13. Gently pushes holder into photometer unit	5						
14. Reads results correctly	5						
15. Records reading accurately	5						
16. Checks patient to be sure finger puncture has stopped bleeding	5						
17. Cleans and replaces all equipment:							
Places used cuvette in sharps container	2						
Wipes photometer with disinfecting solution	2						
Places contaminated disposables in infectious waste bag	2						
Wipes contaminated areas with a disinfectant	2						
18. Removes gloves and washes hands	3						
19. Reports abnormal readings immediately	3						
Totals	100						

* Final Check: Instructor or authorized person evaluates.
** Points Earned: Points possible times each "yes" check.

UNIT 18:6 COUNTING BLOOD CELLS

ASSIGNMENT SHEET

Grade _____ Name _____

INTRODUCTION: This assignment will help you review the main facts regarding diluting pipettes, the counting chamber, and counting erythrocytes and leukocytes.

INSTRUCTIONS: Review the information on Counting Blood Cells. Read the following instructions for help in completing the questions or problems.

1. Why are erythrocyte counts done?

   Why are leukocyte counts done?

2. A diagram of the hemacytometer counting chamber follows.

   A. Label the areas in which white blood cells or leukocytes are counted by marking them with WBC or W.

   B. Label the areas in which red blood cells or erythrocytes are counted by marking them with RBC or R.

3. When counting blood cells, count all cells inside the appropriate squares. Also count all cells that touch the _____ (right or left) side of the outer line and all cells that touch the _____ (top or bottom) outer line.

   Do *not* count cells that touch the _____ (right or left) side of the outer line or cells that touch the _____ (top or bottom) outer line.

Name _____

4. The following counts are for white blood cells or leukocytes. Count the four separate chambers. Write the total number of cells for each chamber in the space provided under the diagram.

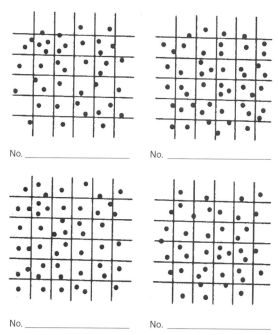

No. _____   No. _____

No. _____   No. _____

5. The following counts are for red blood cells or erythrocytes. Count the number of cells in each of the four separate chambers. Write the total number of cells for each chamber in the space provided under the diagram.

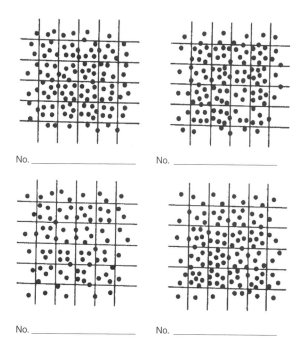

No. _____   No. _____

No. _____   No. _____

6. To do a white blood cell or leukocyte count, count the number of cells in the four outer chambers. Add the four numbers together. Multiply the sum by 50.

Example: Four counts are 35, 40, 38, and 41.

The sum of the four numbers is 154.

Multiplying by 50 gives a WBC count of 7,700.

$$35 + 40 + 38 + 41 = 154 \times 50 = 7,700 \text{ cells total}$$

Since the normal count is 5,000 to 10,000, this count would be in normal limits.

Do the following 5 problems by referring to the preceding example.

   a. The four counts are 35, 42, 45, and 48.

   The total WBC is _____.

   Is this a normal count? (yes–no) _____

   b. The four counts are 38, 42, 44, and 45.

   The total WBC is _____.

   Is this a normal count? _____

   c. The four counts are 40, 45, 47, and 48.

   The total WBC is _____.

   Is this a normal count? _____

   d. The four counts are 40, 48, 52, and 49.

   The total WBC is _____.

   Is this a normal count? _____

   e. The four counts are 50, 55, 58 and 60.

   The total WBC is _____.

   Is this a normal count? _____

7. To do a red blood cell count, count the five RBC chambers. Add the five numbers together. Multiply the sum by 10,000.

Example: Five counts are 89, 90, 92, 94 and 96.

The sum of the five numbers is 461.

Multiplying by 10,000 gives a total count of 4,610,000.

$$89 + 90 + 92 + 94 + 96 = 461 \times 10,000 = 4,610,000$$

Since the normal count is 4 to 6 million, this is normal.

Do the following 4 problems by noting the preceding example.

    a.   The five counts are 89, 92, 95, 97 and 94.

        The total RBC count is _____.

        Is this a normal count? _____

    b.   The five counts are 95, 98, 102, 105 and 100.

        The total RBC is_____.

        Is this a normal count?_____

    c.   The five counts are 100, 102, 105, 105 and 108.

        The total RBC is_____.

        Is this a normal count?_____

    d.   The five counts are 130, 128, 133, 137, and 129.

        The total RBC is _____.

        Is this a normal count? _____

8. Why is it important to select the pipette unit with the proper diluting fluid?

9. What does the diluting fluid for leukocyte counts do to erythrocytes in the blood? Why?

10. How many times does the pipette unit dilute the blood for a leukocyte count?

    How many times does the pipette unit dilute the blood for erythrocyte count?

11. What is the normal count for leukocytes?

12. What is a low leukocyte count called?

    List two (2) causes.

13. What is a high leukocyte count called?

    List two (2) causes.

14. What is the normal count for erythrocytes?

15. What does a low erythrocyte count indicate?

    What does a high erythrocyte count indicate?

UNIT 18:6A Evaluation Sheet

Name ______________________ Date ______________________

Evaluated by ______________________

DIRECTIONS: Practice counting erythrocytes according to the criteria listed. When you are ready for your final check, give this sheet to your instructor.

Counting Erythrocytes	Points Possible	PROFICIENT Peer Check Yes	Peer Check No	Final Check* Yes	Final Check* No	Points Earned**	Comments
1. Assembles equipment and supplies	3						
2. Cleans slide and cover glass with lens paper	3						
3. Washes hands and puts on gloves	3						
4. Introduces self, identifies patient, and explains procedure	3						
5. Performs finger puncture	3						
6. Puts lancet in sharps container	3						
7. Wipes off first drop of blood	3						
8. Fills Unopette:							
Punctures diaphragm	2						
Removes shield	2						
Places tip of pipette in blood	2						
Fills pipette correctly	2						
Wipes off excess blood with gauze pad	2						
9. When sufficient blood is obtained, instructs patient to hold gauze against puncture	5						
10. Mixes blood with diluting fluid:							
Squeezes reservoir slightly to expel air	2						
Puts pipette in reservoir neck	2						
Releases pressure on reservoir and pipette opening	2						
Squeezes reservoir gently to rinse pipette	2						
Inverts reservoir several times to mix blood and diluting fluid	2						
11. Attaches pipette to opposite end of reservoir	5						
12. Discards 3–4 drops from pipette	5						
13. Charges the chamber correctly	6						
14. Finds counting areas under high power	6						
15. Counts five inner squares for RBCs to ± 5 cells accuracy	7						

18:6A (cont.)

Counting Erythrocytes	Points Possible	Peer Check		Final Check*		Points Earned**	Comments
		Yes	No	Yes	No		
16. Adds five totals together	5						
17. Multiplies sum by 10,000	5						
18. Records count correctly	6						
19. Cleans and replaces all equipment:							
Cleans chamber and cover glass with disinfectant	2						
Places contaminated disposables in infectious waste bag	2						
Wipes contaminated areas with a disinfectant	2						
20. Removes gloves and washes hands	3						
Totals	100						

* Final Check: Instructor or authorized person evaluates.
** Points Earned: Points possible times each "yes" check.

UNIT 18:6B Evaluation Sheet

Name _____ Date _____

Evaluated by _____

DIRECTIONS: Practice counting leukocytes according to the criteria listed. When you are ready for your final check, give this sheet to your instructor.

PROFICIENT

Counting Leukocytes	Points Possible	Peer Check Yes	No	Final Check* Yes	No	Points Earned**	Comments
1. Assembles equipment and supplies	3						
2. Cleans slide and cover glass with lens paper	3						
3. Washes hands and puts on gloves	3						
4. Introduces self, identifies patient and explains procedure	3						
5. Performs finger puncture	3						
6. Puts lancet in sharps container	3						
7. Wipes off first drop of blood	3						
8. Fills Unopette:							
Punctures diaphragm	2						
Removes shield	2						
Places tip of pipette in blood	2						
Fills pipette correctly	2						
Wipes off excess blood with gauze pad	2						
9. When sufficient blood is obtained, instructs patient to hold gauze against puncture	5						
10. Mixes blood with diluting fluid:							
Squeezes reservoir slightly to expel air	2						
Puts pipette in reservoir neck	2						
Releases pressure on reservoir and pipette opening	2						
Squeezes reservoir gently to rinse pipette	2						
Inverts reservoir several times to mix blood and diluting fluid	2						
11. Attaches pipette to opposite end of reservoir	5						
12. Discards 3–4 drops from pipette	5						
13. Charges the chamber correctly	6						
14. Finds counting areas under low power	6						

18:6B (cont.)

Counting Leukocytes	Points Possible	Peer Check		Final Check*		Points Earned**	Comments
		Yes	No	Yes	No		
15. Counts four primary outer corner squares to ±5 cells accuracy	7						
16. Adds four totals together	5						
17. Multiplies sum by 50	5						
18. Records count correctly	6						
19. Cleans and replaces all equipment:							
Cleans chamber and cover glass with disinfectant	2						
Places contaminated disposables in infectious waste bag	2						
Wipes contaminated areas with a disinfectant	2						
20. Removes gloves and washes hands	3						
Totals	100						

* Final Check: Instructor or authorized person evaluates.
** Points Earned: Points possible times each "yes" check.

UNIT 18:7 PREPARING AND STAINING A BLOOD FILM OR SMEAR

ASSIGNMENT SHEET

Grade _____ Name _____

INTRODUCTION: This assignment will help you review the main facts on preparing and staining blood films or smears.

INSTRUCTIONS: Read the information on Preparing and Staining a Blood Film or Smear. In the space provided, print the word(s) that best completes the statement or answers the question.

1. How is a blood smear or film prepared?

2. In a differential count, _____ white blood cells are counted. As the count is performed, a _____ is kept of each _____ of leukocyte seen. The _____ of each type is then calculated.

3. Why is a differential count used?

4. The blood smear or film is also used to examine the _____, _____, and _____ of _____, _____, and _____. In addition to abnormal blood counts, abnormal _____ can also be a sign of disease.

5. What do abnormal shapes and an increase in the number of leukocytes indicate?

6. Why must the equipment used for preparing a blood smear or film be extremely clean?

7. What solution can be used to wipe the slide and spreader clean before use?

8. List two (2) purposes or reasons for using Wright's stain on a blood smear or film.

9. For a quick stain, or three-step method, the blood smear slide is dipped into a/an _____ solution for about _____, and then dipped into two separate _____ solutions for approximately _____ each.

10. What is the advantage to using a quick stain method instead of Wright's stain?

UNIT 18:7A Evaluation Sheet

Name _____ Date _____

Evaluated by _____

DIRECTIONS: Practice preparing a blood film or smear according to the criteria listed. When you are ready for your final check, give this sheet to your instructor.

Preparing a Blood Film or Smear	Points Possible	Peer Check Yes	No	Final Check* Yes	No	Points Earned**	Comments
PROFICIENT							
1. Assembles equipment and supplies	3						
2. Washes hands and puts on gloves	3						
3. Cleans slide and spreader with alcohol	3						
4. Introduces self, identifies patient, and explains procedure	3						
5. Performs finger puncture	5						
6. Puts lancet in sharps container	5						
7. Wipes off first drop of blood	5						
8. Centers blood drop ¼ inch from end of slide	7						
9. Avoids touching finger to slide	7						
10. When sufficient blood is obtained, instructs patient to hold gauze against puncture	5						
11. Holds spreader at 30–45 degree angle in front of the blood	7						
12. Pulls spreader back until it touches the blood	7						
13. Allows blood to cover edge of spreader	7						
14. Uses smooth even motion to push blood over slide	7						
15. Prepares smooth film 1½" long, with even margins	7						
16. Allows smear to air dry	6						
17. Checks patient to make sure finger puncture has stopped bleeding	4						
18. Cleans and replaces all equipment:							
Places contaminated disposables in infectious waste bag	3						
Wipes contaminated areas with a disinfectant	3						
19. Removes gloves and washes hands	3						
Totals	100						

* Final Check: Instructor or authorized person evaluates.
** Points Earned: Points possible times each "yes" check.

UNIT 18:7B Evaluation Sheet

Name _____ Date _____

Evaluated by _____

DIRECTIONS: Practice staining a blood film or smear according to the criteria listed. When you are ready for your final check, give this sheet to your instructor.

PROFICIENT

Staining a Blood Film or Smear	Points Possible	Peer Check Yes	No	Final Check* Yes	No	Points Earned**	Comments
1. Assembles equipment and supplies	4						
2. Washes hands and puts on gloves	4						
3. Prepares blood film/smear	5						
4. Places slide on rack with film facing upward and checks that rack is level	5						
5. To stain the slide with Wright's stain:							
Covers slide with stain	6						
Leaves stain in place 1–3 minutes	6						
Covers slide with equal amounts of distilled water or buffer	6						
Blows on slide to mix buffer and stain	6						
Allows mix to remain on slide for 2–4 minutes	6						
6. To stain the slide with a quick stain:							
Reads manufacturer's directions	6						
Dips slide in fix solution for about 1 second	6						
Quickly dips slide in staining solutions for about 1 second each	6						
Repeats three-step process 4 to 5 times	6						
7. Washes slide gently with distilled water	6						
8. Wipes back of slide but allows front to dry in vertical position with heavy side down	6						
9. Checks slide to be sure it is lavender pink in color	6						
10. Cleans and replaces all equipment used:							
Places contaminated disposables in infectious waste bag	3						
Wipes contaminated areas with a disinfectant	3						
11. Removes gloves and washes hands	4						
Totals	100						

* Final Check: Instructor or authorized person evaluates.
** Points Earned: Points possible times each "yes" check.

ASSIGNMENT SHEET

Grade _____ Name _____

INTRODUCTION: In many of the health fields, you will be required to have a basic knowledge of blood types. This assignment will help you review the main facts.

INSTRUCTIONS: Read the information about Testing for Blood Types. In the space provided, print the word(s) that best completes the statement or answers the question.

1. What is the name of the factors located on red blood cells that determine the type of blood?

2. List the type blood that contains the following antigens.

   a. Antigen A: d. Antigen B:

   b. Antigen A and antigen B: e. Rh antigen:

   c. Neither antigen A nor antigen B: f. No Rh antigen:

3. Define the following ways in which antibodies can destroy red blood cells.

   a. hemolyze:

   b. agglutinate:

4. What must be done before any individual can receive a transfusion?

5. What is the difference between a typing and a crossmatch?

6. What is an antibody screen? Why is it done?

7. When does the problem of an Rh incompatibility occur in a pregnant woman?

8. Enter the blood type and Rh status in the last column. (If agglutination occurs with a specific serum, the reaction is shown as positive. If agglutination does not occur, the reaction is shown as negative.)

Anti-A serum	Anti-B serum	Anti-Rh or Anti-D serum	Type
positive	positive	positive	a.
negative	negative	positive	b.
positive	negative	negative	c.
negative	positive	positive	d.

UNIT 18:8 Evaluation Sheet

Name _____ Date _____

Evaluated by _____

DIRECTIONS: Practice typing blood according to the criteria listed. When you are ready for your final check, give this sheet to your instructor.

PROFICIENT

Testing for Blood Types	Points Possible	Peer Check Yes	No	Final Check* Yes	No	Points Earned**	Comments
1. Assembles equipment and supplies	3						
2. Washes hands and puts on gloves	3						
3. Cleans and marks slides	3						
4. Turns on view box	3						
5. Introduces self, identifies patient, and explains procedure	3						
6. Performs finger puncture	3						
7. Puts lancet in sharps container	3						
8. Wipes off first drop of blood	3						
9. Puts blood on slides without touching finger to slide:	3						
Puts two drops on AB slide	3						
Puts third drop on Rh slide	3						
10. When sufficient blood is obtained, instructs patient to hold gauze against puncture	4						
11. Adds anti-A serum to first drop of blood by label "A"	4						
Mixes immediately	4						
12. Adds anti-B serum to second drop of blood by label "B"	4						
Mixes immediately	4						
13. Adds anti-Rh serum to third drop of blood on second slide marked Rh:	4						
Mixes immediately	4						
Places slide on Rh viewbox	4						
14. Rocks AB slide gently for 1–2 minutes	4						
15. Reads AB test correctly	6						
16. Reads Rh test correctly at end of 2 minutes:	6						
17. Records blood type accurately	6						
18. Checks patient to make sure puncture site has stopped bleeding	4						
19. Cleans and replaces all equipment:							
Places contaminated disposables in infectious waste bag	3						
Wipes contaminated areas with a disinfectant	3						
20. Removes gloves and washes hands	3						
Totals	100						

* Final Check: Instructor or authorized person evaluates.
** Points Earned: Points possible times each "yes" check.

UNIT 18:9 PERFORMING AN ERYTHROCYTE SEDIMENTATION RATE

ASSIGNMENT SHEET

Grade _____ Name _____

INTRODUCTION: In many health fields, you may perform an ESR. This sheet will help you review the main facts.

INSTRUCTIONS: Read the information on Performing an Erythrocyte Sedimentation Rate. In the space provided, print the word(s) that best completes the statement or answers the question.

1. What does an erythrocyte sedimentation rate (ESR) measure?

2. What is added to venous blood before an ESR is done? Why is it added?

3. What is the purpose of the special rack used for an ESR?

4. List two (2) time intervals that can be used to measure the sedimentation rate.

5. Give the normal ESR values for the following.

   Adult female:

   Adult male:

6. List five (5) conditions that might show an increased sedimentation rate.

7. Name four (4) medical conditions that can cause a decreased or lower sedimentation rate.

UNIT 18:9 Evaluation Sheet

Name _____ Date _____

Evaluated by _____

DIRECTIONS: Practice performing an erythrocyte sedimentation rate according to the criteria listed. When you are ready for your final check, give this sheet to your instructor.

Performing an Erythrocyte Sedimentation Rate	Points Possible	Peer Check		Final Check*		Points Earned**	Comments
		Yes	No	Yes	No		
1. Assembles equipment and supplies	4						
2. Washes hands and puts on gloves	4						
3. Levels rack	7						
4. Uses anticoagulated blood at room temperature	7						
5. Inverts blood tube 3–5 minutes	7						
6. Places tube in rack with correct alignment	7						
7. Transfers blood to sed tube with pipette	7						
8. Fills sed tube to correct level	7						
9. Avoids air bubbles in sed tube	7						
10. Rechecks level of rack	7						
11. Obtains readings at 15 or 20 minute time intervals with final reading at 60 minutes	8						
12. Reads test to ±1 mm	8						
13. Records correctly	8						
14. Cleans and replaces all equipment:							
Places contaminated disposables in infectious waste bag	4						
Wipes contaminated areas with a disinfectant	4						
15. Removes gloves and washes hands	4						
Totals	100						

* Final Check: Instructor or authorized person evaluates.
** Points Earned: Points possible times each "yes" check.

UNIT 18:10 MEASURING BLOOD-SUGAR (GLUCOSE) LEVEL

ASSIGNMENT SHEET

Grade _____ Name _____

INTRODUCTION: In many different health fields, you may be required to measure the blood sugar (glucose) level. This sheet will help you review the main facts regarding this procedure.

INSTRUCTIONS: Read the information on Measuring Blood-Sugar (Glucose) Level. In the space provided, print the word(s) that best completes the statement or answers the question.

1. The form of sugar that is found in the blood stream is called _____. In diabetes mellitus there is an insufficient amount of _____ to metabolize glucose. Because of this, excess amounts of glucose build up in the _____ and are filtered out by the _____ and eliminated from the body in the _____.

2. Define the following words.

   hyperglycemia:

   glycosuria:

   hypoglycemia:

3. Briefly describe the method for doing a fasting blood sugar (FBS) test.

4. What is the normal fasting blood sugar level?

5. List four (4) advantages to checking blood glucose levels instead of checking glucose levels in the urine.

6. What are reagent strips?

   What happens when glucose in the blood reacts with chemicals on the reagent strip?

7. List two (2) ways the amount of glucose in the blood can be determined using reagent strips.

8. Why is it important to store reagent strips properly?

9. Where should reagent strips be stored?

10. List two (2) reasons why it is important to avoid touching the chemical reagent pad on the strip.

11. Why is it important to read instructions carefully before using reagent strips?

12. How should glucometers be cleaned?

U N I T 18 : 10   E v a l u a t i o n   S h e e t

Name _____   Date _____

Evaluated by _____

DIRECTIONS: Practice measuring a blood-sugar (glucose) level according to the criteria listed. When you are ready for your final check, give this sheet to your instructor.

PROFICIENT

Measuring Blood-Sugar (Glucose) Level	Points Possible	Peer Check Yes	No	Final Check* Yes	No	Points Earned**	Comments
1. Assembles equipment and supplies	3						
2. Washes hands and puts on gloves	4						
3. Calibrates glucometer accurately	5						
4. Introduces self, identifies patient, and explains procedure	4						
5. Performs finger puncture	5						
6. Puts lancet in sharps container	5						
7. Wipes off first drop of blood	5						
8. Presses start button on glucometer or notes time blood placed on strip	5						
9. Places large drop of blood on reagent strip pad without touching the skin to the pad	6						
10. When sufficient blood is obtained, instructs patient to hold gauze against skin puncture	6						
11. Waits correct amount of time	6						
12. If necessary, blots strip correctly	6						
13. Inserts strip into meter correctly or matches strip to color chart	6						
14. Reads test correctly	7						
15. Records glucose level accurately	7						
16. Checks patient to be sure bleeding has stopped	5						
17. Cleans and replaces all equipment:							
Places contaminated disposables in infectious waste bag	3						
Wipes contaminated areas with a disinfectant	3						
18. Removes gloves and washes hands	4						
19. Reports abnormal readings immediately	5						
Totals	100						

* Final Check: Instructor or authorized person evaluates.
** Points Earned: Points possible times each "yes" check.

355

UNIT 18:11 TESTING URINE

ASSIGNMENT SHEET

Grade _____   Name _____

INTRODUCTION: This sheet will help you review the basic facts about the urine before you learn to perform urine tests.

INSTRUCTIONS: Study the information and chart on Testing Urine. Then place the word(s) that best completes the statement or answers the question in the spaces provided.

1. The normal amount daily for urine is _____ cc.

   An increased amount of urine is called _____.

   A decreased amount of urine is called_____.

   No formation of urine is called   _____.

2. The normal color for urine is   _____.

   A pale color of urine indicates _____.

   Clear red urine can mean _____.

   Cloudy red urine indicates_____.

   Yellow or beer brown indicates   _____.

3. What is the normal transparency of urine?

   List three (3) causes of cloudy urine.

4. The normal odor or smell of urine is   _____.

   An ammonia smell or odor indicates _____.

   A fruity or sweet smell indicates _____.

   A foul or putrid smell indicates   _____.

5. The normal pH of urine is _____.

6. What is the normal range for specific gravity of urine?

   List three (3) causes for a high specific gravity.

   List three (3) causes for a low specific gravity.

7. List eight (8) substances that are not normally present in urine. Then briefly list what their presence can indicate.

   a.

   b.

   c.

   d.

   e.

   f.

   g.

   h.

8. Identify the three (3) main areas of testing for a urinalysis.

9. List four (4) points that should be observed and recorded during the physical examination of urine.

10. List six (6) substances that are checked during a chemical testing of urine.

11. Why is urine centrifuged for a microscopic examination?

12. When should a urine specimen be examined for best results?

UNIT 18:12 USING REAGENT STRIPS TO TEST URINE

ASSIGNMENT SHEET

Grade _____ Name _____

INTRODUCTION: Many different types of reagent strips may be used to test the urine. This assignment will help you review the main facts regarding this urine test.

INSTRUCTIONS: Read the information on Using Reagent Strips to Test Urine. In the space provided, print the word(s) that best completes the statement or answers the question.

1. How does the body eliminate excess or abnormal amounts of chemicals?

2. What are urine reagent strips?

3. How are reagent strips used to check for the presence of chemicals in the urine?

4. List three (3) rules for correct storage of urine reagent strips.

5. List two (2) reasons why it is important to avoid skin contact with the chemical reactant pads on the strip?

6. Why is it important to read the expiration date printed on the bottle of reagent strips?

   Should the strips be used after the expiration date? Why or why not?

7. Identify three (3) factors that can change the pH of urine.

8. If the following substances or chemicals are present in the urine, what disease(s) could be present?

   a. protein:

   b. glucose:

   c. ketones (acetones):

   d. blood:

   e. bilirubin:

   f. urobilinogen:

9. Some different chemicals or substances are listed below. List at least three (3) different reagent strips that could be used to test for the presence of each substance.

   a. pH:

   b. glucose:

   c. protein:

   d. ketones:

   e. blood:

10. Identify two (2) reasons why it is important to read the instructions before using any reagent strips.

11. What type of urine specimen should be used for testing urine with reagent strips?

12. When should urine be tested? Why?

UNIT 18:12 Evaluation Sheet

Name _____ Date _____

Evaluated by _____

DIRECTIONS: Practice using reagent strips to test urine according to the criteria listed. When you are ready for your final check, give this sheet to your instructor.

PROFICIENT

Using Reagent Strips to Test Urine	Points Possible	Peer Check		Final Check*		Points Earned**	Comments
		Yes	No	Yes	No		
1. Assembles equipment and supplies	3						
2. Washes hands and puts on gloves	3						
3. Introduces self, identifies patient, and explains procedure	3						
4. Obtains fresh urine specimen	5						
5. Mixes urine well by gently rotating container	5						
6. Holds reagent strip by clear end	5						
7. Immerses strip with reagent areas in urine	5						
8. Removes strip from urine immediately	5						
9. Taps strip to remove excess urine	5						
10. Holds strip horizontally so reagent areas are facing upward	5						
11. Notes the time in seconds	5						
12. Starts reading at center of strip	5						
13. Reads all reagent areas that require an immediate reading	7						
14. Records readings correctly	7						
15. Reads remaining reagent areas at correct time intervals	7						
16. Records all readings correctly	7						
17. Rechecks readings as necessary	4						
18. Cleans and replaces all equipment:							
Discards urine correctly	2						
Discards strip and contaminated disposables in infectious waste bag	2						
Wipes contaminated areas with a disinfectant	2						
19. Removes gloves and washes hands	3						
20. Reports abnormal readings immediately	5						
Totals	100						

* Final Check: Instructor or authorized person evaluates.
** Points Earned: Points possible times each "yes" check.

UNIT 18:13 MEASURING SPECIFIC GRAVITY

ASSIGNMENT SHEET

Grade _____ Name _____

INTRODUCTION: This sheet will prepare you for measuring and recording the specific gravity of urine.

INSTRUCTIONS: Read the information on Measuring Specific Gravity to complete the questions on this paper.

1. What is specific gravity?

2. What is the normal range for specific gravity of urine?

3. What are three (3) reasons or causes of a low specific gravity in urine?

4. What are three (3) reasons or causes of a high specific gravity in urine?

5. Carefully study the following sketch of a urinometer. Look at the line of each meniscus. Enter the correct specific gravity in the space provided to the right of the sketch. The first reading has been entered as an example.

URINOMETER

		Readings
a.	1,000	a. ___1.001___
b.		b. _____
c.		
d.	10	c. _____
e.		d. _____
f.	20	e _____
g.		f. _____
h.		g. _____
i.	30	h. _____
j.	40	i. _____
		j. _____

6. When specific gravity is measured with a refractometer, _____ of well-mixed urine is placed on the refractometer. Specific gravity is read by looking through the _____ or _____.

Name _____ Date _____

Evaluated by _____

DIRECTIONS: Practice measuring specific gravity according to the criteria listed. When you are ready for your final check, give this sheet to your instructor.

PROFICIENT

Measuring Specific Gravity	Points Possible	Peer Check Yes	No	Final Check* Yes	No	Points Earned**	Comments
1. Assembles equipment and supplies	3						
2. Washes hands and puts on gloves	4						
3. Introduces self, identifies patient, and explains procedure	4						
4. Obtains fresh urine specimen	5						
5. Mixes urine well	5						
6. Checks specific gravity with a urinometer:							
Cleans and dries float and jar/cylinder	4						
Pours urine into jar/cylinder to within 1 inch from top	4						
Removes bubbles with paper towel or gauze	4						
Inserts urinometer float by grasping at top and twirling slightly	4						
Checks that float is away from sides and bottom	4						
Reads float at eye level when spinning stops	4						
Reads correctly to ±.001	6						
7. Checks specific gravity with a refractometer:							
Checks refractometer with distilled water	4						
Dries and cleans glass plate with lens paper	4						
Places 1 drop of urine on glass plate	4						
Closes lid gently	4						
Looks through ocular/eyepiece	4						
Reads scale correctly	6						
8. Records reading correctly	6						
9. Rechecks reading if necessary	3						
10. Cleans and replaces all equipment:							
Discards urine correctly	2						
Washes and disinfects urinometer jar and float	2						
Cleans and disinfects refractometer glass with lens paper	2						
Places contaminated disposables in infectious waste bag	2						
Wipes contaminated areas with a disinfectant	2						
11. Removes gloves and washes hands	4						
Totals	100						

* Final Check: Instructor or authorized person evaluates.
** Points Earned: Points possible times each "yes" check.

UNIT 18:14 PREPARING URINE FOR MICROSCOPIC EXAMINATION

ASSIGNMENT SHEET

Grade _____ Name _____

INTRODUCTION: This assignment will help you review the main facts regarding preparing urine for a microscopic examination.

INSTRUCTIONS: Review the information on Preparing Urine for Microscopic Examination. Print the word(s) that best completes the statement or answers the question.

1. Why is a microscopic examination of the urine done?

2. What type of urine specimen is preferred for this test?

   Why is this type of specimen preferred?

3. Why is it important to examine the urine immediately?

4. How can the urine be preserved if it cannot be examined immediately?

5. What does the centrifuge do to the urine specimen?

6. What is the solid material in the bottom of the centrifuge tube called?

7. The size of the drop of urine examined under the microscope is important. If it is too large, what may happen?

   If it is too small, what may happen?

8. Why is it important to examine the urinary sediment immediately after it is placed on the slide?

9. "1pf" stands for _____ and "hpf" stands for _____.

10. What should you do if you are not able to identify elements present in the urine?

Name _____ Date _____

Evaluated by _____

DIRECTIONS: Practice preparing urine for microscopic examination according to the criteria listed. When you are ready for your final check, give this sheet to your instructor.

Preparing Urine for Microscopic Examination	Points Possible	Peer Check		Final Check*		Points Earned**	Comments
		Yes	No	Yes	No		
1. Assembles equipment and supplies	4						
2. Washes hands and puts on gloves	4						
3. Introduces self, identifies patient, and explains procedure	4						
4. Obtains early morning first voided specimen	6						
5. Mixes urine well	6						
6. Pours 10 mL in cup	6						
7. Pours measured urine into clean, dry centrifuge tube	6						
8. Centrifuges 4–5 minutes	6						
9. Pours off 9 mL of clear urine slowly	6						
10. Gently shakes tube to suspend sediment	8						
11. Transfers 1 drop of sediment to clean glass slide	8						
12. Applies cover slip:							
Holds at angle	4						
Drops gently	4						
Avoids air bubbles	4						
13. Focuses slide under microscope	6						
14. Identifies 3 different substances on slide	8						
15. Cleans and replaces all equipment:							
Discards urine correctly	2						
Places contaminated disposables in infectious waste bag	2						
Wipes contaminated areas with a disinfectant	2						
16. Removes gloves and washes hands	4						
Totals	100						

* Final Check: Instructor or authorized person evaluates.
** Points Earned: Points possible times each "yes" check.

UNIT 19:1 MEASURING/RECORDING HEIGHT AND WEIGHT

ASSIGNMENT SHEET

Grade _____ Name _____

INTRODUCTION: To record height-weight measurements correctly, you must read all scales accurately. In addition, you must be able to convert inches into feet and ounces into pounds. This sheet will help you master these skills.

INSTRUCTIONS: Put your name on this paper. Read each section carefully before doing any of the work.

1. Some diagrams of the adult weight scale follow. Read the scales correctly. Place your answers in the space provided. A sample answer is provided in each case.

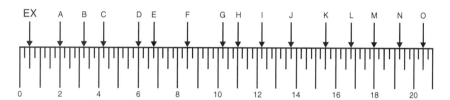

NOTE: This is the top scale. It goes from 0 to 50 pounds. Each small line represents 1/4 pound. The scale is read 1/4, 1/2, 3/4, 1, etc. Each long line represents 1 pound (1 lb).

Example: The first arrow is pointing to the second small line. This would be read as 1/2 pound (1/2 lb).

Place a ruler or straightedge to the right of each arrow to determine what line the arrow is pointing to. Then read the scale and record your readings.

A.	F.	K.
B.	G.	L.
C.	H.	M.
D.	I.	N.
E.	J.	O.

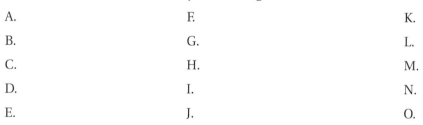

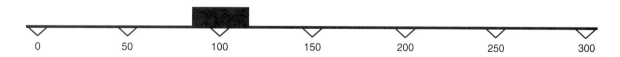

NOTE: The second diagram represents the lower scale on the adult beam-balance scale. For a patient who weighs more than 50 pounds, the lower scale is used first. It is adjusted in 50-pound amounts. The sample drawn is set at 100 pounds. A patient would weigh 100 pounds plus the amount shown on the top scale. Therefore, in the preceding example, the patient would show a weight of 100 pounds on the lower scale plus 1/2 pound on the upper scale. The total weight would be 100 and 1/2 (100 1/2 or 100.5 lb).

2. Re-read problems A–E as though the lower weight scale was set at 50 pounds. This means you must add 50 pounds to each of the original weights.

A.   C.   E.

B.   D.

Re-read problems F–J as though the lower weight scale was set at 200 pounds.

F.   H.   J.

G.   I.

Re-read problems K–O as though the lower weight scale was set at 250 pounds.

K.   M.   O.

L.   N.

3. The following illustration represents the height beam on the adult scale. Each small line represents 1/4 inch. Each long line represents 1 inch. From the bottom to the break, readings are taken in an upward direction. If a patient is taller than 50 inches, readings are taken in a downward direction and recorded directly at the break in the scale.

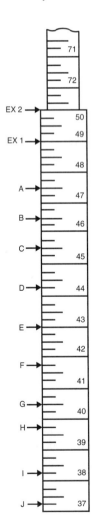

Example 1:   The arrow is pointing to the long line marked 49 inches; the patient is 49 inches tall (49 in).

Example 2:   The arrow is at the break; the patient is over 50 inches tall. Readings are taken downward to the break, which is 3 marks below the 72 mark. Therefore, the height is 72 and 3/4 inches (72 3/4 in).

Read the readings by the arrows. Record:

A.   E.   H.

B.   F.   I.

C.   G.   J.

D.

The following readings are at the break. Read and record.

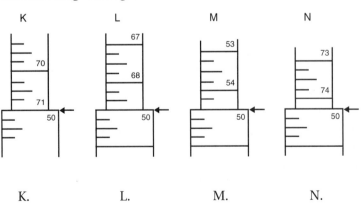

K.   L.   M.   N.

4. Height for an adult is recorded in feet and inches. Therefore, inches must be converted. An example follows:

Example 1:   Measurement is recorded as 52 inches.

Divide this by 12 (12 inches = 1 foot).

$$12\overline{)52} \quad = \quad 12\overline{)\,52}^{\,4} \qquad = \qquad 4 \text{ ft } 4 \text{ in}$$
$$\underline{-48}$$
$$4$$

Example 2: Measurement is recorded as 62 and 1/2 inches.

$$12\overline{)62\,{}^{1}\!/_{2}} \quad = \quad 12\overline{)\,62\,{}^{1}\!/_{2}}^{\,5} \qquad = \qquad 5 \text{ ft } 2\,{}^{1}\!/_{2} \text{ in}$$
$$\underline{-60}$$
$$2\,{}^{1}\!/_{2}$$

Follow the preceding examples to convert inches to feet and inches. Work out the problems and show how you got your answers. Circle your final answer if necessary.

A. 48 inches equals _____

B. 54 inches equals _____

C. 39 inches equals _____

D. 58 inches equals _____

E. 62 inches equals _____

F   68 inches equals _____

G. 74 inches equals _____

H. 30 inches equals _____

I.   18 inches equals _____

J.   78 inches equals _____

K. 42 1/2 inches equals _____

L. 54 1/4 inches equals _____

M. 61 3/4 inches equals _____

N. 55 1/4 inches equals _____

O. 73 1/2 inches equals _____

5. A tape measure is used to record infant height. It is read like a ruler. Each small line is 1/8 inch; the readings are 1/8, 2/8 (1/4), 3/8, 4/8 (1/2), 5/8, 6/8 (3/4), 7/8, and 8/8 (1).

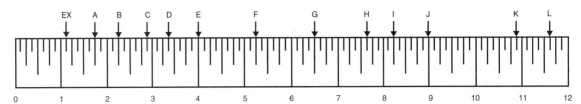

Example: The arrow is pointing to the first line past 1 inch. The reading is 1 1/8 inches (1 1/8 in). Read and record. Use a ruler or straightedge to note the line the arrow is pointing to.

A.	D.	G.	J.
B.	E.	H.	K.
C.	F.	I.	L.

6. The infant scale is read in one ounce increments. Each short line represents 1 ounce. Each long line is 1 pound.

NOTE: There are 16 ounces per pound.

The following sample scale is commonly used to weigh infants.

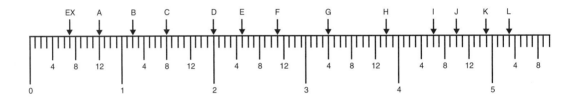

Example: The arrow points to the 7th line; it is read as 7 ounces (7 oz).

Read the other lines the arrows are pointing to. Record your answers after the letters that follow.

A.	D.	G.	J.
B.	E.	H.	K.
C.	F.	I.	L.

7. At times, infant weight is recorded in pounds and ounces. For example: 3 pounds 6 ounces (3 lb 6 oz)

At other times, the weight is recorded in pounds and fractions of pounds.

For example: 3 1/2 pounds (3 1/2 lb)

To convert the ounces to pounds, divide by 16.

Example 1: 8 ounces converted to fractions of a pound

$$8/16 = \frac{8/8}{16/8} = 1/2$$

Example 2: 3 pounds 4 ounces converted to pounds

$$4/16 = \frac{4/4}{16/4} = 1/4$$

Thus 3 1/4 pounds

NOTE: Only the ounces are converted. The pound number remains unchanged.

Use the previous examples to convert the following to fractions of a pound. Show your work. Circle your final answer.

A. 2 ounces equals _____

B. 4 ounces equals _____

C. 6 ounces equals _____

D. 8 ounces equals _____

E. 10 ounces equals_____

F. 12 ounces equals_____

G. 14 ounces equals_____

H. 16 ounces equals_____

I. 2 pounds 4 ounces equals_____

J. 6 pounds 8 ounces equals_____

K. 8 pounds 3 ounces equals_____

L. 10 pounds 7 ounces equals _____

M. 12 pounds 12 ounces equals_____

N. 11 pounds 15 ounces equals_____

O. 15 pounds 10 ounces equals_____

U N I T 19 : 1 A   E v a l u a t i o n   S h e e t

Name _____   Date _____

Evaluated by _____

DIRECTIONS: Practice measuring height and weight according to the criteria listed. When you are ready for your final check, give this sheet to your instructor.

PROFICIENT

Measuring/Recording Height and Weight	Points Possible	Peer Check Yes	No	Final Check* Yes	No	Points Earned**	Comments
1. Assembles equipment and supplies	3						
2. Washes hands	3						
3. Places paper towel on foot platform of scale	3						
4. Balances scale at zero	3						
5. Introduces self, identifies patient, and explains procedure	3						
6. Tells patient to remove shoes, jackets, heavy outer clothing, purses, and heavy objects in pocket	3						
7. Positions patient on scale:							
Assists as needed	2						
Positions in center of platform	2						
Positions feet slightly apart	2						
Checks that patient is standing unassisted	2						
8. Balances scale correctly	4						
9. Reads weight accurately	6						
10. Records weight correctly	6						
11. Assists patient off of scale	4						
12. Raises height bar	4						
13. Assists patient back onto scale with back toward scale	4						
14. Asks patient to stand as erect as possible	4						
15. Moves measuring bar without hitting patient	4						
16. Positions bar correctly	4						
17. Accurately reads measurement in inches	6						
18. Assists patient off scale after elevating height bar	4						
19. Converts height measurement to feet and inches	6						
20. Records height correctly	6						
21. Replaces all equipment	3						
22. Returns weight beams to zero	3						
23. Lowers measurement bar	3						
24. Washes hands	3						
Totals	100						

* Final Check: Instructor or authorized person evaluates.
** Points Earned: Points possible times each "yes" check.

UNIT 19:1B Evaluation Sheet

Name _____ Date _____

Evaluated by _____

DIRECTIONS: Practice measuring an infant's height and weight according to the criteria listed. When you are ready for your final check, give this sheet to your instructor.

Measuring/Recording Height and Weight of an Infant	Points Possible	Peer Check		Final Check*		Points Earned**	Comments
		Yes	No	Yes	No		
1. Assembles equipment and supplies	3						
2. Washes hands	3						
3. Prepares scale:							
Covers with tissue paper	3						
Balances at zero	3						
4. Introduces self, identifies infant, and explains procedure to parent	4						
5. Asks parent to undress infant	4						
6. Picks up infant correctly	5						
7. Places infant on scale	4						
8. Keeps hand by infant at all times	5						
9. Balances weight beams	5						
10. Reads scale correctly	5						
11. Records weight correctly	5						
12. Places infant on flat surface	4						
13. Measures height:							
Uses tape measure	3						
Places zero mark at infant's head	3						
Places other end of tape by infant's heel	3						
Keeps tape positioned in straight line	3						
Watches infant closely	3						
14. Reads height correctly	5						
15. Records height correctly	5						
16. Measures head circumference:							
Holds zero mark of tape against infant's forehead just above the eyes	2						
Brings tape around infant's head, above ears, and back to forehead	2						
Pulls tape snug, but not too tight	2						
Reads head circumference correctly	2						
Records head circumference correctly	2						
17. Returns infant to crib or parent	3						
18. Cleans and replaces all equipment and disinfects scale	2						
19. Sets scale weights at zero	2						
20. Folds up tape measure	2						
21. Washes hands	3						
Totals	100						

* Final Check: Instructor or authorized person evaluates.

** Points Earned: Points possible times each "yes" check.

UNIT 19:2 POSITIONING A PATIENT

ASSIGNMENT SHEET

Grade _____   Name _____

INTRODUCTION: To position patients correctly for various procedures, you must know the different positions and their uses. This sheet will help you review the facts.

INSTRUCTIONS: Review the information on Positioning a Patient. Then, read each fact in column A. Determine what position listed in column B applies to the fact. Enter the appropriate letter or letters before the fact. Letters may be used once, more than once, or not at all.

Column A	Column B
_____ 1. Used to examine the breasts and abdomen	A. Dorsal Recumbent
_____ 2. Used for enemas and rectal temperatures	B. Fowler's
_____ 3. Used for sigmoidoscopic examinations	C. Horizontal Recumbent
_____ 4. Used for rectal surgery	D. Jackknife
_____ 5. Used for breathing problems	E. Knee-chest
_____ 6. Head elevated at 25, 45, or 90 degrees	F. Lithotomy
_____ 7. Patient lying flat on abdomen	G. Prone
_____ 8. Patient lying on left side	H. Sims'
_____ 9. Used for pap tests or vaginal examinations	I. Trendelenburg
_____ 10. Used for pelvic surgery	
_____ 11. Used for circulatory shock	
_____ 12. Used to examine the back and spine	
_____ 13. Also called supine position	
_____ 14. Patient lying flat on back	
_____ 15. Used to encourage drainage	
_____ 16. Feet elevated in stirrups	
_____ 17. Also called left lateral position	
_____ 18. Patient rests body weight on knees and chest	
_____ 19. Used for rectal examinations and treatments	
_____ 20. Used to examine the chest	

21. How can you learn how to operate an examination table before positioning a patient?

22. List two (2) ways to avoid exposing a patient during any examination or procedure.

372

UNIT 19:2 Evaluation Sheet

Name _____ Date _____

Evaluated by _____

DIRECTIONS: Practice positioning a patient according to the criteria listed. When you are ready for your final check, give this sheet to your instructor.

PROFICIENT

Positioning a Patient	Points Possible	Peer Check Yes	No	Final Check* Yes	No	Points Earned**	Comments
Horizontal Recumbent							
1. Assembles equipment and supplies	4						
2. Washes hands	4						
3. Introduces self, identifies patient, and explains procedure	5						
4. Asks patient to put on gown and to empty bladder	5						
5. Assists patient onto table	5						
6. Lies patient flat on back	10						
7. Positions arms at side	10						
8. Positions legs flat and slightly separated	10						
9. Uses small pillow for head	10						
10. Drapes with 1 sheet/drape	10						
11. Allows sheet/drape to hang loose	10						
12. Assists patient off of table correctly	5						
13. Cleans and replaces all equipment	4						
14. Washes hands	4						
15. Records required information	4						
Totals	100						
Prone							
1. Assembles equipment and supplies	4						
2. Washes hands	4						
3. Introduces self, identifies patient, and explains procedure	5						
4. Asks patient to put on gown and to empty bladder	5						
5. Assists patient onto table	5						
6. Turns patient towards self	10						
7. Positions patient on abdomen	10						
8. Positions head to side on small pillow	10						
9. Flexes arms by head	10						
10. Drapes with one large sheet/drape	10						
11. Allows drape/sheet to hang loose	10						
12. Assists patient off of table correctly	5						
13. Cleans and replaces all equipment	4			.			
14. Washes hands	4						
15. Records required information	4						
Totals	100						

* Final Check: Instructor or authorized person evaluates.
** Points Earned: Points possible times each "yes" check.

Positioning a Patient	Points Possible	Peer Check		Final Check*		Points Earned**	Comments
		Yes	No	Yes	No		
Sims'or Left Lateral							
1. Assembles equipment and supplies	4						
2. Washes hands	4						
3. Introduces self, identifies patient, and explains procedure	5						
4. Asks patient to put on gown and to empty bladder	5						
5. Assists patient onto table	5						
6. Turns patient on left side	8						
7. Positions left arm behind back	8						
8. Turns head to side on small pillow	8						
9. Flexes left leg slightly	8						
10. Flexes right leg to abdomen	8						
11. Positions right arm bent at elbow in front of body	8						
12. Drapes correctly with 1 or 2 sheets/drapes	6						
13. Allows drape to hang loose	6						
14. Assists patient off of table correctly	5						
15. Cleans and replaces all equipment	4						
16. Washes hands	4						
17. Records required information	4						
Totals	100						
Knee-Chest							
1. Assembles equipment and supplies	4						
2. Washes hands	4						
3. Introduces self, identifies patient, and explains procedure	4						
4. Asks patient to put on gown and to empty bladder	4						
5. Assists patient onto table	5						
6. Turns patient to prone position	8						
7. Supports weight on knees and chest	9						
8. Positions thighs at right angles to table	9						
9. Flexes arms by head	8						
10. Rests head on small pillow	8						
11. Drapes with 1 or 2 sheets or drapes correctly	6						
12. Allows drape to hang loose	6						
13. Remains with patient at all times	8						
14. Assists patient off of table correctly	5						
15. Cleans and replaces all equipment	4						
16. Washes hands	4						
17. Records required information	4						
Totals	100						

* Final Check: Instructor or authorized person evaluates.
** Points Earned: Points possible times each "yes" check.

19:2 (cont.)

Positioning a Patient	Points Possible	Peer Check		Final Check*		Points Earned**	Comments
		Yes	No	Yes	No		
Fowler's Positions							
1. Assembles equipment and supplies	4						
2. Washes hands	4						
3. Introduces self, identifies patient, and explains procedure	4						
4. Asks patient to put on gown and to empty bladder	4						
5. Assists patient onto table	4						
6. Positions patient on back	8						
7. Places small pillow under head	8						
8. Elevates head and back 25° for low-Fowler's	8						
9. Elevates head and back 45° for semi-Fowler's	8						
10. Elevates head and back 90° for high-Fowler's	8						
11. Flexes knees slightly and supports with pillow	8						
12. Drapes correctly with 1 large sheet/drape	8						
13. Allows sheet/drape to hang loose	8						
14. Assists patient off of table correctly	4						
15. Cleans and replaces all equipment	4						
16. Washes hands	4						
17. Records required information	4						
Totals	100						
Lithotomy							
1. Assembles equipment and supplies	4						
2. Washes hands	4						
3. Introduces self, identifies patient, and explains procedure	4						
4. Asks patient to put on gown and to empty bladder	4						
5. Assists patient onto table	4						
6. Positions patient on back	7						
7. Positions arms at sides	7						
8. Positions buttocks at end of table	7						
9. Places pillow under head	7						
10. Flexes and separates knees	7						
11. Places feet in stirrups	7						
12. Uses diamond shaped draping procedure	7						
13. Pushes in extension or drops lower end of table	7						
14. Pulls out extension or raises end of table and removes patient from position correctly	7						
15. Assists patient off of table correctly	5						
16. Cleans and replaces all equipment	4						
17. Washes hands	4						
18. Records required information	4						
Totals	100						

* Final Check: Instructor or authorized person evaluates.
** Points Earned: Points possible times each "yes" check.

Positioning a Patient	Points Possible	Peer Check Yes	No	Final Check* Yes	No	Points Earned**	Comments
Trendelenburg							
1. Assembles equipment and supplies	4						
2. Washes hands	4						
3. Introduces self, identifies patient, and explains procedure	5						
4. Asks patient to put on gown and to empty bladder	5						
5. Assists patient onto table	5						
6. Positions patient on back	10						
7. Inclines table/bed so head is lower than rest of body	10						
8. Inclines legs downward for surgical trendelenburg	10						
9. Drapes correctly with 1 or 2 sheets/drape or surgical sheet with hole	10						
10. Uses straps to secure patient	10						
11. Remains with patient at all times	10						
12. Assists patient off of table correctly	5						
13. Cleans and replaces all equipment	4						
14. Washes hands	4						
15. Records required information	4						
Totals	100						
Jackknife							
1. Assembles equipment and supplies	4						
2. Washes hands	4						
3. Introduces self, identifies patient, and explains procedure	5						
4. Asks patient to put on gown and to empty bladder	5						
5. Assists patient onto table	5						
6. Positions patient in prone position	10						
7. Secures safety straps	10						
8. Inclines table so head and upper body are down	10						
9. Inclines opposite end of table so legs down	10						
10. Drapes correctly with 1 or 2 sheets/drapes or surgical sheet with hole	10						
11. Remains with patient at all times	10						
12. Assists patient off of table correctly	5						
13. Cleans and replaces all equipment	4						
14. Washes hands	4						
15. Records required information	4						
Totals	100						

* Final Check: Instructor or authorized person evaluates.
** Points Earned: Points possible times each "yes" check.

UNIT 19:3 SCREENING FOR VISION PROBLEMS

ASSIGNMENT SHEET

Grade _____ Name _____

INTRODUCTION: As an assistant, you may be required to screen vision with a Snellen chart. This assignment will help you review the main facts.

INSTRUCTIONS: Review the information on Screening for Vision Problems. In the space provided, print the word(s) that best completes the statement or answers the question.

1. Name three (3) types of Snellen charts.

2. Characters on the Snellen chart have specific _____, which progress from small to large figures. A patient with normal vision should be able to see figures _____ millimeters high while standing _____ feet from the chart.

3. When referring to 20/20 vision, what does the top number represent?

4. When referring to 20/20 vision, what does the bottom number represent?

5. If a patient has 20/50 vision, this means that the patient can see figures _____ millimeters high while standing _____ feet from the chart. A person with normal vision could see the same figures while standing _____ feet from the chart.

6. What vision defect is tested with the Snellen chart?

7. What test is used for defects in color vision?

   How is this test done?

8. List the meaning of the following abbreviations.

   OD

   OS

   OU

9. What is myopia?

10. What is hyperopia?

Name _____ Date _____

Evaluated by _____

DIRECTIONS: Practice screening vision according to the criteria listed. When you are ready for your final check, give this sheet to your instructor.

Screening for Vision Problems	Points Possible	Peer Check Yes	Peer Check No	Final Check* Yes	Final Check* No	Points Earned**	Comments
PROFICIENT							
1. Assembles equipment and supplies	3						
2. Positions Snellen chart	4						
3. Places tape 20 feet from chart	5						
4. Washes hands	3						
5. Introduces self, identifies patient, and explains procedure	4						
6. Tells patient to stand with toes on tape line	5						
7. Screens both eyes:							
Points to figures without blocking them	5						
Points to large figures first	5						
Selects figures at random	5						
Checks patient for squinting or leaning forward	5						
Records correct reading	5						
8. Screens right eye:							
Instructs patient on covering left eye	5						
Selects figures at random	5						
Checks patient for squinting or leaning forward	5						
Records correct reading	5						
9. Screens left eye:							
Instructs patient to cover right eye	5						
Selects figures at random	5						
Checks patient for squinting or leaning forward	5						
Records correct reading	5						
10. Dismisses patient when test complete	4						
11. Cleans and replaces all equipment and disinfects eye shield if not disposable	3						
12. Washes hands	4						
Totals	100						

* Final Check: Instructor or authorized person evaluates.
** Points Earned: Points possible times each "yes" check.

UNIT 19:4 ASSISTING WITH PHYSICAL EXAMINATIONS

ASSIGNMENT SHEET

Grade _____ Name _____

INTRODUCTION: Assisting with examinations will be part of the medical assistant's responsibilities. This sheet will help you review some of the key points of this procedure.

INSTRUCTIONS: Read the information on Assisting with Physical Examinations. In the space provided, print the word(s) that best completes the statement or answers the question.

1. Name the main areas examined in each of the following examinations.
    a. EENT:
    b. gyn:
    c. general physical:

2. Why is a Papanicolaou test performed?

3. dentify the following techniques used during a physical examination.
    a. Physician uses hands and fingers to feel various parts of the body:
    b. Physician uses fingers to tap various body parts and listen to sounds emitted:
    c. Physician looks at patient closely:
    d. Physician uses stethoscope to listen to sounds produced by body organs:

4. Why is it important for the patient to void (urinate) before a physical examination?

5. List four (4) tests that may be performed before the physical examination is done.

6. List the use of each of the following pieces of equipment.
    a. ophthalmoscope
    b. otoscope
    c. tonometer
    d. laryngeal mirror
    e. percussion hammer
    f. Ayer blade
    g. rectal speculum
    h. sigmoidoscope

7. Why is it important to explain all procedures to a patient while preparing the patient for a physical examination?

8. List three (3) specific standard precautions that must be followed at all times while assisting with a physical examination.

Name _____ Date _____

Evaluated by _____

DIRECTIONS: Practice assisting with an eye, ear, nose, and throat examination according to the criteria listed. When you are ready for your final check, give this sheet to your instructor.

PROFICIENT

Assisting with an Eye, Ear, Nose, and Throat Examination	Points Possible	Peer Check Yes	Peer Check No	Final Check* Yes	Final Check* No	Points Earned**	Comments
1. Assembles equipment and supplies	3						
2. Washes hands and puts on gloves if needed	3						
3. Introduces self, identifies patient, and explains procedure	3						
4. Screens vision with Snellen chart and records results	4						
5. Places patient in sitting position	4						
6. Asks patient to remove glasses and/or hearing aid	4						
7. Notifies physician that patient is ready	4						
8. Hands ophthalmoscope:							
Turns on light	3						
Hands in correct position	3						
Turns off light when done	2						
9. Hands tonometer	4						
10. Hands nasal speculum:							
Passes correctly	3						
Turns on flashlight and hands correctly	3						
Prepares applicators for use if needed	3						
11. Hands otoscope:							
Turns on light and applies otoscope tip	2						
Hands in correct position	2						
Prepares applicators	2						
Turns off light when done	2						
Places used tip in basin	2						
12. Passes tuning fork correctly	4						
13. Hands tongue blade/depressor correctly:	4						
Turns on flashlight before handing to physician	4						

Name _____

19:4A (cont.)

Assisting with an Eye, Ear, Nose, and Throat Examination	Points Possible	Peer Check		Final Check*		Points Earned**	Comments
		Yes	No	Yes	No		
14. Passes culture tubes as needed	3						
15. Hands laryngeal mirror:							
Places in warm water	2						
Dries before use	2						
Passes in correct position	2						
Places in basin after use	2						
16. Discards used tongue blade correctly	3						
17. When examination complete, assists patient off examining table	3						
18. Labels all specimens and completes requisition form correctly	3						
19. Cleans and replaces all equipment:							
Cleans and sterilizes instruments	2						
Places contaminated disposables in infectious waste bag	2						
Wipes contaminated areas with disinfectant	2						
20. Removes gloves and washes hands	3						
21. Records all required information	3						
Totals	100						

* Final Check: Instructor or authorized person evaluates.
** Points Earned: Points possible times each "yes" check.

Name _____ Date _____

Evaluated by _____

DIRECTIONS: Practice assisting with a gynecological examination according to the criteria listed. When you are ready for your final check, give this sheet to your instructor.

PROFICIENT

Assisting with a Gynecological Examination	Points Possible	Peer Check Yes	Peer Check No	Final Check* Yes	Final Check* No	Points Earned**	Comments
1. Assembles equipment and supplies	3						
2. Washes hands and puts on gloves	3						
3. Introduces self, identifies patient, and explains procedure	3						
4. Asks patient to put on examining gown and to void	4						
5. Positions patient in sitting position on exam table	4						
6. Notifies physician that patient is ready	3						
7. Assists with breast examination	4						
8. Positions patient in lithotomy position and drapes correctly	4						
9. Positions examining light	4						
10. Hands gloves to physician	4						
11. Warms speculum	4						
Passes it in closed position	4						
Applies lubricant to speculum	4						
12. Passes culture sticks as needed	4						
13. Assists with Pap test:							
Transmits Ayer blade or cytology brush correctly	4						
Prepares slide(s) for use	4						
Spreads smear thinly	4						
Puts Ayer blade or cytology brush in infectious waste bag	4						
Applies fixative to slide	4						
14. When physician removes speculum, places speculum in basin	3						
15. Applies lubricant to physician's gloved fingers correctly	4						
16. When examination complete, offers tissues to patient and assists patient off table	4						
17. Labels all cultures and specimens and completes requisition form correctly	4						
18. Cleans and replaces all equipment:							
Cleans and sterilizes instruments	2						
Places contaminated disposables in infectious waste bag	2						
Wipes contaminated areas with disinfectant	2						
19. Removes gloves and washes hands	3						
20. Records all required information	4						
Totals	100						

* Final Check: Instructor or authorized person evaluates.
** Points Earned: Points possible times each "yes" check.

UNIT 19:4C Evaluation Sheet

Name _____ Date _____

Evaluated by _____

DIRECTIONS: Practice assisting with a physical examination according to the criteria listed. When you are ready for your final check, give this sheet to your instructor.

Assisting with a General Physical Examination	Points Possible	Peer Check Yes	No	Final Check* Yes	No	Points Earned**	Comments
PROFICIENT							
1. Assembles all equipment and supplies	3						
2. Washes hands and puts on gloves	3						
3. Introduces self, identifies patient, and explains procedure	3						
4. Tells patient to remove clothes and put on gown	3						
Asks patient to void	3						
5. Performs the following tests:							
Ht. and Wt.	3						
TPR and BP	3						
Vision screening	3						
6. Seats patient on examination table and drapes correctly	4						
7. Assists with eye, ear, nose and throat exam	4						
8. Hands stethoscope and/or sphygmomanometer to physician	3						
9. Remains quiet during lung examination	3						
10. Positions patient in horizontal recumbent and drapes correctly	4						
11. Assists as needed with breast exam	3						
12. Assists as needed with abdominal examination	3						
13. Assists with examination of legs and feet:							
Passes percussion hammer	3						
Passes open safety pin or sensory wheel	3						
14. Positions patient in prone and drapes correctly	4						
15. Assists with examination of back and spine	3						
16. Positions patient correctly and assists with examination of genital organs	4						

19:4C (cont.)

Assisting with a General Physical Examination	Points Possible	Peer Check		Final Check*		Points Earned**	Comments
		Yes	No	Yes	No		
17. Assists with rectal examination:							
Positions male in Sims'	3						
Positions female in Sims' or lithotomy	3						
Passes gloves and lubricant	3						
Passes rectal speculum	3						
18. Assists patient off of table at end of examination and informs patient how and when he/she will be notified of test results	3						
19. Labels specimens and completes requisition form with all required information	4						
20. Cleans and replaces all equipment:							
Cleans and sterilizes instruments	3						
Places contaminated disposables in infectious waste bag	3						
Wipes contaminated areas with disinfectant	3						
21. Removes gloves and washes hands	3						
22. Records all required information	4						
Totals	100						

* Final Check: Instructor or authorized person evaluates.
** Points Earned: Points possible times each "yes" check.

UNIT 19:5 ASSISTING WITH MINOR SURGERY AND SUTURE REMOVAL

ASSIGNMENT SHEET

Grade _____ Name _____

INTRODUCTION: You may assist with minor surgery or suture removal in many health fields. This sheet will help you review the main facts.

INSTRUCTIONS: Read the information on Assisting with Minor Surgery and Suture Removal. In the space provided, print the word(s) that best completes the statement or answers the question.

1. List three (3) examples of minor surgery.

2. What is meant by suture removal?

3. Why must sterile technique be followed while performing minor surgery or suture removal?

4. List the main purpose for each of the following instruments:

   a. Scalpel:

   b. Surgical scissors:

   c. Hemostats:

   d. Tissue forceps:

   e. Retractors:

   f. Needle holder:

5. List the two (2) instruments that are used as a suture removal set.

6. Why do suture scissors have a curved cutting edge?

7. If a patient has specific questions about the surgery, what should you do?

8. What must be done with tissues and other specimens that are removed during minor surgery?

9. Because contamination by blood and body fluids is likely during minor surgery, _____ must be observed at all times.

UNIT 19:5A Evaluation Sheet

Name _____ Date _____

Evaluated by _____

DIRECTIONS: Practice assisting with minor surgery according to the criteria listed. When you are ready for your final check, give this sheet to your instructor.

Assisting with Minor Surgery	Points Possible	Peer Check Yes	Peer Check No	Final Check* Yes	Final Check* No	Points Earned**	Comments
PROFICIENT							
1. Assembles all equipment and supplies	2						
2. Washes hands	2						
3. Checks sterilization indicators and dates on sterile supplies	3						
4. Positions tray/stand conveniently and places sterile towel on tray/stand correctly	2						
5. Places following equipment on sterile field without contamination:							
Sterile drapes	3						
Needle and syringe	3						
Basin	3						
Gauze	3						
Antiseptic solution	3						
Scalpel	3						
Surgical scissors	3						
Hemostats: straight and curved	3						
Tissue forceps	3						
Needle and suture material	3						
Needle holder	3						
Retractors	3						
Dressings in order of use	3						
6. Places following equipment by tray:							
2–3 pairs sterile gloves	3						
Infectious waste bag	3						
Tape	3						
Anesthetic solution	3						
7. Introduces self, identifies patient, and explains procedure	3						
8. Confirms patient observed pre-operative instructions	3						
9. Positions and drapes patient for procedure	3						
10. Assists with surgery as needed:							
Uncovers tray	2						
Gives gloves to physician	2						
Assists with anesthetic	2						
Obtains additional supplies	2						

19:5A (cont.)

Assisting with Minor Surgery	Points Possible	Peer Check		Final Check*		Points Earned**	Comments
		Yes	No	Yes	No		
11. Assists with placement of dressings and bandages	3						
12. Reviews post-operative orders with patient	3						
13. Assists patient off of table after surgery	2						
14. Puts all specimens in correct containers, labels all specimens correctly, and completes requisition form	3						
15. Cleans and replaces all equipment:							
Cleans and sterilizes instruments	2						
Places sharp objects in sharps container	2						
Places contaminated disposables in infectious waste bag	2						
Wipes contaminated areas with disinfectant	2						
16. Removes gloves and washes hands	2						
17. Records all required information	2						
Totals	100						

* Final Check: Instructor or authorized person evaluates.
** Points Earned: Points possible times each "yes" check.

UNIT 19:5B Evaluation Sheet

Name _____ Date _____

Evaluated by _____

DIRECTIONS: Practice assisting with suture removal according to the criteria listed. When you are ready for your final check, give this sheet to your instructor.

PROFICIENT

Assisting with Suture Removal	Points Possible	Peer Check Yes	No	Final Check* Yes	No	Points Earned**	Comments
1. Assembles equipment and supplies	4						
2. Washes hands	4						
3. Checks sterilization indicator and date on all sterile supplies	4						
4. Places sterile towel on tray or stand	4						
5. Places following equipment on sterile field without contamination:							
Basin	6						
Gauze	6						
Antiseptic solution	6						
Suture removal set	6						
Dressings in order of use	6						
6. Places following equipment by tray:							
Sterile gloves	6						
Infectious waste bag	6						
Tape	6						
7. Introduces self, identifies patient, and explains procedure	4						
8. Positions and drapes patient correctly	4						
9. Assists with suture removal as necessary	4						
10. Places dressing on site if necessary	4						
11. Instructs patient on wound care	3						
12. Assists patient off of table after procedure	3						
13. Cleans and replaces all equipment:							
Cleans and sterilizes instruments	2						
Places contaminated disposables in infectious waste bag	2						
Wipes contaminated areas with disinfectant	2						
14. Removes gloves and washes hands	4						
15. Records all required information	4						
Totals	100						

* Final Check: Instructor or authorized person evaluates.
** Points Earned: Points possible times each "yes" check.

UNIT 19:6 RECORDING AND MOUNTING AN ELECTROCARDIOGRAM

ASSIGNMENT SHEET

Grade _____ Name _____

INTRODUCTION: In order to record an electrocardiogram correctly, the assistant must know certain information. This sheet will help with review of this information.

INSTRUCTIONS: Read the information on this topic. In the space provided, print the word(s) that best completes the statement or answers the question.

1. Briefly describe the pathway followed by the electrical conduction pattern in the heart.

2. What is occurring in the heart when the following waves of the PQRST complex appear on the electrocardiogram?

    a. P wave:

    b. QRS wave:

    c. T wave:

3. How many heartbeats does each PQRST complex represent?

4. Why does a physician note electrical disturbances in the various leads of the ECG?

5. How many leads are normally recorded on an ECG?

6. State the area where each of the following coded electrodes is placed.

    RA   LL

    RL   LA

7. List the correct marking code for each of the following leads.

V_1	V_4	1	aVR
V_2	V_5	2	aVL
V_3	V_6	3	aVF

8. Differentiate between a single-channel and a multiple-channel ECG.

9. How would an assistant correct the following problems that could occur while running an ECG?

    a. Tracing line is very light

    b. Standard is 8 blocks high when sensitivity is at 1

    c. Complexes are very tiny

    d. Complexes are very fast and close together (rate 200)

10. For a normal ECG, the standard should be _____ small squares high or _____ large squares high when the sensitivity is set at 1.

11. The normal sensitivity setting for an ECG is _____. The usual paper run speed is _____.

12. Why is it important for the patient to be relaxed during an ECG?

    List two (2) ways to encourage a patient to relax.

UNIT 19:6 Evaluation Sheet

Name _____   Date _____

Evaluated by _____

DIRECTIONS: Practice recording and mounting an ECG according to the criteria listed. When you are ready for your final check, give this sheet to your instructor.

PROFICIENT

Recording and Mounting an Electrocardiogram	Points Possible	Peer Check Yes	No	Final Check* Yes	No	Points Earned**	Comments
1. Assembles equipment and supplies	2						
2. Washes hands	2						
3. Introduces self, identifies patient, and explains procedure	2						
4. Prepares patient as follows:							
Stresses that patient will not experience discomfort	2						
Asks patient to lie still	2						
Places in supine position with body parts supported	2						
Drapes with bath blanket or drape	2						
5. Positions ECG machine conveniently and attaches cord pointing away from patient	3						
6. Applies limb electrodes correctly:							
Prepares skin at area of application	3						
Applies gel for metal or suction bulb electrodes	3						
Positions on fleshy outer part of arms or legs	3						
7. Attaches chest electrodes correctly:							
Locates correct area for each electrode	3						
Uses electrode pad or gel if necessary	3						
8. Connects cable correctly:							
Attaches cable ends to correct electrodes	3						
Follows body contour	3						
Coils excess wire	3						
9. Turns on main switch	3						
10. Sets sensitivity at one	3						
11. Checks standard on run 25	3						
12. Checks color of line and adjusts as necessary	3						

Recording and Mounting an Electrocardiogram	Points Possible	Peer Check		Final Check*		Points Earned**	Comments
		Yes	No	Yes	No		
13. Records the leads:							
Sets at run 25	3						
Centers on paper	3						
Inserts standard marks as required	3						
Records sufficient amounts of each lead	3						
Adjusts size of complexes as required by changing sensitivity	3						
Changes speed to run 50 if complexes too close	3						
14. When ECG recorded, turns selector to ST'D and record switch to off	3						
15. Cleans skin electrode sites with water	3						
16. Assists patient off table after procedure	3						
17. Cleans electrodes correctly or discards disposable electrodes	2						
18. Coils all wires	2						
19. Mounts ECG correctly:							
Labels with required information	4						
Attaches ECG to mount correctly	4						
Checks that all leads are in correct location	4						
20. Replaces all equipment	2						
21. Washes hands	2						
Totals	100						

* Final Check: Instructor or authorized person evaluates.
** Points Earned: Points possible times each "yes" check.

UNIT 19:7 USING THE *PHYSICIANS' DESK REFERENCE (PDR)*

ASSIGNMENT SHEET #1

Grade _____ Name _____

INTRODUCTION: This assignment will help you learn to use the *Physicians' Desk Reference.*

INSTRUCTIONS: Use the *PDR* to locate the following information. Record the information in the space provided.

1. Find the address of the main office of Bristol-Myers-Squibb Company.

   List the area code and phone number.

   To whom should inquiries be addressed?

2. List three (3) drugs produced by Bristol-Myers-Squibb.

3. The following two drugs are brand names. Find the information required for each of these drugs.
   a. Dalmane: Manufacturer

      Action

      Adverse reactions

      Oral dosage
   b. Hydrodiuril: Manufacturer

      Action

      Precautions

      Adverse reactions

      Adult oral dosage

4. The following two drugs are generic or chemical names. List three (3) brand names available for each of these products.

   a. Meperidine Hydrochloride:

   b. Vitamin C:

5. List three (3) drugs that can be used to treat hemorrhoids.

UNIT 19:7 USING THE *PHYSICIANS' DESK REFERENCE (PDR)*

ASSIGNMENT SHEET #2

Grade _____ Name _____

INTRODUCTION: Note corrections made on *PDR* assignment number 1. Then complete this assignment to learn correct use of the *PDR*.

INSTRUCTIONS: Use the *PDR* to locate the following information. Record the information in the space provided.

1. Find the manufacturer of the drug Bufferin.

   Name

   List the following information on this manufacturer.

   Address

   Telephone

2. Find the following information for each of the drugs listed.

   a. Demerol Hydrochloride: Action

   Warning

   Adverse reactions

   Adult oral dose

   b. Erythromycin Tablets: Action

   Adverse reactions

   Adult oral dose

   c. Motrin: Action

   Warnings

   Adverse reactions

   Oral dose

3. A patient is taking a pink and white capsule marked *Lilly 3110*. Where in the *PDR* would you find help to identify what it is?

4. List four (4) products that are classified as tetracyclines.

5. List four (4) drugs that may be used to treat thyroid disease.

UNIT 19:7 USING THE *PHYSICIANS' DESK REFERENCE (PDR)*

ASSIGNMENT SHEET #3

Grade _____ Name _____

INTRODUCTION: Study corrections on assignments 1 and 2. Then complete this assignment.

INSTRUCTIONS: Use the *PDR* to locate the following information. Record in the space provided.

1. Find the address of the nearest office for the Upjohn Company.

    Address…

2. List two drugs produced by the Upjohn Company.

3. Find the following information for the drugs listed.

    a. Vibramycin Capsules: Action

       Adverse reactions

       Adult maintenance dosage

    b. Lanoxin: Action

       Precautions

       Maintenance dose

    c. Darvon Compound: Action

       Adverse reactions

       Adult dosage

4. The doctor ordered Butazolidin, which is currently marketed as a white and orange capsule. What name and/or number is on this capsule? _____

    What is the action of this drug? _____

    Usual dosage range _____

    Highest maintenance dosage _____

    Can it be given to children under 14? _____ To pregnant women ?_____

5. List four (4) drugs that can be used to treat coughs and colds.

395

UNIT 19:8 WORKING WITH MATH AND MEDICATIONS

ASSIGNMENT SHEET

Grade _____ Name _____

INTRODUCTION: This sheet will help you review some facts about medications.

INSTRUCTIONS: Read the information sheet on Working with Math and Medications. In the space provided, print the word(s) that best completes the statement or answers the question.

1. List three (3) forms of liquid medications.

2. List three (3) forms of solid medications.

3. List three (3) forms of semisolid medications.

4. Briefly describe the following routes of administration for medications.

    a. oral:

    b. rectal:

    c. subcutaneous:

    d. intramuscular:

    e. intravenous:

    f. topical:

    g. sublingual:

5. List the five (5) "rights" or five main points to watch each and every time a medication is prepared.

6. How many times should the label on any medication container be read? When should it be read?

7. Where should medications be stored?

8. If a medication bottle is not labeled, or if the label is not clear, what should be done?

9. What is the best method to discard old medications?

10. How are expired controlled substances, such as narcotics, discarded?

UNIT 19:8A USING ROMAN NUMERALS

ASSIGNMENT SHEET

Grade _____ Name _____

INTRODUCTION: Roman numerals are used in some medications and also when ordering some supplies. This worksheet will help you practice using Roman numerals.

INSTRUCTIONS: Read the information sheet on Using Roman Numerals. Then complete the following problems. Place your answer in the space provided.

1. Write the Roman numeral symbol for the following numbers.

1 _____	72 _____	343 _____
7 _____	88 _____	510 _____
11 _____	99 _____	622 _____
13 _____	104 _____	990 _____
18 _____	110 _____	1015 _____
22 _____	129 _____	1987 _____
54 _____	150 _____	1999 _____

2. Insert the Arabic number represented by each of the following Roman numerals in the space provided next to it.

XXVI _____	XCVII _____	CMLXXI _____
XI _____	CXXII _____	MCL _____
IX _____	CXLIV _____	MCML _____
LIV _____	CDIII _____	MCMLXXX _____
LXXV _____	CDLVI _____	MMM _____

3. The following medications have been ordered. Write the correct dosage in Arabic numbers.

Aspirin Gr X _____	Aspirin Gr XXV _____
Aspirin Gr V _____	Aspirin Gr XXX _____
Aspirin Gr XV _____	Aspirin Gr VII _____

4. You are ordering supplies for the doctor. What do the following codes mean?

C for $9.00 _____	L for $2 _____
D for $16.00 _____	C for $3 _____
M for $25.00 _____	D for $8 _____
MM for $40.00 _____	DCCL for $10 _____

UNIT 19:8B CONVERTING METRIC MEASUREMENTS

ASSIGNMENT SHEET

Grade _____ Name _____

INTRODUCTION: Because you may have to convert from one measurement in the metric system to another measurement, the following assignment will provide practice.

INSTRUCTIONS: Read the information sheet on Converting Metric Measurements. Show your answers to the following problems in the space provided.

NOTE: Remember to list each scale from largest to smallest as follows:

kilo _____ hecto _____ deka _____ Base unit deci _____ centa _____ milli _____

1. Convert the following milligrams to grams.

   1000 mg =   500 mg =

   1500 mg =   3500 mg =

   5000 mg =   250 mg =

2. Convert the following grams to kilograms.

   2000 g =   3500 g =

    500 g =   2500 g =

   1850 g =   100 g =

3. Convert the following millliliters to liters.

   1000 mL =   750 mL =

    250 mL =   2550 mL =

   4000 mL =   10,000 mL =

4. Convert the following grams to milligrams.

    5 g =   3 g =

   2.5 g =   6.25 g =

   l0 g =   8.875 g =

5. Convert the following liters to milliliters.

    2 L =   0.1 L =

   5.5 L =   3.5 L =

   10 L =   7 L =

6. Convert the following hectometers to centimeters.

      7 hm =   2.23 hm =

    3.524 hm =   88.5 hm =

     118 hm =   0.006432 hm =

7. Convert the following decigrams to dekagrams.

     228 dg =   27.32 dg =

   8,921 dg =   540 dg =

    8.32 dg =   0.23 dg =

8. Convert the following centaliters to kiloliters.

  64,000 cL =   4,200,000 cL =

     228 cL =   10,000 cL =

 980,000 cL =   554.32 cL =

9. Convert the following kilometers to meters.

    580 km =   0.0425 km =

     47 km =   1.52 km =

  0.381 km =   296 km =

10. Convert the following as indicated.

  3000 mg =   g   4.5 g =   mg

  2500 cc=   L   3.25 kg =   g

    5.6 L =   mL   500 dkg =   mg

 82.64 dm=   hm   32,000 cc =   kL

 32,114 mL=   dL   42,500 cm =   dkm

UNIT 19:8C CONVERTING HOUSEHOLD (ENGLISH) MEASUREMENTS

ASSIGNMENT SHEET

Grade _____ Name _____

INTRODUCTION: The following assignment will provide practice in converting household or English measurements. (A cubic centimeter is equivalent to a milliliter; the terms are interchangeable.)

INSTRUCTIONS: Read the information sheet on Converting Household or English Measurements. In the space provided, show your answer to the following problems.

1. How many ounces are in the following number of milliliters?

   300 mL =   60 mL =

   240 mL =   135 mL =

   900 mL =   45 mL =

2. How many cubic centimeters or millimeters are in the following numbers of ounces?

   4 oz =   5 1/2 oz =

   8 oz =   7 oz =

   10 oz =   12 oz =

3. How many teaspoons are in the following numbers of milliliters?

   15 mL =   7 1/2 mL =

   40 mL =   20 mL =

   25 mL =   30 mL =

4. How many cubic centimeters or millimeters are in the following number of teaspoons?

   5 tsp =   10 tsp =

   2 tsp =   8 tsp =

   1 tsp =   7 tsp =

5. How many tablespoons (tbsp) are in the following numbers of milliliters?

   15 mL =   30 mL =

   60 mL =   150 mL =

   45 mL =   135 mL =

6. How many drops (gtts) are in the following numbers of mLs?

    1 mL =   3 mL =

    5 mL =   7 mL =

    15 mL =   80 mL =

7. How many kilograms (kg) are in the following number of pounds (lb)?

    122 lb =   243 lb =

    208 lb =   108 lb =

    143 lb =   92 lb =

8. How many ounces (oz) are in the following number of kilograms (kg)?

    0.224 kg =   1.12 kg =

    0.896 kg =   0.336 kg =

    0.448 kg =   0.238 kg =

9. How many meters (m) are in the following measurements?

    18 in =   6 ft =

    30 in =   60 miles =

    5 yd =   103 miles =

10. Convert the following as indicated.

500 mL =	pt	4000 mL =	qt
1500 mL =	qt	2500 mL =	pt
3000 mL =	qt	750 mL =	pt
480 mL =	oz	270 mL =	tbsp
60 mL =	tsp	1230 mL =	oz

UNIT 20:1 ADMITTING, TRANSFERRING, AND DISCHARGING PATIENTS

ASSIGNMENT SHEET

Grade _____ Name _____

INTRODUCTION: This assignment will help you review the main facts about admitting, transferring, or discharging patients.

INSTRUCTIONS: Read the information on Admitting, Transferring, and Discharging Patients. In the space provided, print the word(s) that best completes the statement or answers the question.

1. Admission to a health care facility can cause _____ and _____ for many patients/residents and their families.

2. Identify three (3) ways a health care assistant can create a positive first impression and alleviate a patient's fears and anxiety.

3. If a patient is unable to answer questions for an admission form, who can you ask for the information?

4. List at least three (3) rules to follow while handling a patient's valuables.

5. List at least six (6) areas or things that should be explained while orientating a patient to the health care facility.

6. What are two (2) main reasons for transferring a patient?

7. List two (2) items that must be transferred with the patient.

8. What is required before a patient/resident can be discharged from a health care facility?

9. When you enter Mr. O'Shea's room, he is packing his suitcase and states he is leaving and going home. What should you do?

10. Why do health care agencies use forms or checklists for admissions, transfers, and discharges?

UNIT 20:1A Evaluation Sheet

Name _____ Date _____

Evaluated by _____

DIRECTIONS: Practice admitting the patient according to the criteria listed. When you are ready for your final check, give this sheet to your instructor.

Admitting the Patient	Points Possible	PROFICIENT Peer Check Yes	No	Final Check* Yes	No	Points Earned**	Comments
1. Checks orders or obtains authorization	3						
2. Washes hands	3						
3. Assembles equipment and supplies	3						
4. Prepares room for admission:							
Opens the bed	2						
Unpacks admission kit	2						
Places supplies/equipment in bedside stand	2						
5. Greets and identifies patient	4						
6. Introduces self and other patient	4						
7. Asks family/visitors to wait in lounge/lobby	4						
8. Closes door and screens unit	4						
9. Assists patient into gown/pajamas	4						
10. Positions patient comfortably in bed/chair	4						
11. Completes admission form/checklist	4						
12. Measures and records vital signs	4						
13. Weighs and measures patient	4						
14. Completes clothing list:	2						
Lists personal items	2						
Obtains proper signatures	2						
Hangs up clothes and puts items away	2						
15. Completes valuables list:	2						
Obtains proper signatures	2						
Places valuables in safe	2						
16. Obtains routine urine specimen if required	4						
17. Orientates patient to facility	4						
18. Fills water pitcher if allowed	4						
19. Positions patient in correct alignment	4						

20:1A (cont.)

Admitting the Patient	Points Possible	Peer Check Yes	Peer Check No	Final Check* Yes	Final Check* No	Points Earned**	Comments
20. Elevates siderail if indicated and lowers bed before leaving patient	3						
21. Places call signal and supplies in patient's reach	3						
22. Replaces equipment and leaves area neat and clean	3						
23. Washes hands	3						
24. Allows family/visitors to return to unit	3						
25. Records or reports required information	4						
Totals	100						

* Final Check: Instructor or authorized person evaluates.
** Points Earned: Points possible times each "yes" check.

U N I T 20 : 1 B E v a l u a t i o n S h e e t

Name _____ Date _____

Evaluated by _____

DIRECTIONS: Practice transferring the patient according to the criteria listed. When you are ready for your final check, give this sheet to your instructor.

PROFICIENT

Transferring the Patient	Points Possible	Peer Check Yes	Peer Check No	Final Check* Yes	Final Check* No	Points Earned**	Comments
1. Checks orders or obtains authorization	3						
2. Determines following information:							
New room number or unit	3						
Unit is ready for transfer	3						
Method of transport	3						
3. Assembles equipment and supplies	3						
4. Knocks on door and pauses before entering	3						
5. Introduces self, identifies patient, and explains procedure	4						
6. Washes hands	3						
7. Collects clothing and personal items	4						
Checks items on admission checklist	4						
Puts items in bag or on cart	4						
8. Places equipment to be transferred on cart	4						
9. Checks valuables to be transferred	4						
10. Transfers patient to wheelchair or stretcher	4						
11. Transports patient and belongings to new unit/room	4						
12. Introduces patient to new staff members	4						
13. Orientates patient if required	4						
14. Checks belongings with new staff member	4						
15. Puts away clothing and personal items	4						
16. Positions patient comfortably and in correct alignment before leaving	4						
17. Elevates siderails if indicated and lowers bed to lowest level	3						
18. Places call signal and supplies in patient's reach	3						
19. Replaces equipment and leaves area neat and clean	3						
20. Washes hands	3						
21. Completes transfer list	4						
22. Returns to previous room/unit and cleans unit as required	4						
23. Washes hands	3						
24. Records or reports required information	4						
Totals	100						

* Final Check: Instructor or authorized person evaluates.
** Points Earned: Points possible times each "yes" check.

UNIT 20:1C Evaluation Sheet

Name _____ Date _____

Evaluated by _____

DIRECTIONS: Practice discharging the patient according to the criteria listed. When you are ready for your final check, give this sheet to your instructor.

Discharging the Patient	Points Possible	Peer Check Yes	No	Final Check* Yes	No	Points Earned**	Comments
		PROFICIENT					
1. Checks orders or obtains authorization	3						
2. Determines time of discharge	3						
3. Assembles equipment and supplies	3						
4. Knocks on door and pauses before entering	3						
5. Introduces self, identifies patient, and explains procedure	3						
6. Closes door and screens unit	3						
7. Washes hands	3						
8. Assists patient with dressing	4						
9. Assembles patient's belongings	4						
Checks items against clothing list	4						
Obtains proper signatures	5						
10. Assembles equipment given to patient	4						
11. Checks that patient has received discharge instructions	5						
12. Obtains valuables from safe	4						
Checks valuables with list	4						
Obtains proper signatures	5						
13. Completes discharge checklist	5						
14. Places items on cart or gives to relative	4						
15. Transfers patient to wheelchair	4						
16. Transports patient to business office and/or car	4						
17. Assists patient into car	4						
18. Places belongings in car	4						
19. Says good-bye to patient	4						
20. Returns to unit and cleans as required	4						
21. Washes hands	3						
22. Records or reports required information	4						
Totals	100						

* Final Check: Instructor or authorized person evaluates.
** Points Earned: Points possible times each "yes" check.

UNIT 20:2 POSITIONING, TURNING, MOVING, AND TRANSFERRING PATIENTS

ASSIGNMENT SHEET

Grade _____ Name _____

INTRODUCTION: Correct alignment, moving, and transfer techniques help prevent injury to both the patient and the health assistant. This assignment will help you review the main points on these procedures.

INSTRUCTIONS: Review the information on Positioning, Turning, Moving, and Transferring Patients. In the space provided, print the word(s) that best completes the statement or answers the question.

1. Define *alignment*.

2. List two (2) complications that may be prevented by correct alignment.

3. Bedridden patients should have their position changed at least every _____ hours. Give three (3) reasons why bed patients should be turned frequently.

4. Define *contracture*.

5. Define *pressure ulcer*.

6. Briefly describe the appearance of each of the four (4) stages of a pressure ulcer.

7. List the three (3) times the patient's pulse must be checked during the dangling procedure.

8. Why is the pulse checked during the dangling procedure?

9. List five (5) points you should observe or check on a patient during any move or transfer.

10. Before a patient is moved or transferred, the health assistant must obtain _____ or _____ from his/her _____. _____ move or transfer a patient without correct authorization.

UNIT 20:2A Evaluation Sheet

Name _____   Date _____

Evaluated by _____

DIRECTIONS: Practice aligning the patient according to the criteria listed. When you are ready for your final check, give this sheet to your instructor.

PROFICIENT

Aligning the Patient	Points Possible	Peer Check		Final Check*		Points Earned**	Comments
		Yes	No	Yes	No		
1. Checks orders or obtains authorization	2						
2. Assembles supplies	2						
3. Knocks on door and pauses before entering	2						
4. Introduces self, identifies patient, and explains procedure	2						
5. Closes door and screens unit	2						
6. Washes hands	2						
7. Raises bed and lowers siderail if elevated	2						
8. Positions patient on back:							
Places head in straight line with spine	3						
Places pillow under head and shoulders	3						
Places pillow or rolled blanket under lower legs	3						
Places feet at right angle	3						
Positions arms and legs	3						
Supports all body parts	3						
Protects bony areas	3						
9. Positions patient on side:							
Supports head and shoulders	3						
Flexes arms at elbows	3						
Positions lower arm in line with face	3						
Supports upper arm on pillow or rolled blanket	3						
Places pillow between flexed knees	3						
Places feet at right angles	3						
Protects bony areas	3						
Supports back and/or abdomen	3						
Avoids twisting body	3						
10. Aligns patient in prone position:							
Places head in line with spine	3						
Supports head with pillow	3						
Supports waist with pillow	3						
Flexes knees	3						
Puts pillow under lower legs	3						
Puts feet at right angles	3						

409

Aligning the Patient	Points Possible	Peer Check		Final Check*		Points Earned**	Comments
		Yes	No	Yes	No		
Flexes elbows slightly	3						
Positions arms in line to either side of head	3						
Protects bony areas	3						
11. Elevates siderail if indicated and lowers bed before leaving patient	2						
12. Checks patient for comfort and places call signal and supplies in reach	2						
13. Replaces all equipment and leaves area neat and clean	2						
14. Washes hands	2						
15. Records or reports required information	3						
Totals	100						

* Final Check: Instructor or authorized person evaluates.
** Points Earned: Points possible times each "yes" check.

UNIT 20:2B Evaluation Sheet

Name _____ Date _____

Evaluated by _____

DIRECTIONS: Practice moving a patient up in bed according to the criteria listed. When you are ready for your final check, give this sheet to your instructor.

PROFICIENT

Moving the Patient Up in Bed	Points Possible	Peer Check Yes	No	Final Check* Yes	No	Points Earned**	Comments
1. Checks order or obtains authorization	3						
2. Knocks on door and pauses before entering	3						
3. Introduces self, identifies patient, and explains procedure	3						
4. Closes door and screens unit	3						
5. Washes hands	3						
6. Locks bed to prevent movement and raises bed to correct height	4						
7. Lowers head of bed to lowest level	4						
8. Lowers nearest siderail if elevated	4						
9. Removes pillow and places it against headboard	4						
10. Observes patient for respiratory distress	5						
11. Instructs or assists patient to flex knees and brace feet on bed	8						
12. Places one arm under shoulders and other arm under hips	8						
13. Gives signal to patient	8						
14. Slides patient to head of bed shifting weight at the same time	8						
15. Gets help if unable to move patient	6						
16. Positions patient in good alignment	6						
17. Elevates siderail if indicated and lowers bed	4						
18. Places call signal and necessary supplies within reach	4						
19. Replaces equipment and leaves area neat and clean	4						
20. Washes hands	3						
21. Records or reports required information	5						
Totals	100						

* Final Check: Instructor or authorized person evaluates.
** Points Earned: Points possible times each "yes" check.

Name _____   Date _____

Evaluated by _____

DIRECTIONS: Practice turning a patient away according to the criteria listed. When you are ready for your final check, give this sheet to your instructor.

PROFICIENT

Turning the Patient Away to Change Position	Points Possible	Peer Check Yes	No	Final Check* Yes	No	Points Earned**	Comments
1. Checks order or obtains authorization	3						
2. Knocks on door and pauses before entering	3						
3. Introduces self, identifies patient, and explains procedure	3						
4. Closes door and screens unit	3						
5. Washes hands	3						
6. Locks bed to prevent movement and raises bed to correct height	3						
7. Lowers nearest siderail if elevated	3						
8. Checks opposite siderail to make sure it is elevated	4						
9. Crosses patient's arms on chest	6						
10. Crosses nearest leg over other leg	6						
11. Moves patient toward near edge of bed:							
Slides upper body toward near edge of bed, with hands under head and upper back	5						
Slides hips toward near edge of bed, with hands under hips	5						
Slides legs toward near edge of bed, with hands under legs	5						
12. Positions hands under shoulder and hip	6						
13. Rolls patient away with smooth even motion	6						
14. Moves head and shoulders back to center of bed	5						
15. Moves hips back to center	5						
16. Moves legs back to center	5						
17. Positions patient in correct alignment using pillows to support back, legs, and upper arm	4						
18. Elevates siderail if indicated and lowers bed	3						
19. Places call signal and supplies in patient's reach	3						
20. Replaces equipment and leaves area neat and clean	3						
21. Washes hands	3						
22. Records or reports required information	5						
Totals	100						

* Final Check: Instructor or authorized person evaluates.
** Points Earned: Points possible times each "yes" check.

UNIT 20:2D Evaluation Sheet

Name _____ Date _____

Evaluated by _____

DIRECTIONS: Practice turning the patient toward you according to the criteria listed. When you are ready for your final check, give this sheet to your instructor.

Turning the Patient Inward to Change Position	Points Possible	Peer Check Yes	Peer Check No	Final Check* Yes	Final Check* No	Points Earned**	Comments
1. Checks order or obtains authorization	3						
2. Knocks on door and pauses before entering	3						
3. Introduces self, identifies patient, and explains procedure	3						
4. Closes door and screens unit	3						
5. Washes hands	3						
6. Locks bed to prevent movement and raises bed to correct height	3						
7. Lowers nearest siderail if elevated	3						
8. Crosses patient's arms on chest	5						
9. Places patient's farthest leg on top of other leg	5						
10. Moves patient to opposite side of bed:							
Slides upper body, with hands under head and shoulders	4						
Slides hips, with hands under hips	4						
Slides legs, with hands under legs	4						
11. Places hands on far shoulder and hip	5						
12. Rolls patient toward self with smooth motion	5						
13. Elevates siderail if indicated	5						
14. Goes to opposite side and lowers siderail if elevated	5						
15. Places hands under head and shoulders to move to center of bed	5						
16. Places hands under hips to position hips in center of bed	5						
17. Places hands under legs to move to center of bed	5						
18. Positions patient in correct alignment using pillows to support back, legs, and upper arm	5						
19. Elevates siderail if indicated and lowers bed	3						
20. Places call signal and other supplies in patient's reach	3						
21. Replaces equipment and leaves area neat and clean	3						
22. Washes hands	3						
23. Records or reports required information	5						
Totals	100						

* Final Check: Instructor or authorized person evaluates.
** Points Earned: Points possible times each "yes" check.

Name _____ Date _____

Evaluated by _____

DIRECTIONS: Practice dangling the patient according to the criteria listed. When you are ready for your final check, give this sheet to your instructor.

PROFICIENT

Sitting Up to Dangle	Points Possible	Peer Check Yes	No	Final Check* Yes	No	Points Earned**	Comments
1. Checks orders or obtains authorization	2						
2. Assembles equipment and suppplies	2						
3. Knocks on door and pauses before entering	3						
4. Introduces self, identifies patient, and explains procedure	3						
5. Closes door and screens unit	3						
6. Washes hands	2						
7. Locks bed to prevent movement	3						
8. Lowers bed to lowest level	3						
9. Lowers siderail (if elevated) on side patient is to dangle	3						
10. Checks radial pulse	5						
11. Elevates head of bed slowly	3						
12. Assists patient to put on robe	3						
13. Places one arm under shoulders and other arm under knees	4						
14. Bends at knees and maintains broad base of support to get close to patient	4						
15. Turns patient onto side and then to sitting position slowly and smoothly	4						
16. Covers legs with bath blanket and puts on slippers	4						
17. Places feet on stool	4						
18. Checks radial pulse and notes any signs of distress	5						
19. Instructs patient to flex and extend legs and feet	4						
20. Places call signal within reach and dangles for proper length of time	4						

20:2E (cont.)

Sitting Up to Dangle	Points Possible	Peer Check		Final Check*		Points Earned**	Comments
		Yes	No	Yes	No		
21. Removes slippers and bath blanket	3						
22. Places one arm by shoulders and other by knees to move patient from sitting to supine position slowly and smoothly	4						
23. Assists patient to remove robe	3						
24. Lowers head of bed slowly	3						
25. Positions in correct alignment	2						
26. Checks radial pulse	5						
27. Elevates siderail if indicated and lowers bed to lowest level	2						
28. Places call signal and supplies in patient's reach	2						
29. Replaces equipment and leaves area neat and clean	2						
30. Washes hands	2						
31. Records or reports required information	4						
Totals	100						

* Final Check: Instructor or authorized person evaluates.
** Points Earned: Points possible times each "yes" check.

UNIT 20:2F Evaluation Sheet

Name _____ Date _____

Evaluated by _____

DIRECTIONS: Practice transferring a patient to a chair/wheelchair according to the criteria listed. When you are ready for your final check, give this sheet to your instructor.

PROFICIENT

Transferring a Patient to a Chair or Wheelchair	Points Possible	Peer Check Yes	No	Final Check* Yes	No	Points Earned**	Comments
1. Checks order or obtains authorization	3						
2. Assembles equipment and supplies	2						
3. Knocks on door and pauses before entering	2						
4. Introduces self, identifies patient, and explains procedure	2						
5. Closes door and screens unit	2						
6. Washes hands	3						
7. Prepares wheelchair/chair:							
Positions correctly	2						
Locks wheels or secures against wall	2						
Elevates footrests	2						
8. Locks bed to prevent movement	2						
9. Lowers bed to lowest level	2						
10. Elevates head slowly	2						
11. Lowers siderail (if elevated) on side patient will exit bed	2						
12. Assists patient to put on robe	2						
13. Assists patient to sitting position - dangles	3						
14. Puts transfer belt on patient	3						
15. Helps with slippers or shoes	2						
16. Stands close to patient with broad base of support	3						
17. Grasps each side of belt with underhand grasp	3						
18. Gives signal	3						
19. Assists to standing position by lifting up on belt while patient pushes up from the bed	4						
20. Allows patient to adjust to upright position	4						

Name _____

20:2F (cont.)

Transferring a Patient to a Chair or Wheelchair	Points Possible	Peer Check		Final Check*		Points Earned**	Comments
		Yes	No	Yes	No		
21. Turns patient to chair slowly and provides support for patient's leg(s) as needed	4						
22. Lowers gently into chair when patient's legs touch seat of chair	4						
23. Covers with blanket	3						
24. Observes for signs of distress	3						
25. Transports patient in wheelchair correctly:							
Directs wheelchair to right of hallway	3						
Watches intersections	3						
Pulls backward into elevator	3						
Walks backward down ramp	3						
Uses weight of body to push chair	3						
26. Returns patient to bed correctly	3						
27. Positions patient in correct alignment	2						
28. Elevates siderails if indicated and lowers bed to lowest level	2						
29. Places call signal and other supplies within reach of patient	2						
30. Replaces all equipment and leaves area neat and clean	2						
31. Washes hands	2						
32. Records or reports required information	3						
Totals	100						

* Final Check: Instructor or authorized person evaluates.
** Points Earned: Points possible times each "yes" check.

Name _____ Date _____

Evaluated by _____

DIRECTIONS: Practice transferring a patient from a bed to a stretcher according to the criteria listed. When you are ready for your final check, give this sheet to your instructor.

PROFICIENT

Transferring a Patient to a Stretcher	Points Possible	Peer Check Yes	No	Final Check* Yes	No	Points Earned**	Comments
1. Checks order or obtains authorization	2						
2. Assembles equipment and supplies	2						
3. Knocks on door and pauses before entering	2						
4. Introduces self, identifies patient, and explains procedure	2						
5. Closes door and screens unit	2						
6. Washes hands	2						
7. Elevates bed to level of stretcher	2						
8. Locks bed to prevent movement	2						
9. Lowers siderail (if elevated) on side of transfer	2						
10. Drapes patient with bath blanket	2						
11. Positions stretcher parallel to bed	3						
12. Locks wheels on stretcher	3						
13. If patient is conscious and capable of moving unassisted: Holds stretcher against bed with weight of body	4						
Holds up bath blanket	4						
Asks patient to slide across to stretcher	4						
Assists patient as needed	4						
14. If patient cannot assist with transfer: Positions a lift sheet/blanket under patient	4						
Obtains assistance of 3 to 4 people, positioning 2 to 3 people on stretcher side and 1 to 2 people on open side of bed	4						
Instructs all assistants to roll sides of lift sheet/blanket close to patient's body	4						
Gives signal	4						
Using overhand grasps, all assistants lift sheet to gently slide patient to stretcher	4						
15. Positions patient in correct alignment	3						
16. Locks safety belt(s)	3						

Name _____

20:2G (cont.)

Transferring a Patient to a Stretcher	Points Possible	Peer Check Yes	No	Final Check* Yes	No	Points Earned**	Comments
17. Elevates siderails of stretcher	3						
18. Transports with 2 team members:							
One at head and one at foot	2						
Moves slowly	2						
Directs to right of hall	2						
Moves patient's feet forward only	2						
Watches intersections	2						
Braces foot of stretcher on inclines	2						
19. Returns to bed correctly	4						
20. Positions in correct alignment	2						
21. Elevates siderails if indicated and lowers bed to lowest level	2						
22. Places call signal and supplies in patient's reach	2						
23. Replaces equipment and leaves area neat and clean	2						
24. Washes hands	2						
25. Records or reports required information	3						
Totals	100						

* Final Check: Instructor or authorized person evaluates.
** Points Earned: Points possible times each "yes" check.

UNIT 20:2H Evaluation Sheet

Name _____ Date _____

Evaluated by _____

DIRECTIONS: Practice transferring a patient with a mechanical lift according to the criteria listed. When you are ready for your final check, give this sheet to your instructor.

Using a Mechanical Lift to Transfer a Patient	Points Possible	Peer Check Yes	No	Final Check* Yes	No	Points Earned**	Comments
1. Obtains authorization or checks orders and facility policy for use of lift	3						
2. Assembles equipment and supplies	2						
3. Checks straps, sling, and clasps on lift for defects	3						
4. Checks hydraulic unit for oil leaks	3						
5. Knocks on door and pauses before entering	2						
6. Introduces self, identifies patient, and explains procedure	3						
7. Closes door and screens unit	3						
8. Washes hands	2						
9. Positions wheelchair correctly and locks wheels	3						
10. Locks bed to prevent movement	3						
11. Lowers siderail (if elevated) on side of transfer	3						
12. Positions sling under patient correctly	4						
13. Attaches suspension straps to sling properly	4						
14. Positions mechanical lift over the bed	4						
15. Attaches straps to frame of lift	4						
16. Positions patient's arms across chest and inside the straps	4						
17. Warns patient of any movement	4						
18. Operates lift to raise patient slightly above the bed	4						
19. Checks straps, sling, and lift to make sure patient suspended securely	4						

20:2H (cont.)

Using a Mechanical Lift to Transfer a Patient	Points Possible	Peer Check		Final Check*		Points Earned**	Comments
		Yes	No	Yes	No		
20. Raises patient above bed and turns lift to move patient slowly and smoothly into position over wheelchair or chair	4						
21. Lowers lift to position patient in chair/wheelchair	4						
22. Unhooks suspension straps from the sling	4						
23. Moves lift away from patient	4						
24. Covers patient with blanket	3						
25. Positions patient comfortably in chair observing all safety points	3						
26. Reverses procedure to return patient to bed	3						
27. Positions patient in correct alignment	2						
28. Raises siderail if indicated and lowers bed	2						
29. Positions call signal and other supplies	2						
30. Replaces all equipment and leaves area neat and clean	2						
31. Washes hands	2						
32. Records or reports required information	3						
Totals	100						

* Final Check: Instructor or authorized person evaluates.
** Points Earned: Points possible times each "yes" check.

UNIT 20:3 BEDMAKING

ASSIGNMENT SHEET

Grade _____ Name _____

INTRODUCTION: This sheet will help you review the main facts regarding correct bedmaking techniques.

INSTRUCTIONS: Review the information on Bedmaking. In the space provided, print the word(s) that completes the statement or answers the question.

1. Why is it important to avoid wrinkles in the bed linen?

2. Why are mitered corners used on all types of beds?

3. List two (2) purposes for making an open bed.

4. What is the difference between a closed bed and an occupied bed?

5. What is the purpose of a bed cradle?

6. List five (5) disorders or conditions that might require a bed cradle.

7. What are draw sheets?

   Why are they used?

8. Why is it important to unfold the sheets rather than to shake them out?

9. Why do you complete one entire side of the bed before going to the opposite side?

10. How is the pillow placed on the bed? Why is it placed in this position?

Name _____   Date _____

Evaluated by _____

DIRECTIONS: Practice making a closed bed according to the criteria listed. When you are ready for your final check, give this sheet to your instructor.

PROFICIENT

Making a Closed Bed	Points Possible	Peer Check Yes	No	Final Check* Yes	No	Points Earned**	Comments
1. Assembles equipment and supplies	2						
2. Washes hands	2						
3. Places linen on chair in order of use	2						
4. Elevates bed	2						
5. Locks bed to prevent movement	2						
6. Removes dirty sheets properly and wears gloves if necessary	3						
7. Applies bottom sheet:							
Unfolds sheet and positions	3						
Places right side up	3						
Lines up small hem even with bottom of mattress	3						
Centers on bed	3						
Makes mitered corner	3						
Tucks from top to bottom	3						
8. Applies drawsheet:							
Unfolds sheet	3						
Places 14–16 inches from top of mattress	3						
Places right side up	3						
Tucks top to bottom	3						
9. Applies top sheet:							
Unfolds sheet	3						
Places wrong side up	3						
Lines up large hem even with top of mattress	3						
Makes mitered corner after tucking in at foot of bed	3						
Tucks to center of bed	3						

Making a Closed Bed	Points Possible	Peer Check		Final Check*		Points Earned**	Comments
		Yes	No	Yes	No		
10. Applies spread:							
Unfolds spread	3						
Places right side up	3						
Lines up top edge even with top of mattress	3						
Makes mitered corner after tucking in at foot of bed	3						
11. Moves to opposite side of the bed	3						
12. Completes bottom sheet	3						
13. Completes drawsheet(s)	3						
14. Completes top sheet	3						
15. Completes spread	3						
16. Removes all wrinkles	2						
17. Inserts pillow in case correctly	3						
18. Places pillow with open end away from door	2						
19. Lowers bed to lowest level	2						
20. Replaces all equipment and leaves area neat and clean	2						
21. Washes hands	2						
22. Records or reports required information	2						
Totals	100						

* Final Check: Instructor or authorized person evaluates.
** Points Earned: Points possible times each "yes" check.

Name _____ Date _____

Evaluated by _____

DIRECTIONS: Practice making an occupied bed according to the criteria listed. When you are ready for your final check, give this sheet to your instructor.

Making an Occupied Bed	Points Possible	Peer Check Yes	No	Final Check* Yes	No	Points Earned**	Comments
1. Assembles equipment and supplies	2						
2. Knocks on door, introduces self, identifies patient, and explains procedure	2						
3. Closes door and screens unit	2						
4. Washes hands and puts on gloves if needed	2						
5. Puts linen in order of use	2						
6. Locks bed to prevent movement	2						
7. Elevates bed to working level	2						
8. Lowers head and foot of bed	2						
9. Lowers siderail (if elevated) – checks opposite rail to be sure it is elevated	2						
10. Covers patient with bath blanket	3						
11. Removes top linen	3						
12. Places linen in hamper/bag/cart	2						
13. Turns patient to opposite side of bed	3						
14. Fanfolds dirty bottom linen to center parallel to patient	3						
15. Applies bottom sheet:							
Places right side up	1						
Lines small hem even with bottom of mattress	1						
Fanfolds at center of bed	1						
Makes mitered corner after tucking in at top	1						
Tucks top to bottom	1						
16. Applies drawsheet:							
Places right side up	1						
Positions 14–16 inches from top of mattress	1						
Fanfolds at center	1						
Tucks securely at side	1						

Making an Occupied Bed	Points Possible	Peer Check		Final Check*		Points Earned**	Comments
		Yes	No	Yes	No		
17. Turns patient after warning about fanfolded linen	3						
18. Elevates siderail if indicated	2						
19. Goes to opposite side of bed	3						
20. Lowers siderail	2						
21. Removes dirty bottom linen	2						
22. Places linen in hamper/bag/cart	2						
23. Completes bottom sheet	3						
24. Completes drawsheet	3						
25. Positions patient in center of bed on back	3						
26. Positions top sheet:							
Places wrong side up	2						
Centers with large hem at top of mattress	2						
27. Removes bath blanket	3						
28. Positions blanket and/or spread	3						
29. Tucks in sheet, blanket, spread at bottom	3						
30. Makes toepleat	3						
31. Makes mitered corner	3						
32. Inserts pillow in pillowcase properly	2						
33. Places pillow on bed with open end away from door	2						
34. Positions patient in correct alignment	2						
35. Elevates siderails (if indicated) and lowers bed to lowest level	2						
36. Places call signal and supplies within patient's reach	2						
37. Replaces equipment and leaves area neat and clean	2						
38. Removes gloves if worn and washes hands	2						
39. Records or reports required information	3						
Totals	100						

* Final Check: Instructor or authorized person evaluates.
** Points Earned: Points possible times each "yes" check.

U N I T 20 : 3 C E v a l u a t i o n S h e e t

Name _____   Date _____

Evaluated by _____

DIRECTIONS: Practice opening a closed bed according to the criteria listed. When you are ready for your final check, give this sheet to your instructor.

Opening a Closed Bed	Points Possible	Peer Check Yes	No	Final Check* Yes	No	Points Earned**	Comments
1. Washes hands	5						
2. Checks closed bed to be sure it is made correctly	6						
3. Locks and elevates bed	6						
4. Puts pillow on chair or overbed table	6						
5. Makes cuff in top linen at head of bed	8						
6. Faces foot of bed	8						
7. Grasps top linen with both hands	8						
8. Fanfolds linen to foot of bed	8						
9. Forms three even layers of folds	8						
10. Positions top fold to face head of bed	8						
11. Places pillow back on bed with open end away from door	7						
12. Checks area before leaving:							
Places call signal within reach	3						
Lowers bed to lowest level	3						
Locks wheels on bed	3						
Leaves area neat and clean	3						
13. Washes hands	5						
14. Records or reports required information	5						
Totals	100						

PROFICIENT

* Final Check: Instructor or authorized person evaluates.
** Points Earned: Points possible times each "yes" check.

Name _____ Date _____

Evaluated by _____

DIRECTIONS: Practice making a bed with a cradle according to the criteria listed. When you are ready for your final check, give this sheet to your instructor.

Placing a Bed Cradle	Points Possible	Peer Check Yes	No	Final Check* Yes	No	Points Earned**	Comments
PROFICIENT							
1. Assembles all equipment and supplies	3						
2. Knocks on door, introduces self, identifies patient, and explains procedure	3						
3. Closes door and screens unit	3						
4. Washes hands and puts on gloves if needed	3						
5. Locks bed to prevent movement	3						
6. Elevates bed to working height	3						
7. Lowers siderail (if elevated) – checks opposite rail to be sure it is elevated	3						
8. Drapes patient with bath blanket	4						
9. Removes soiled top linen	4						
10. Places linen in hamper/bag/cart	4						
11. Places clean bottom sheet and/or drawsheet on bed and completes on both sides	4						
12. Positions cradle correctly	6						
13. Anchors cradle to bed with clamps, gauze, or straps	6						
14. Places top sheet, spread, and/or blanket over the top of the cradle	4						
15. Removes bath blanket	4						
16. Tucks top linen in place	4						
17. Makes fold by lower edge of cradle	4						
18. Makes mitered corner	4						
19. Makes cuff in top linen at head of bed	4						
20. Places clean pillowcase on pillow	3						

Name _____

20:3D (cont.)

Placing a Bed Cradle	Points Possible	Peer Check Yes	No	Final Check* Yes	No	Points Earned**	Comments
21. Positions pillow with open end away from door	3						
22. Positions patient in correct alignment	3						
23. Elevates siderails if indicated and lowers bed to lowest level	3						
24. Places call signal and supplies within reach	3						
25. Checks cradle to be sure linen is away from patient	3						
26. Replaces all equipment and leaves area neat and clean	3						
27. Removes gloves if worn and washes hands	3						
28. Records or reports required information	3						
Totals	100						

* Final Check: Instructor or authorized person evaluates.
** Points Earned: Points possible times each "yes" check.

UNIT 20:4 ADMINISTERING PERSONAL HYGIENE

ASSIGNMENT SHEET

Grade _____ Name _____

INTRODUCTION: Personal hygiene is a term used to describe many aspects of patient care. This assignment will help you review the main facts on the various procedures.

INSTRUCTIONS: Read the information section on Administering Personal Hygiene. In the space provided, print the word(s) that best completes the statement or answers the question.

1. List six (6) types of care that can be included in personal hygiene.

2. What is meant by the term *complete bed bath?*

3. Briefly describe two (2) explanations for a *partial bed bath.*

4. List three (3) reasons for providing oral hygiene.

5. What type of patient is given special oral hygiene?

6. List two (2) reasons for brushing the hair.

7. Why is it important to keep nails clean and filed?

8. If you are permitted to cut fingernails, use _____, not _____, and clip the nails _____.

9. Why is it important to *never* clip toenails?

10. What two (2) types of razors can be used to shave a patient?

   What determines the type razor used?

11. List three (3) purposes for a backrub.

12. If a patient has an injured or weak arm, or if an IV (intravenous solution) is infusing in one arm, how should you remove the gown or pajama top?

13. List five (5) important areas of observations the health assistant should note while administering personal hygiene.

14. Define the following terms.

a. erythema:

b. cyanosis:

c. jaundice:

d. vertigo:

e. dyspnea:

f. diaphoresis:

g. lethargy:

15. List three (3) specific standard precautions that must be observed at all times while administering personal hygiene.

16. Identify three (3) ways to provide privacy for a patient while administering personal hygiene.

17. What would you do in the following situations?

a. While you are giving Mr. McNeil a backrub, you notice a red rash covering his entire back.

b. Mrs. Sanchez is a post-operative patient who had back surgery and is confined to bed for two days. She wants her hair shampooed.

c. Mr. Mollica is on an anticoagulant because he has a blood clot in his leg. Your supervisor told you to shave him with an electric razor. However, Mr. Mollica insists that he wants to use his straight razor because he hates electric razors.

UNIT 20:4A Evaluation Sheet

Name _____ Date _____

Evaluated by _____

DIRECTIONS: Practice administering routine oral hygiene according to the criteria listed. When you are ready for your final check, give this sheet to your instructor.

Providing Routine Oral Hygiene	Points Possible	PROFICIENT Peer Check Yes	No	Final Check* Yes	No	Points Earned**	Comments
1. Checks order or obtains authorization	2						
2. Assembles equipment and supplies	2						
3. Knocks on door, introduces self, identifies patient, and explains procedure	2						
4. Closes door and screens unit for privacy	3						
5. Washes hands and puts on gloves	2						
6. Elevates bed to working level and locks bed	3						
7. Raises head of bed	3						
8. Arranges equipment conveniently	3						
9. Lowers siderail if elevated	3						
10. Drapes patient with bath towel or disposable bed protector	3						
11. Prepares toothbrush:							
Puts water on brush	3						
Puts toothpaste on brush	3						
12. Allows patient to brush but assists as needed:							
Inserts brush carefully	4						
Places brush at angle	4						
Cleans teeth with vibrating motion	4						
13. Assists with rinsing of mouth:							
Offers water to patient	4						
Holds emesis basin under chin	4						
Tells patient to expectorate	4						
Offers tissue to wipe mouth and chin	4						
14. Allows patient to floss or helps with flossing:							
Inserts floss gently	4						
Curves floss to C shape	4						
Uses up and down motion to clean sides of teeth	4						

20:4A (cont.)

Providing Routine Oral Hygiene	Points Possible	Peer Check		Final Check*		Points Earned**	Comments
		Yes	No	Yes	No		
15. Offers mouthwash:							
Mixes mouthwash correctly	4						
Gives mouthwash to patient	4						
Assists with emesis basin and tissues	4						
16. Positions patient in proper body alignment	3						
17. Elevates siderails if indicated and lowers bed to lowest level	3						
18. Places call signal and supplies in reach of patient	3						
19. Cleans and replaces all equipment	2						
20. Removes gloves and washes hands	2						
21. Reports or records required information	3						
Totals	100						

* Final Check: Instructor or authorized person evaluates.
** Points Earned: Points possible times each "yes" check.

UNIT 20:4B Evaluation Sheet

Name _____ Date _____

Evaluated by _____

DIRECTIONS: Practice administering denture care according to the criteria listed. When you are ready for your final check, give this sheet to your instructor.

		PROFICIENT					
Cleaning Dentures	Points Possible	Peer Check Yes	No	Final Check* Yes	No	Points Earned**	Comments
1. Checks orders or obtains authorization	3						
2. Assembles equipment and supplies	3						
3. Knocks on door, introduces self, identifies patient, and explains procedure	3						
4. Closes door and screens unit	3						
5. Washes hands and puts on gloves	3						
6. Elevates bed to working height and locks bed	3						
7. Raises head of bed	3						
8. Lowers siderail if elevated	3						
9. Obtains dentures from patient – assists as needed	5						
10. Places dentures in cup	5						
11. Elevates siderail if indicated	3						
12. Lines sink with paper towels	5						
13. Uses warm water to clean dentures	5						
14. Brushes all surfaces	5						
15. Handles dentures carefully	5						
16. Rinses dentures in cool water	5						
17. Places clean dentures in cool water in denture cup	5						
18. Returns to bedside and lowers siderail if elevated	3						
19. Assists patient with mouthwash and allows patient to brush gums if desired	5						
20. Returns dentures to patient or stores in labeled cup	5						
21. Positions patient in correct alignment	3						
22. Elevates siderails if indicated and lowers bed to lowest level	3						
23. Places supplies and call signal within reach	3						
24. Cleans and replaces all equipment	3						
25. Removes gloves and washes hands	3						
26. Reports or records required information	5						
Totals	100						

* Final Check: Instructor or authorized person evaluates.
** Points Earned: Points possible times each "yes" check.

UNIT 20:4C Evaluation Sheet

Name _____ Date _____

Evaluated by _____

DIRECTIONS: Practice administering special mouth care according to the criteria listed. When you are ready for your final check, give this sheet to your instructor.

	Points Possible	Peer Check Yes	Peer Check No	Final Check* Yes	Final Check* No	Points Earned**	Comments
Giving Special Mouth Care (PROFICIENT)							
1. Checks order or obtains authorization	3						
2. Assembles equipment and supplies	3						
3. Knocks on door, introduces self, identifies patient, and explains procedure	3						
4. Closes door and screens unit	3						
5. Washes hands and puts on gloves	4						
6. Elevates bed to working level, locks bed, lowers siderail if elevated, and raises head of bed	4						
7. Positions patient with head to side	5						
8. Drapes area with bath towel or underpad	5						
9. Opens prepackaged swabs	5						
10. Cleans the following areas of the mouth:							
Teeth	5						
Gums	5						
Tongue	5						
Roof of mouth	5						
11. Uses gentle motion to clean	5						
12. Discards used swabs in plastic bag and uses fresh swabs as needed until entire mouth is clean	5						
13. Uses applicators with water or mouthwash to rinse mouth	5						
14. Discards used applicators in plastic bag	5						
15. Applies lubricant to lips and tongue	5						
16. Positions patient in correct alignment	3						
17. Elevates siderails if indicated and lowers bed to lowest level	3						

20:4C (cont.)

Giving Special Mouth Care	Points Possible	Peer Check		Final Check*		Points Earned**	Comments
		Yes	No	Yes	No		
18. Places call signal within reach	3						
19. Cleans and replaces all equipment	3						
20. Removes gloves and washes hands	4						
21. Reports or records required information	4						
Totals	100						

* Final Check: Instructor or authorized person evaluates.
** Points Earned: Points possible times each "yes" check.

Name _____   Date _____

Evaluated by _____

DIRECTIONS: Practice administering hair care according to the criteria listed. When you are ready for your final check, give this sheet to your instructor.

PROFICIENT

Administering Daily Hair Care	Points Possible	Peer Check Yes	No	Final Check* Yes	No	Points Earned**	Comments
1. Checks orders or obtains authorization	2						
2. Assembles supplies	2						
3. Knocks on door, introduces self, identifies patient, and explains procedure	3						
4. Closes door and screens unit	3						
5. Washes hands	3						
6. Elevates bed to working level and locks bed	3						
7. Raises head of bed	3						
8. Lowers siderail if elevated	3						
9. Covers pillow with towel	4						
10. Positions patient	4						
11. Parts or sections hair	5						
12. Combs or brushes thoroughly	5						
13. Combs with hand between comb and scalp	5						
14. Uses alcohol to remove tangles from oily hair	5						
15. Uses petroleum jelly to remove tangles from dry hair	5						
16. Combs all parts of head:							
Combs both sides	4						
Combs top	4						
Combs back	4						
17. Arranges hair attractively or braids long hair	5						
18. Observes condition of hair and scalp	5						
19. Positions patient in correct alignment	3						
20. Elevates siderails if indicated and lowers bed to lowest level	3						

Name _____

20:4D (cont.)

Administering Daily Hair Care	Points Possible	Peer Check		Final Check*		Points Earned**	Comments
		Yes	No	Yes	No		
21. Places call signal and supplies within reach	3						
22. Cleans and replaces all equipment	3						
23. Washes comb and brush as necessary	3						
24. Washes hands	3						
25. Records or reports required information	5						
Totals	100						

* Final Check: Instructor or authorized person evaluates.
** Points Earned: Points possible times each "yes" check.

Name _____ Date _____

Evaluated by _____

DIRECTIONS: Practice administering nail care according to the criteria listed. When you are ready for your final check, give this sheet to your instructor.

PROFICIENT

Providing Nail Care	Points Possible	Peer Check Yes	No	Final Check* Yes	No	Points Earned**	Comments
1. Checks order or obtains authorization and checks agency policy for cutting fingernails	4						
2. Assembles all equipment and supplies	3						
3. Knocks on door, introduces self, identifies patient, and explains procedure	3						
4. Closes door and screens unit	3						
5. Washes hands	3						
6. Elevates bed to working level and locks bed	3						
7. Lowers siderail if elevated	3						
8. Soaks nails in soapy water	7						
9. Cleans nails with blunt end of orange stick	7						
10. If allowed, uses nails clippers to cut long fingernails straight across, but never cuts toenails	7						
11. Files nails:							
Uses short strokes	6						
Works from side to top	6						
Files straight across	6						
Smooths rough edges with smooth side of emeryboard	6						
12. Applies lotion or other emollient to nails	7						
13. Applies lotion to hands and feet	7						
14. Positions patient in correct alignment	3						
15. Elevates siderails if indicated and lowers bed to lowest level	3						
16. Places call signal and supplies within reach	3						
17. Cleans and replaces all equipment	3						
18. Washes hands	3						
19. Records or reports required information	4						
Totals	100						

* Final Check: Instructor or authorized person evaluates.
** Points Earned: Points possible times each "yes" check.

UNIT 20:4F Evaluation Sheet

Name _____ Date _____

Evaluated by _____

DIRECTIONS: Practice administering a backrub according to the criteria listed. When you are ready for your final check, give this sheet to your instructor.

PROFICIENT

Giving a Backrub	Points Possible	Peer Check Yes	No	Final Check* Yes	No	Points Earned**	Comments
1. Obtains authorization or checks orders	3						
2. Assembles equipment and supplies	2						
3. Knocks on door, introduces self, identifies patient, and explains procedure	3						
4. Closes door and screens unit	2						
5. Washes hands and puts on gloves if necessary	2						
6. Elevates bed to working level and locks bed	2						
7. Lowers siderail if elevated	2						
8. Positions patient in prone position or on side	4						
9. Places towel lengthwise to protect linen	4						
10. Washes and dries back	4						
11. Warms lotion in hand or places in basin of warm water	4						
12. Performs 1st motion:							
Applies long strokes from base of spine up back	3						
Goes around shoulders and down back	3						
Goes around buttocks to starting point	3						
Repeats four times	3						
13. Performs 2nd motion:							
Repeats long upward stroke	3						
Uses circular motion on downward strokes	3						
Goes around buttocks and back to starting point	3						
Repeats four times	3						

Giving a Backrub	Points Possible	Peer Check		Final Check*		Points Earned**	Comments
		Yes	No	Yes	No		
14. Performs 3rd motion one time:							
Repeats long upward stroke	3						
Uses small circles on downward strokes	3						
Goes around buttocks and back to starting point	3						
Uses palms of hands and applies firm pressure	3						
15. Performs 4th motion:							
Repeats initial strokes in first motion	3						
Rubs 3–5 minutes	3						
16. Performs 5th motion:							
Uses up and down motion	3						
Continues for 1–2 minutes	3						
17. Dries back with towel	3						
18. Changes gown if necessary and straightens linen	3						
19. Positions patient in correct alignment	3						
20. Elevates siderails if indicated and lowers bed to lowest level	2						
21. Places call signal and supplies in reach	2						
22. Cleans and replaces all equipment	2						
23. Removes gloves if worn and washes hands	2						
24. Records or reports required information	4						
Totals	100						

* Final Check: Instructor or authorized person evaluates.
** Points Earned: Points possible times each "yes" check.

U N I T 20:4G E v a l u a t i o n S h e e t

Name _____ Date _____

Evaluated by _____

DIRECTIONS: Practice shaving a patient according to the criteria listed. When you are ready for your final check, give this sheet to your instructor.

	Shaving a Patient	Points Possible	Peer Check Yes	Peer Check No	Final Check* Yes	Final Check* No	Points Earned**	Comments
				PROFICIENT				
1.	Checks order or obtains authorization	2						
2.	Assembles equipment and supplies	2						
3.	Checks razor for nicks or damaged edge	4						
4.	Knocks on door, introduces self, identifies patient, and explains procedure	2						
5.	Closes door and screens unit	2						
6.	Washes hands and puts on gloves if needed	2						
7.	Elevates bed to working height and locks bed	2						
8.	Elevates head of bed	2						
9.	Lowers siderail if elevated	2						
10.	Positions patient	2						
11.	Drapes shoulders and chest with towel	3						
12.	Moistens area with warm water	4						
13.	Applies lather to small area	4						
14.	Shaves as follows:							
	Holds skin taut	4						
	Shaves in direction of hair growth	4						
	Uses firm, short strokes	4						
	Rinses razor	4						
15.	Shaves both cheeks	4						
16.	Shaves chin area	4						
17.	Shaves nostril area	4						
18.	Washes and dries face	4						
19.	Applies aftershave if desired	4						

Shaving a Patient	Points Possible	Peer Check		Final Check*		Points Earned**	Comments
		Yes	No	Yes	No		
20. Uses electric razor:							
Reads directions	4						
Holds skin taut	4						
Uses circular or short stroke type motion	4						
Cleans razor with brush	3						
21. Positions patient in correct alignment	2						
22. Elevates siderails if indicated and lowers bed to lowest level	2						
23. Places call signal and supplies within reach	2						
24. Discards blade or disposable razor in sharps container	2						
25. Cleans and replaces equipment	2						
26. Removes gloves if worn and washes hands	2						
27. Records or reports required information	4						
Totals	100						

* Final Check: Instructor or authorized person evaluates.
** Points Earned: Points possible times each "yes" check.

Name _____ Date _____

Evaluated by _____

DIRECTIONS: Practice changing bedclothes according to the criteria listed. When you are ready for your fina
check, give this sheet to your instructor.

Changing a Patient's Gown or Pajamas	Points Possible	Peer Check Yes	No	Final Check* Yes	No	Points Earned**	Comments
1. Checks orders or obtains authorization	3						
2. Assembles equipment and supplies	2						
3. Knocks on door, introduces self, identifies patient, and explains procedure	3						
4. Closes door and screens unit	3						
5. Washes hands and puts on gloves if needed	3						
6. Elevates bed to correct working level and locks bed	3						
7. Lowers siderail if elevated	3						
8. Drapes patient with towel or bath blanket	4						
9. Unties or unbuttons soiled bedclothes	4						
10. Loosens bedclothes	4						
11. Removes sleeve from unaffected arm first	5						
12. Removes sleeve from affected arm last	5						
13. Removes pajama pants correctly	5						
14. Unfolds clean bedclothes and places over patient	5						
15. Puts sleeve on affected arm first	5						
16. Puts sleeve on unaffected arm last	5						
17. Smooths bedclothes and removes wrinkles	5						
18. Ties or buttons correctly	4						
Avoids knots on bony areas	4						
19. Puts on pajama pants correctly	5						
20. Positions patient in correct alignment	3						
21. Elevates siderails if indicated and lowers bed to lowest level	3						
22. Places call signal and supplies within reach	3						
23. Places soiled clothes in hamper or area designated by patient	3						
24. Removes gloves if worn and washes hands	3						
25. Records or reports required information	5						
Totals	100						

PROFICIENT

* Final Check: Instructor or authorized person evaluates.
** Points Earned: Points possible times each "yes" check.

UNIT 20:4I Evaluation Sheet

Name _____ Date _____

Evaluated by _____

DIRECTIONS: Practice administering a complete bed bath according to the criteria listed. When you are ready for your final check, give this sheet to your instructor.

PROFICIENT

Giving a Complete Bed Bath	Points Possible	Peer Check Yes	No	Final Check* Yes	No	Points Earned**	Comments
1. Obtains authorization or checks order	2						
2. Assembles equipment and supplies	2						
3. Knocks on door, introduces self, identifies patient, and explains procedure	2						
4. Closes door and screens unit	2						
5. Arranges all equipment and supplies conveniently	2						
6. Washes hands and puts on gloves if needed	2						
7. Elevates bed to correct working level and locks bed	2						
8. Lowers siderail if elevated	2						
9. Drapes patient with bath blanket	2						
10. Administers oral hygiene	3						
11. Shaves patient if needed	3						
12. Obtains basin of bath water at 105°F or 40.6°C	3						
13. Removes bedclothes properly	2						
14. Makes wash mitten	3						
15. Washes body correctly:							
Washes eyes	4						
Washes face, neck, and ears	4						
Washes arms	4						
Gives nail care to fingernails	3						
Washes chest	4						
Washes abdomen	4						
Washes legs and feet	4						
Administers nail care to toenails	3						
16. Changes water after elevating siderails if indicated	3						

20:4I (cont.)

Giving a Complete Bed Bath	Points Possible	Peer Check		Final Check*		Points Earned**	Comments
		Yes	No	Yes	No		
17. Lowers siderails if elevated	2						
18. Washes back	4						
19. Administers backrub	3						
20. Washes or helps patient wash perineal area:							
Positions patient on back	2						
Washes with front to back direction on female	2						
Washes penis top to bottom and washes under scrotal area in male	2						
21. Replaces bedclothes	2						
22. Administers hair care	3						
23. Changes linen on bed	2						
24. Positions patient in proper alignment	2						
25. Elevates siderails if indicated and lowers bed to lowest level	2						
26. Places call signal and other supplies within reach of patient	2						
27. Cleans and replaces all equipment	2						
28. Removes gloves if worn and washes hands	2						
29. Records or reports required information	3						
Totals	100						

* Final Check: Instructor or authorized person evaluates.
** Points Earned: Points possible times each "yes" check.

UNIT 20:4J Evaluation Sheet

Name _____   Date _____

Evaluated by _____

DIRECTIONS: Practice assisting with a tub bath/shower according to the criteria listed. When you are ready for your final check, give this sheet to your instructor.

Helping a Patient Take a Tub Bath or Shower	Points Possible	Peer Check Yes	No	Final Check* Yes	No	Points Earned**	Comments
1. Obtains authorization or checks order	4						
2. Assembles equipment and supplies	3						
3. Knocks on door, introduces self, identifies patient, and explains procedure	3						
4. Washes hands	3						
5. Prepares tub/shower area:							
Takes supplies to area	5						
Wears gloves to clean and disinfect tub/shower	5						
Places bathmat on floor	5						
Fills tub 1/2 full with water at 105°F or 40.6°C	5						
6. Assists patient to tub/shower area	5						
7. Assists patient with undressing and helps into tub or shower	5						
8. Instructs patient on how to use call signal	5						
9. Remains with patient or checks at frequent intervals	5						
10. Dries patient as needed	5						
11. Helps patient to dress if necessary	5						
12. Takes patient back to bedside area	5						
13. Administers backrub	5						
14. Assists with hair and/or nail care if necessary	5						
15. Positions patient in correct alignment	3						
16. Elevates siderails if indicated and lowers bed to lowest level	3						
17. Places call signal and supplies within reach	3						
18. Wears gloves to clean and disinfect tub/shower area	3						
19. Replaces all equipment	3						
20. Removes gloves and washes hands	3						
21. Records or reports required information	4						
Totals	100						

* Final Check: Instructor or authorized person evaluates.
** Points Earned: Points possible times each "yes" check.

UNIT 20:5A MEASURING AND RECORDING INTAKE AND OUTPUT

ASSIGNMENT SHEET

Grade _____ Name _____

INTRODUCTION: The purpose of this assignment is to help you become familiar with measurement of liquids. Because many measurements in the health fields are done in the metric system, it is important that you know how to use this system.

INSTRUCTIONS: Use separate measuring containers provided to determine how much liquid is in the following listed containers. All containers are marked. Be sure you have the correct container. Measure as accurately as possible. Each problem ends with the metric measures (milliliter and cubic centimeter).

1. Measure the liquid in a teaspoon and tablespoon to see how many cubic centimeters or milliliters each one contains.

    1 teaspoon   = _____ cc or mL

    1 tablespoon   = _____ cc or mL

2. Measure the liquid in a juice glass to determine the following:

    1 juice glass   = _____ ounces

                  or _____ cc or mL

3. Measure the liquid in a medium glass to determine the following:

    1 medium glass   = _____ ounces

                  or _____ cc or mL

4. Measure the liquid in a large glass to determine the following:

    1 large glass   = _____ ounces

                  or _____ cc or mL

5. Measure the liquid in a coffee cup to determine the following:

    1 coffee cup   = _____ ounces

                  or _____ cc or mL

6. Measure the liquid in a small bowl to determine the following:

    1 small bowl   = _____ ounces

                  or _____ cc or mL

449

7. Measure the liquid in a large bowl to determine the following:

    1 large bowl   = _____ ounces

                      or _____ cc or mL

8. Measure the liquid in a milk carton to determine the following:

    1 milk carton   = _____ cups

                      or _____ ounces

                      or _____ cc or mL

9. Measure the liquid in a water pitcher and determine the following:

    1 water pitcher   = _____ ounces

                      or _____ cups

                      or _____ pints

                      or _____ quarts

                      or _____ cc or mL

10. Measure the liquid in a gallon jug to determine the following:

    1 gallon jug   = _____ cups

                      or _____ pints

                      or _____ quarts

                      or _____ ounces

                      or _____ cc or mL

11. Measure the liquid in an alcohol bottle to determine the following:

    1 alcohol bottle = _____ cups

                      or _____ pints

                      or _____ ounces

                      or _____ cc or mL

12. Measure the liquid in an eye-dropper bottle to determine the following:

    1 eye-dropper bottle = _____ gtts (drops)

                      or _____ Tbsp (tablespoons)

                      or _____ ounces

                      or _____ cc or mL

UNIT 20:5B RECORDING INTAKE AND OUTPUT

ASSIGNMENT SHEET # 1

Grade _____ Name _____

INTRODUCTION: Dr. Marandez admitted Sam Jones for stomach surgery. Mr. Jones was admitted to room 236 of Ram Hospital. After surgery, Mr. Jones was placed on I and O. The following things occurred during the first 24 hours.

INSTRUCTIONS: Using the text procedure sheet and the measurements on the metric conversion chart as references, enter the following information on an I and O record. Check all figures carefully. Total all 8 hr and 24 hr columns.

UNIT AND MEASUREMENT			CONTAINER AND MEASUREMENT		
15 drops	=	1 cc	1 juice glass	=	120 cc
1 teaspoon	=	5 cc	1 water glass	=	180 cc
1 tablespoon	=	15 cc	1 large glass	=	240 cc
1 ounce	=	30 cc	1 coffee cup	=	120 cc
1 pint	=	500 cc	1 small bowl	=	120 cc
1 quart	=	1000 cc	1 soup bowl	=	200 cc

8 AM:	Ate breakfast	2 cups coffee (Sanka)	5 PM:	Supper	1 small bowl jello
		1 glass juice			1/2 soup bowl broth
		1 small bowl cereal			2 crackers
		1 small bowl jello	6 PM:	Drank 1 large glass of juice	
10 AM:	Used bedpan	Urine 400 cc	8 PM:	Used bedpan	Urine 480 cc
12 Noon:	Ate lunch	1 large glass milk	10 PM:	Drank 1 glass water	
		1 soup bowl broth	11 PM:	IV had absorbed 750 cc since 3 PM	
		1 small bowl custard	2 AM:	Drank 1 glass water	
		1 small bowl jello	4 AM:	Used bedpan twice	Urine 550 cc
1 PM:	Drank 1 glass water				Liquid BM 300 cc –
2 PM:	Used bedpan	550 cc urine			light brown
		1 formed BM	6 AM:	Drank 1 glass water	
3 PM:	Drank 1 glass water			IV Had absorbed 850 cc since 11 PM	
	IV - had absorbed 800 cc since 7 AM				
4 PM:	Vomited 550 cc dark green liquid				

Grade _____ Name _____

INTAKE AND OUTPUT RECORD													
Family Name				**First Name**		**Attending Physician**			**Room No.**		**Hosp. No.**		
Date	**INTAKE**				**OUTPUT**					**OTHER**			**REMARKS**
TIME	Oral	I.V.	Blood		Urine	Tube	Emesis	Feces					
7 - 8 a.m.													
8 - 9 a.m.													
9 - 10 a.m.													
10 - 11 a.m.													
11 - 12 noon													
12 - 1 p.m.													
1 - 2 p.m.													
2 - 3 p.m.													
8 HOUR TOTAL													
3 - 4 p.m.													
4 - 5 p.m.													
5 - 6 p.m.													
6 - 7 p.m.													
7 - 8 p.m.													
8 - 9 p.m.													
9 - 10 p.m.													
10 - 11 p.m.													
8 HOUR TOTAL													
11 - 12 p.m.													
12 - 1 a.m.													
1 - 2 a.m.													
2 - 3 a.m.													
3 - 4 a.m.													
4 - 5 a.m.													
5 - 6 a.m.													
6 - 7 a.m.													
8 HOUR TOTAL													
24 HOUR TOTAL	**TOTAL INTAKE**				**TOTAL OUTPUT**								

UNIT 20:5B RECORDING INTAKE AND OUTPUT

ASSIGNMENT SHEET # 2

Grade _____ Name _____

INTRODUCTION: Mr. Fred Wray is a patient who had bowel surgery. A catheter is in place for urine. His urinary output is measured every hour. He has an IV in place. He is allowed ice chips and ginger ale in small sips. Otherwise he is NPO. A nasogastric tube is in place to drain stomach fluids. It is connected to a suction machine and drained into a jar. At times the tube is irrigated so it will not clog. Mr. Wray is under the care of Dr. Pease, and he is in room 2851.

INSTRUCTIONS: Using the measurements on the metric conversion chart, record all of the following on an I and O record. Total all 8 hr and 24 hr columns.

UNIT AND MEASUREMENT			CONTAINER AND MEASUREMENT		
15 drops	=	1 cc	1 juice glass	=	120 cc
1 teaspoon	=	5 cc	1 water glass	=	180 cc
1 tablespoon	=	15 cc	1 large glass	=	240 cc
1 ounce	=	30 cc	1 coffee cup	=	120 cc
1 pint	=	500 cc	1 small bowl	=	120 cc
1 quart	=	1000 cc	1 soup bowl	=	200 cc

1. Urine measured hourly:

7 AM	30 cc		7 PM	40 cc
8	40 cc		8	30 cc
9	25 cc		9	25 cc
10	30 cc		10	30 cc
11	35 cc		11	10 cc
12 Noon	40 cc		12 MN	None
1 PM	25 cc		1 AM	5 cc
2	25 cc		2	5 cc
3	15 cc		3	None
4	30 cc		4	10 cc
5	10 cc		5	15 cc
6 PM	20 cc		6 AM	20 cc

2. The nasogastric tube was irrigated with normal saline (NS):

7 AM	20 cc		12 MN	20 cc
12 Noon	30 cc		2 AM	10 cc
4 PM	10 cc		4 AM	10 cc
8 PM	20 cc		6 AM	10 cc

453

3. Nasogastric tube drainage measured:

2 PM	750 cc greenish
10 PM	990 cc greenish
6 AM	650 cc golden

4. IV intake recorded:

2 PM	1000 cc
10 PM	950 cc
6 AM	1050 cc

5. Intake in ice cubes (Note: 1 ice cube equals 5 cc)

7 AM	2 ice cubes		7 PM	2 ice cubes
9 AM	1 ice cube		12 MN	3 ice cubes
12 Noon	3 ice cubes		4 AM	2 ice cubes
3 PM	2 ice cubes			

6. Ginger ale: small sips as follows:

1 tablespoon at each of the following times:

8 AM, 11 AM, 1 PM, 5 PM, 10 PM, 1 AM, 3 AM, and 5 AM

7. Vomited 100 cc clear liquid at 1 PM

Grade _____ Name _____

INTAKE AND OUTPUT RECORD													
Family Name				**First Name**			**Attending Physician**		**Room No.**			**Hosp. No.**	
Date	**INTAKE**				**OUTPUT**					**OTHER**			**REMARKS**
TIME	Oral	I.V.	Blood		Urine	Tube	Emesis	Feces					
7 - 8 a.m.													
8 - 9 a.m.													
9 - 10 a.m.													
10 - 11 a.m.													
11 - 12 noon													
12 - 1 p.m.													
1 - 2 p.m.													
2 - 3 p.m.													
8 HOUR TOTAL													
3 - 4 p.m.													
4 - 5 p.m.													
5 - 6 p.m.													
6 - 7 p.m.													
7 - 8 p.m.													
8 - 9 p.m.													
9 - 10 p.m.													
10 - 11 p.m.													
8 HOUR TOTAL													
11 - 12 p.m.													
12 - 1 a.m.													
1 - 2 a.m.													
2 - 3 a.m.													
3 - 4 a.m.													
4 - 5 a.m.													
5 - 6 a.m.													
6 - 7 a.m.													
8 HOUR TOTAL													
24 HOUR TOTAL													
	TOTAL INTAKE				**TOTAL OUTPUT**								

UNIT 20:5B RECORDING INTAKE AND OUTPUT

ASSIGNMENT SHEET # 3

Grade _____ Name _____

INTRODUCTION: Tamika Perry, a patient of Dr. Kowalski, had a gastrectomy (removal of the stomach). A nasogastric tube is in site to drain all fluids. It is connected to suction and irrigated at times. Intake is limited to sips of ginger ale and ice cubes.

INSTRUCTIONS: Using the measurements on the metric conversion chart, record the following information on an I and O record. Record all 8 hr and 24 hr totals.

UNIT AND MEASUREMENT			CONTAINER AND MEASUREMENT		
15 drops	=	1 cc	1 juice glass	=	120 cc
1 teaspoon	=	5 cc	1 water glass	=	180 cc
1 tablespoon	=	15 cc	1 large glass	=	240 cc
1 ounce	=	30 cc	1 coffee cup	=	120 cc
1 pint	=	500 cc	1 small bowl	=	120 cc
1 quart	=	1000 cc	1 soup bowl	=	200 cc

1. Nasogastric tube irrigated with normal saline (N.S.) as follows:

7 AM	10 cc	1 AM	10 cc
11 AM	10 cc	4 AM	15 cc
4 PM	10 cc		
9 PM	15 cc		

2. IV was absorbed as follows:

12 Noon	400 cc	10 PM	200 cc
2 PM	150 cc	3 AM	400 cc
8 PM	500 cc	6 AM	200 cc

3. Urine output was as follows:

9 AM	400 cc	9 PM	550 cc
1 PM	250 cc	1 AM	400 cc
5 PM	375 cc	5 AM	200 cc

4. The patient had greenish liquid stool as follows:

11 AM	300 cc	5 PM	200 cc	3 AM	750 cc

5. The nasogastric tube suction jar was emptied on each shift. Measurements are as follows:

2 PM	780 cc greenish liquid
10 PM	550 cc golden brown liquid
6 AM	625 cc golden brown liquid

6. Water intake was as follows:

8 AM	2 Tbsp	5 PM	3 Tbsp	3 AM	1 Tbsp
1 PM	1 Tbsp	12 MN	2 Tbsp		

7. Sips of ginger ale were taken as follows:

9 AM	1/2 juice glass	8 PM	1 ounce
12 Noon	1/2 large glass	1 AM	2 ounces
6 PM	1 juice glass	4 AM	1/2 water glass

8. The patient vomited several times. Amounts as follows:

2 PM	100 cc clear liquid
9 PM	130 cc reddish brown liquid
5 AM	200 cc golden green liquid

9. Ice cubes were given as follows: (Note: 1 cube = 5 cc)

2 ice cubes at 7 AM, 12 N, 4 PM, 10 PM and 2 AM

Grade _____ Name _____

INTAKE AND OUTPUT RECORD													
Family Name			**First Name**		**Attending Physician**			**Room No.**			**Hosp. No.**		
Date	**INTAKE**				**OUTPUT**				**OTHER**				**REMARKS**
TIME	Oral	I.V.	Blood		Urine	Tube	Emesis	Feces					
7 - 8 a.m.													
8 - 9 a.m.													
9 - 10 a.m.													
10 - 11 a.m.													
11 - 12 noon													
12 - 1 p.m.													
1 - 2 p.m.													
2 - 3 p.m.													
8 HOUR TOTAL													
3 - 4 p.m.													
4 - 5 p.m.													
5 - 6 p.m.													
6 - 7 p.m.													
7 - 8 p.m.													
8 - 9 p.m.													
9 - 10 p.m.													
10 - 11 p.m.													
8 HOUR TOTAL													
11 - 12 p.m.													
12 - 1 a.m.													
1 - 2 a.m.													
2 - 3 a.m.													
3 - 4 a.m.													
4 - 5 a.m.													
5 - 6 a.m.													
6 - 7 a.m.													
8 HOUR TOTAL													
24 HOUR TOTAL													
	TOTAL INTAKE				**TOTAL OUTPUT**								

UNIT 20:5B RECORDING INTAKE AND OUTPUT

ASSIGNMENT SHEET # 4

Grade _____ Name _____

NOTE: Anyone who gets this 100% correct will not be required to do anymore I and O records.

INTRODUCTION: Mr. John Wreckless was admitted to room 1835 of Ram Hospital by Dr. Santoro after being in an automobile accident. After emergency surgery, he was admitted to intensive care. Two IVs were infusing. A Hemovac drainage unit was in the surgical site to remove drainage. A nasogastric tube was in place and connected to suction drainage. A Foley catheter was in place to drain urine.

INSTRUCTIONS: Using the measurements on the metric conversion chart, record the following information on an I and O record. Record all 8 hr and 24 hr totals.

UNIT AND MEASUREMENT			CONTAINER AND MEASUREMENT		
15 drops	=	1 cc	1 juice glass	=	120 cc
1 teaspoon	=	5 cc	1 water glass	=	180 cc
1 tablespoon	=	15 cc	1 large glass	=	240 cc
1 ounce	=	30 cc	1 coffee cup	=	120 cc
1 pint	=	500 cc	1 small bowl	=	120 cc
1 quart	=	1000 cc	1 soup bowl	=	200 cc

1. IV number 1 was absorbed as follows:

10 AM	1 pint blood	2 AM	1 pint plasma
2 PM	500 cc saline	6 AM	200 cc saline
8 PM	100 cc saline		

2. IV number 2 was absorbed as follows:

2 PM	400 cc	10 PM	600 cc	6 AM	600 cc

3. The nasogastric tube was irrigated with normal saline:

   10 cc at 10 AM, 5 PM, 9 PM, 4 AM

   15 cc at 1 PM, 1 AM, and 5 AM

4. Nasogastric tube drainage was as stated:

2 PM	800 cc reddish brown	6 AM	400 cc greenish
10 PM	750 cc golden brown		

5. Meals were as follows:

8 AM	Breakfast:	1 cup tea, 1/2 glass juice, and 1 small bowl broth
12 Noon	Lunch:	1/2 cup tea, 1/2 soup bowl broth, and 1 small bowl jello
5 PM	Supper:	1 glass juice, 1 small bowl jello, and 1/2 small bowl broth

6. Hemovac drainage was measured as follows:

2 PM	20 cc reddish	6 AM	10 cc pink serous
10 PM	15 cc pink serous		

7. Ice cubes were given as follows: (Note: 1 cube = 5 cc)

1 cube at 9 AM, 1 PM, 3 PM, 7 PM, and 2 AM

2 cubes at 11 AM, 4 PM, 10 PM, and 4 AM

8. Ginger ale was given as follows:

1 juice glass at 10 AM, 2 PM, and 9 PM

1/2 large glass at 6 PM and 5 AM

9. Water was given as follows:

1 juice glass at 8 PM and 3 AM

1/2 water glass at 7 AM, 4 PM, and 12 MN

10. Urine drainage was as follows:

10 AM	800 cc	10 PM	940 cc	6 AM	160 cc
2 PM	600 cc	2 AM	850 cc		

11. Emesis occurred as follows:

12 Noon	200 cc	clear liquid
3 AM	350 cc	greenish liquid

12. Liquid stool, light brown:

4 PM	300 cc	11 PM	250 cc

Grade _____ Name _____

INTAKE AND OUTPUT RECORD														
Family Name				**First Name**			**Attending Physician**		**Room No.**		**Hosp. No.**			
Date	**INTAKE**				**OUTPUT**					**OTHER**				**REMARKS**
TIME	Oral	I.V.	Blood		Urine	Tube	Emesis	Feces						
7 - 8 a.m.														
8 - 9 a.m.														
9 - 10 a.m.														
10 - 11 a.m.														
11 - 12 noon														
12 - 1 p.m.														
1 - 2 p.m.														
2 - 3 p.m.														
8 HOUR TOTAL														
3 - 4 p.m.														
4 - 5 p.m.														
5 - 6 p.m.														
6 - 7 p.m.														
7 - 8 p.m.														
8 - 9 p.m.														
9 - 10 p.m.														
10 - 11 p.m.														
8 HOUR TOTAL														
11 - 12 p.m.														
12 - 1 a.m.														
1 - 2 a.m.														
2 - 3 a.m.														
3 - 4 a.m.														
4 - 5 a.m.														
5 - 6 a.m.														
6 - 7 a.m.														
8 HOUR TOTAL														
24 HOUR TOTAL	**TOTAL INTAKE**				**TOTAL OUTPUT**									

UNIT 20:5B RECORDING INTAKE AND OUTPUT

ASSIGNMENT SHEET # 5

Grade _____ Name _____

INTRODUCTION: Maranda O'Connor, a patient of Dr. Schmidt, was admitted to intensive care at Ram Hospital with a high fever and nausea and vomiting. A nasogastric tube was inserted and connected to suction drainage. An IV was started. She was allowed clear liquids and ice chips by mouth.

INSTRUCTIONS: Using the measurements on the metric conversion chart, record the following information on an I and O record. Record all 8 hr and 24 hr totals.

UNIT AND MEASUREMENT	CONTAINER AND MEASUREMENT
15 drops = 1 cc	1 juice glass = 120 cc
1 teaspoon = 5 cc	1 water glass = 180 cc
1 tablespoon = 15 cc	1 large glass = 240 cc
1 ounce = 30 cc	1 coffee cup = 120 cc
1 pint = 500 cc	1 small bowl = 120 cc
1 quart = 1000 cc	1 soup bowl = 200 cc

1. IV of 5% D/W was absorbed as follows:

   | 10 AM | 200 cc | 8 PM | 450 cc | 2 AM | 100 cc |
   | 2 PM | 550 cc | 10 PM | 100 cc | 6 AM | 200 cc |

2. The nasogastric tube was irrigated with normal saline as follows:

   | 10 AM | 10 cc | 5 PM | 15 cc | 2 AM | 10 cc |
   | 1 PM | 10 cc | 9 PM | 10 cc | 5 AM | 10 cc |

3. Nasogastric tube drainage was measured as follows:

   | 2 PM | 550 cc greenish brown | 6 AM | 450 cc greenish |
   | 10 PM | 200 cc golden brown | | |

4. Meals were as follows:

8 AM	Breakfast:	1 glass juice, 1/2 small bowl broth, 1 small bowl jello
12 Noon	Lunch:	1 large glass juice, 1 soup bowl broth, and 2 small bowls jello
5 PM	Supper:	1 glass juice, 1 soup bowl broth, and 1 small bowl jello

5. Ice cubes were given as follows: (Note: 1 ice cube = 5 cc)

   1 ice cube at 9 AM, 11 AM, 3 PM, and 10 PM

   2 ice cubes at 12 N, 4 PM, 12 MN, and 2 AM

   3 ice cubes at 2 PM and 5 PM

6. Ginger ale as follows:

   1 juice glass at 10 AM and 7 PM

   1/2 water glass at 1 PM and 9 PM

7. Water as follows:

    1/2 water glass at 7 AM and 6 PM

    1 water glass at 1 AM and 5 AM

8. Urine output was as follows:

10 AM	400 cc	10 PM	qs Patient incontinent
1 PM	550 cc	1 AM	500 cc
5 PM	400 cc	4 AM	650 cc

9. Emesis was as follows:

9 AM	200 cc clear liquid
7 PM	300 cc brownish liquid

10. Stool was as follows:

8 AM	1 formed brown stool
7 PM	200 cc brown liquid
2 AM	300 cc brown liquid

Grade _____ Name _____

INTAKE AND OUTPUT RECORD													
Family Name				**First Name**		**Attending Physician**			**Room No.**		**Hosp. No.**		
Date	**INTAKE**				**OUTPUT**					**OTHER**			**REMARKS**
TIME	Oral	I.V.	Blood		Urine	Tube	Emesis	Feces					
7 - 8 a.m.													
8 - 9 a.m.													
9 - 10 a.m.													
10 - 11 a.m.													
11 - 12 noon													
12 - 1 p.m.													
1 - 2 p.m.													
2 - 3 p.m.													
8 HOUR TOTAL													
3 - 4 p.m.													
4 - 5 p.m.													
5 - 6 p.m.													
6 - 7 p.m.													
7 - 8 p.m.													
8 - 9 p.m.													
9 - 10 p.m.													
10 - 11 p.m.													
8 HOUR TOTAL													
11 - 12 p.m.													
12 - 1 a.m.													
1 - 2 a.m.													
2 - 3 a.m.													
3 - 4 a.m.													
4 - 5 a.m.													
5 - 6 a.m.													
6 - 7 a.m.													
8 HOUR TOTAL													
24 HOUR TOTAL													
	TOTAL INTAKE				**TOTAL OUTPUT**								

UNIT 20:6 FEEDING A PATIENT

ASSIGNMENT SHEET

Grade _____ Name _____

INTRODUCTION: Since good nutrition is an important part of a patient's treatment, this sheet will help you review the main facts on feeding a patient.

INSTRUCTIONS: Read the information about Feeding a Patient. In the space provided, print the word(s) that best completes the statement or answers the question.

1. List six (6) things you should do to prepare a patient for mealtime.

2. What should you do if a patient's meal will be delayed due to X rays or other treatments?

3. If you question an item on a patient's tray (example: salt on a low salt diet), what should you do?

4. If a patient does not like a particular food, what should you do?

5. List three (3) things you should check on the patient's tray.

6. Mr. Mendez is blind but must be encouraged to feed himself. How can you assist?

7. How can you test hot foods or liquids before feeding them to a patient?

8. Identify three (3) principles that should be followed while feeding a patient.

9. When a patient is finished eating, why should you note the amount of food eaten?

10. Identify two (2) ways to prevent the patient from choking while being fed.

Name _____ Date _____

Evaluated by _____

DIRECTIONS: Practice feeding a patient according to the criteria listed. When you are ready for your final check, give this sheet to your instructor.

Feeding a Patient	Points Possible	Peer Check Yes	Peer Check No	Final Check* Yes	Final Check* No	Points Earned**	Comments
PROFICIENT							
1. Checks orders or obtains authorization	2						
2. Assembles equipment and supplies	2						
3. Knocks on door, introduces self, identifies patient, and explains procedure	2						
4. Washes hands and puts on gloves if needed	2						
5. Prepares patient for meal:							
Provides oral hygiene if desired	2						
Offers bedpan	2						
Washes hands and face	2						
Places in sitting position	2						
Positions overbed table	2						
6. Checks tray:							
Notes patient's name	2						
Checks type diet	2						
Checks foods present	2						
Substitutes or removes food only after checking	2						
7. Places tray on overbed table	2						
8. Positions napkin/towel under patient's chin	2						
9. Assists patient as needed:							
Cuts meat, butters bread	2						
Opens cartons	2						
Arranges conveniently	2						
10. Tests hot liquids or foods on wrist	4						
11. Uses separate straw for each liquid	4						
12. Holds utensil at right angle	4						
13. Feeds patient from tip of utensil	4						
14. Places small amounts on utensil	4						

20:6 (cont.)

Feeding a Patient	Points Possible	Peer Check Yes	No	Final Check* Yes	No	Points Earned**	Comments
15. Tells patient what he/she is eating	4						
16. Provides time to chew	4						
17. Alternates solids and liquids	4						
18. Wipes mouth properly	3						
19. Encourages patient to eat as much as possible	3						
20. Watches patient closely to make sure patient is swallowing	3						
21. Allows patient to wash hands when done	3						
22. Provides oral hygiene	3						
23. Observes following checks before leaving patient:							
Patient in alignment	1						
Siderails elevated if indicated	1						
Bed at lowest level	1						
Call signal and supplies in reach	1						
Area neat and clean	1						
24. Notes and records amount of food patient ate	3						
25. Measures and records liquid amounts if patient is on I and O record	3						
26. Cleans and replaces all equipment	2						
27. Removes gloves if worn and washes hands	2						
28. Records or reports required information	2						
Totals	100						

* Final Check: Instructor or authorized person evaluates.
** Points Earned: Points possible times each "yes" check.

UNIT 20:7 ASSISTING WITH A BEDPAN/URINAL

ASSIGNMENT SHEET

Grade _____ Name _____

INTRODUCTION: Caring for the basic need of elimination is one of your responsibilities as a health assistant. This sheet will help you review the main points.

INSTRUCTIONS: Read the information about Assisting with a Bedpan/Urinal. In the space provided, print the word(s) that best completes the statement or answers the question.

1. Define *urinate, micturate,* and *void.*

    Define *defecate.*

2. What will occur if wastes are not eliminated from the body?

3. List the two (2) main types of bedpans.

4. Identify two (2) ways to provide privacy for a patient who is using a bedpan or urinal.

5. List three (3) observations a health assistant should make about the contents of a bedpan.

6. Before emptying or discarding a urine specimen, the health assistant should make sure that the patient is not on _____ records. If the patient is, the urine must be _____ and _____ first.

7. If you note an abnormal observation in the urine or stool, what two (2) actions should you take?

8. Many patients are _____ about using the bedpan or urinal. It is important that the assistant provide _____, make the patient as _____ as possible, and provide the bedpan or urinal _____ when the patient requests it.

9. List four (4) specific standard precautions that must be observed at all times while assisting a patient with a bedpan or urinal.

UNIT 20:7A Evaluation Sheet

Name _____ Date _____

Evaluated by _____

DIRECTIONS: Practice assisting with a bedpan according to the criteria listed. When you are ready for your final check, give this sheet to your instructor.

Assisting with a Bedpan	Points Possible	Peer Check Yes	No	Final Check* Yes	No	Points Earned**	Comments
1. Checks orders or obtains authorization	2						
2. Assembles equipment and supplies	2						
3. Knocks on door, introduces self, identifies patient, and explains procedure	2						
4. Closes door and screens unit	2						
5. Washes hands and puts on gloves	2						
6. Elevates bed to correct working level and locks bed	2						
7. Lowers headrest	2						
8. Warms bedpan	3						
9. Lowers siderail if elevated	2						
10. Folds top covers at an angle	3						
11. Assists with bedclothes	3						
12. Instructs patient to flex knees and put weight on feet and arranges signal	4						
13. Gives signal	4						
14. Raises hips with hand by small of back	4						
15. Slides pan into place	4						
16. If patient too heavy to lift, assists if needed by turning patient on side and positioning pan	4						
17. Supports patient on pan correctly	4						
18. Places call signal and toilet tissue in reach	4						
19. Elevates siderail if indicated	2						
20. Answers signal immediately	3						
21. Removes bedpan correctly	3						

PROFICIENT

Assisting with a Bedpan	Points Possible	Peer Check		Final Check*		Points Earned**	Comments
		Yes	No	Yes	No		
22. Places covered pan on chair	3						
23. Assists with cleaning perineal area as necessary	3						
24. Allows patient to wash hands	3						
25. Positions patient in correct alignment	2						
26. Elevates siderails if indicated and lowers bed to lowest level	2						
27. Places call signal and supplies within reach	2						
28. Takes bedpan to bathroom	2						
29. Checks contents of pan	3						
30. Saves specimen or measures amount as necessary	3						
31. Empties bedpan	2						
32. Uses paper towel to turn on faucet or flush toilet	2						
33. Rinses bedpan with cold water and a disinfectant	2						
34. Rinses and dries pan	2						
35. Replaces pan in patient's unit and leaves area neat and clean	2						
36. Removes gloves and washes hands	3						
37. Records/reports required information	3						
Totals	100						

* Final Check: Instructor or authorized person evaluates.
** Points Earned: Points possible times each "yes" check.

Name _____ Date _____

Evaluated by _____

DIRECTIONS: Practice assisting with a urinal according to the criteria listed. When you are ready for your final check, give this sheet to your instructor.

Assisting with a Urinal	Points Possible	Peer Check		Final Check*		Points Earned**	Comments
		Yes	No	Yes	No		
1. Checks orders or obtains authorization	3						
2. Assembles equipment and supplies	3						
3. Knocks on door, introduces self, identifies patient, and explains procedure	3						
4. Closes door and screens unit	3						
5. Washes hands and puts on gloves	3						
6. Locks and elevates bed and lowers siderail if elevated	3						
7. Lifts top bed linen	3						
8. Places urinal under covers so patient can grasp handle	4						
9. Assists with placement of urinal if necessary	4						
10. Places call signal and toilet tisssue in reach	4						
11. Elevates siderail if indicated before leaving	3						
12. Answers signal immediately	4						
13. Lowers siderail if elevated	3						
14. Receives urinal from patient or reaches under covers to grasp handle	4						
15. Places covered urinal on a chair	3						
16. Assists with toilet tissue	4						
17. Assists patient in washing hands and perineal area if necessary	4						
18. Positions patient in correct alignment	3						
19. Elevates siderails if indicated and lowers bed to lowest level	3						
20. Places call signal and supplies within reach	3						
21. Takes urinal to bathroom	3						

Over the table heading: PROFICIENT

Assisting with a Urinal	Points Possible	Peer Check		Final Check*		Points Earned**	Comments
		Yes	No	Yes	No		
22. Observes appearance of urine	4						
23. Measures amount or saves specimen as necessary	4						
24. Empties urinal	3						
25. Rinses with cool water	3						
26. Cleans with a disinfectant	3						
27. Rinses and dries	3						
28. Replaces urinal in unit or in urinal holder	3						
29. Removes gloves and washes hands	3						
30. Records/reports required information	4						
Totals	100						

* Final Check: Instructor or authorized person evaluates.
** Points Earned: Points possible times each "yes" check.

UNIT 20:8 PROVIDING CATHETER AND URINARY DRAINAGE UNIT CARE

ASSIGNMENT SHEET

Grade _____ Name _____

INTRODUCTION: It is essential to use correct techniques while working with catheters or urinary drainage units in order to prevent infections. This sheet will help you review the main facts.

INSTRUCTIONS: Read the information about Providing Catheter and Urinary Drainage Unit Care. In the space provided, print the word(s) that completes the statement or answers the question.

1. Hollow, narrow tubes made of soft rubber or plastic are called _____.

2. Foley catheters have a _____ at the end. This is inflated with _____ to keep _____.

3. List six (6) points that should be checked frequently when a catheter and urinary drainage unit are in place.

4. What can occur if the drainage bag is raised above the level of the bladder?

5. If a catheter and drainage unit are in place, how would you obtain a fresh urine specimen for a urine test?

6. When the catheter is disconnected from the drainage unit, why is it important to use sterile technique?

7. What is the purpose of catheter care?

8. List three (3) observations that should be noted about the urine in the drainage bag.

9. What would you do if you noted bright red drainage in the urinary drainage bag?

10. What is the purpose of a bladder training program?

Name _____ Date _____

Evaluated by _____

DIRECTIONS: Practice providing catheter care according to the criteria listed. When you are ready for your final check, give this sheet to your instructor.

PROFICIENT

Providing Catheter Care	Points Possible	Peer Check Yes	Peer Check No	Final Check* Yes	Final Check* No	Points Earned**	Comments
1. Obtains authorization or checks order	2						
2. Assembles equipment and supplies	2						
3. Knocks on door, introduces self, identifies patient, and explains procedure	2						
4. Closes door and screens unit	2						
5. Washes hands	2						
6. Locks and elevates bed to correct working level	2						
7. Lowers siderail if elevated	2						
8. Drapes patient with bath blanket	3						
9. Positions in dorsal recumbent and drapes correctly	3						
10. Positions plastic waste bag conveniently	3						
11. Positions underpad under buttocks and upper legs	3						
12. Puts on gloves	3						
13. Obtains sterile applicator with antiseptic solution or uses soap and water	3						
14. Cleanses female correctly:							
Separates labia to expose urinary meatus	2						
Wipes with front to back motion	2						
Places used applicator in plastic waste bag	2						
Repeats procedure using clean sterile applicator each time	2						
15. Cleanses male correctly:							
Draws foreskin back gently	2						
Wipes from meatus down shaft of penis	2						
Places used applicator in plastic waste bag	2						
Repeats procedure using clean sterile applicator each time	2						
Gently returns foreskin to normal position	2						

Name _____

20:8A (cont.)

Providing Catheter Care	Points Possible	Peer Check Yes	Peer Check No	Final Check* Yes	Final Check* No	Points Earned**	Comments
16. Cleans catheter correctly:							
Wipes from meatus down about 4 inches	3						
Places used applicator in plastic waste bag	2						
Repeats as needed using clean sterile applicator each time	2						
17. Observes area carefully for:							
Signs of irritation	3						
Abnormal discharges	3						
Crusting	3						
18. Removes underpad and places in plastic waste bag	3						
19. Removes gloves and washes hands	3						
20. Checks catheter to be sure it is strapped or taped properly	3						
21. Checks that there is no strain or pull on catheter	3						
22. Positions patient in correct alignment	2						
23. Replaces bedcovers and removes bath blanket	2						
24. Elevates siderails if indicated and lowers bed	2						
25. Places call signal and supplies within reach	2						
26. Checks catheter and urinary drainage unit	3						
27. Cleans and replaces equipment:							
Places disposable supplies in plastic waste bag	2						
Seals bag correctly	2						
Cleans and replaces equipment	2						
28. Washes hands thoroughly	2						
29. Records or reports required information	3						
Totals	100						

* Final Check: Instructor or authorized person evaluates.
** Points Earned: Points possible times each "yes" check.

Name _____ Date _____

Evaluated by _____

DIRECTIONS: Practice emptying a urinary drainage unit according to the criteria listed. When you are ready for your final check, give this sheet to your instructor.

Emptying a Urinary Drainage Unit	Points Possible	Peer Check Yes	Peer Check No	Final Check* Yes	Final Check* No	Points Earned**	Comments
1. Obtains authorization or checks order	2						
2. Assembles equipment and supplies	2						
3. Knocks on door, introduces self, identifies patient, and explains procedure	3						
4. Washes hands and puts on gloves	2						
5. Places measuring graduate on paper towels on floor	4						
6. Puts drainage outlet in graduate	5						
7. Releases clamp	5						
8. Tilts bag as necessary to empty urine	5						
9. Clamps drainage outlet when bag is empty	5						
10. Wipes drainage outlet with antiseptic/ disinfectant	5						
11. Replaces outlet in unit	5						
12. Checks patient for following points before leaving:							
Patient in correct alignment	2						
Siderails elevated if indicated	2						
Bed at lowest level	2						
Call signal and supplies within reach of patient	2						
Area neat and clean	2						
13. Checks catheter and drainage unit for following points before leaving:							
Catheter strapped or taped to leg	2						
Tubing free of kinks, bends	2						
Tubing does not loop below drainage bag	2						
Drainage bag attached to bedframe	2						
Drainage bag below level of bladder	2						
Drainage tubing above level of urine in bag	2						
Urine flowing into bag	2						

20:8B (cont.)

Emptying a Urinary Drainage Unit	Points Possible	Peer Check		Final Check*		Points Earned**	Comments
		Yes	No	Yes	No		
14. Takes urine to bathroom	2						
15. Measures amount in graduate	4						
16. Records amount correctly	5						
17. Reports unusual observations immediately	4						
18. Empties graduate in the toilet	2						
19. Rinses in cold water	2						
20. Washes with warm soapy water	2						
21. Cleans with a disinfectant	2						
22. Rinses and dries pitcher	2						
23. Replaces equipment	2						
24. Removes gloves and washes hands	2						
25. Records/reports required information	4						
Totals	100						

* Final Check: Instructor or authorized person evaluates.
** Points Earned: Points possible times each "yes" check.

UNIT 20:9 PROVIDING OSTOMY CARE

ASSIGNMENT SHEET

Grade _____ Name _____

INTRODUCTION: As a health care assistant, you may be responsible for providing care to patients with ostomies. This sheet will help you review the main facts regarding ostomy care.

INSTRUCTIONS: Read the information on Providing Ostomy Care. In the space provided, print the word(s) that best completes the statement or answers the question.

1. What is an ostomy?

2. List four (4) reasons why an ostomy may be created.

3. What is the correct name for each of the following types of ostomies?

    a. Ureter is brought to surface of abdomen to drain urine:

    b. Section of large intestine is brought to surface of abdomen to drain stool:

    c. Section of ileum is brought to surface of abdomen to drain stool:

4. How is the stool expelled through an ascending colostomy different from the stool expelled from a sigmoid colostomy? What is the reason for this difference?

5. Describe three (3) problems that can occur when an ostomy or pouch is placed over the stoma.

6. Why are skin barriers used on the skin around the stoma?

    Identify three (3) types of skin barriers.

7. How can a health care assistant help a patient who is afraid and depressed after an ostomy has been created?

8. Describe the appearance of a normal stoma.

9. What do the following abnormal appearances of a stoma indicate?

    a. Pale or pink color:

    b. Dry or dull appearance:

    c. Blue to black color:

10. Identify three (3) factors that should be observed in regards to the drainage in the ostomy bag or pouch.

Name _____ Date _____

Evaluated by _____

DIRECTIONS: Practice providing ostomy care according to the criteria listed. When you are ready for your final check, give this sheet to your instructor.

		PROFICIENT						
Providing Ostomy Care	**Points Possible**	**Peer Check**		**Final Check***		**Points Earned****	**Comments**
		Yes	**No**	**Yes**	**No**		
1. Checks order or obtains authorization	2						
2. Assembles equipment and supplies	2						
3. Knocks on door, introduces self, identifies patient, and explains procedure	2						
4. Closes door and screens unit	2						
5. Washes hands	2						
6. Locks and elevates bed and lowers siderail if elevated	2						
7. Drapes patient with bath blanket	2						
8. Positions underpad under patient's hips on side of stoma	2						
9. Fills basin with water at temperature of 105°–110° F (40.6°–43.3° C)	3						
10. Positions bedpan and infectious waste bag conveniently	3						
11. Puts on disposable gloves	3						
12. Opens belt and removes ostomy bag carefully	4						
13. Notes amount, color, and type of drainage in bag	4						
14. Places bag in bedpan or infectious waste bag	4						
15. Wipes stoma area gently with toilet tissue and discards tissue in bedpan or infectious waste bag	4						
16. Checks stoma area carefully for:							
Irritated areas	2						
Bleeding	2						
Edema or swelling	2						
Discharge	2						
17. Washes ostomy area with soap and water in a circular motion	4						

20:9 (cont.)

Providing Ostomy Care	Points Possible	Peer Check		Final Check*		Points Earned**	Comments
		Yes	No	Yes	No		
18. Rinses and dries area completely	4						
19. Uses measuring chart to determine correct size wafer	4						
20. Applies wafer and stoma paste correctly or applies skin barrier if wafer not used	4						
21. Positions belt around patient	4						
22. Applies ostomy bag to stoma and makes sure bag is sealed tightly	4						
23. If pouch has a drainage area, clamps or clips securely	4						
24. Removes underpad and straightens or replaces bed linen	3						
25. Checks patient for following points before leaving:							
Patient in correct alignment	1						
Siderails elevated if indicated	1						
Bed at lowest level	1						
Call signal and supplies within reach of patient	1						
26. Takes bedpan and waste bag to bathroom	2						
27. Follows agency policy for disposal of ostomy bag	2						
28. Cleans and disinfects bedpan correctly	2						
29. Discards any contaminated disposable supplies in infectious waste bag	2						
30. Replaces bedpan in patient's unit and leaves area neat and clean	2						
31. Removes gloves and washes hands	2						
32. Records/reports all required information	4						
Totals	100						

* Final Check: Instructor or authorized person evaluates.
** Points Earned: Points possible times each "yes" check.

UNIT 20:10 COLLECTING STOOL/URINE SPECIMENS

ASSIGNMENT SHEET

Grade _____ Name _____

INTRODUCTION: Stool and urine specimens are often used to aid a doctor in making a diagnosis. This sheet will help you review the main facts regarding collection of specimens.

INSTRUCTIONS: Read the information on Collecting Stool/Urine Specimens. In the space provided, print the word(s) that best completes the statement or answers the question.

1. List two (2) reasons why a first-voided AM specimen is used for many urine tests.

2. How much urine is usually collected for a routine specimen? _____ cc. What should you do if a patient is not able to void this amount?

3. If a urine specimen cannot be sent to the laboratory immediately, what should you do with the specimen?

4. Why is a clean catch or midstream voided specimen done?

5. Briefly describe how the genital area of both females and males should be cleaned before a midstream specimen is collected.

6. What type of specimen container is needed for a midstream specimen?

7. How can a sterile urine specimen be obtained?

8. Why is the first urine voided in a twenty-four hour specimen discarded or thrown away?

9. List two (2) ways to preserve urine for a 24-hour specimen.

10. Why is it important to immediately send the stool specimen being examined for ova and parasites to the laboratory?

11. If an occult blood test on stool is positive, what does this indicate?

12. Why are all stool and urine specimens placed in a special biohazard bag before being transported to the laboratory for testing?

481

UNIT 20:10A Evaluation Sheet

Name _____ Date _____

Evaluated by _____

DIRECTIONS: Practice collecting a routine urine specimen according to the criteria listed. When you are ready for your final check, give this sheet to your instructor.

PROFICIENT

Collecting a Routine Urine Specimen	Points Possible	Peer Check Yes	No	Final Check* Yes	No	Points Earned**	Comments
1. Checks order or obtains authorization	3						
2. Assembles equipment and supplies	3						
3. Knocks on door, introduces self, identifies patient, and explains procedure	3						
4. Washes hands and puts on gloves	3						
5. Tells patient not to put tissue in bedpan/urinal or specimen collector	5						
6. Assists with bedpan/urinal or specimen collector	5						
7. Allows patient to wash hands	5						
8. Observes following checks before leaving patient:							
Patient comfortable and in correct alignment	2						
Siderails elevated if indicated	2						
Bed at lowest level	2						
Call signal and supplies within reach of patient	2						
Area neat and clean	2						
9. Pours urine into graduate	5						
10. Measures and records amount if patient is on I and O record	5						
11. Pours 120 cc into specimen container	5						
12. Washes outside of container	5						
13. Removes gloves and washes hands	5						
14. Covers specimen container	5						

20:10A (cont.)

Collecting a Routine Urine Specimen	Points Possible	Peer Check		Final Check*		Points Earned**	Comments
		Yes	No	Yes	No		
15. Labels specimen and completes lab requisition with:							
Type specimen	2						
Test ordered	2						
Patient's name	2						
Date/time	2						
Room number/address	2						
Physician's name	2						
16. Cleans and replaces equipment	3						
17. Places specimen in biohazard bag for transport	5						
18. Takes or sends specimen to laboratory or refrigerates	5						
19. Washes hands	3						
20. Records/reports all required information	5						
Totals	100						

* Final Check: Instructor or authorized person evaluates.
** Points Earned: Points possible times each "yes" check.

Name _____ Date _____

Evaluated by _____

DIRECTIONS: Practice collecting a midstream urine specimen according to the criteria listed. When you are ready for your final check, give this sheet to your instructor.

PROFICIENT

Collecting a Midstream Urine Specimen	Points Possible	Peer Check Yes	No	Final Check* Yes	No	Points Earned**	Comments
1. Checks order or obtains authorization	3						
2. Assembles equipment and supplies	3						
3. Knocks on door, introduces self, identifies patient, and explains procedure	3						
4. Washes hands	3						
5. Closes door, screens unit, locks and elevates bed, and lowers siderail if elevated or assists patient to bathroom	3						
6. Washes genital area or instructs patient:							
Puts on gloves	3						
Uses gauze and antiseptic	3						
Cleans female from front to back; from outer folds to inner folds to center	3						
Cleans male with circular motions from meatus out and down	3						
Discards each gauze after one use in plastic waste bag	3						
7. Collects midstream specimen:							
Uses sterile container	3						
Allows first urine to escape	3						
Catches middle urine in specimen container	3						
Allows last urine to escape	3						
Catches first and last urine in bedpan if I and O record or amount measured	3						
8. Places sterile cap on container immediately without contaminating container or cap	4						
9. Allows patient to wash hands	3						

20:10B (cont.)

Collecting a Midstream Urine Specimen	Points Possible	Peer Check		Final Check*		Points Earned**	Comments
		Yes	No	Yes	No		
10. Observes following checks before leaving patient:							
Patient in correct alignment	2						
Siderails elevated if indicated	2						
Bed at lowest level	2						
Call signal and supplies within reach	2						
Area neat and clean	2						
11. Washes outside of container	4						
12. Removes gloves and washes hands	4						
13. Labels specimen and lab requisition with:							
Type specimen	2						
Test ordered	2						
Patient's name	2						
Date/time	2						
Room number/address	2						
Physician's name	2						
14. Cleans and replaces all equipment	3						
15. Places specimen in biohazard bag for transport	4						
16. Takes or sends specimen to laboratory or refrigerates	4						
17. Washes hands	3						
18. Records/reports all required information	4						
Totals	100						

* Final Check: Instructor or authorized person evaluates.
** Points Earned: Points possible times each "yes" check.

UNIT 20 : 10 C Evaluation Sheet

Name _____ Date _____

Evaluated by _____

DIRECTIONS: Practice collecting a 24-hour urine specimen according to criteria listed. When you are ready for your final check, give this sheet to your instructor.

PROFICIENT

Collecting a 24-Hour Urine Specimen	Points Possible	Peer Check Yes	No	Final Check* Yes	No	Points Earned**	Comments
1. Checks order or obtains authorization	3						
2. Checks on type container and preservative	4						
3. Assembles equipment and supplies	3						
4. Labels container and lab requisition with:							
Patient's name	2						
Room number/address	2						
Test ordered	2						
Type specimen	2						
Date/time	2						
Physician's name	2						
5. Knocks on door, introduces self, identifies patient, and explains procedure	3						
6. Stresses importance of saving all urine	5						
7. Washes hands	3						
8. Puts on gloves	3						
9. Allows patient to void; discards	5						
10. Records amount if on I and O	4						
11. Notes time of voiding as start of 24-hour test	5						
12. Removes gloves and washes hands	3						
13. Places sign on bed	5						
14. Puts all urine voided in 24-hour period in special container	5						
15. Asks patient to void at end of 24-hour period	5						
16. Puts final urine into specimen container	5						
17. Removes sign	5						
18. Checks label and lab requisition for accuracy	4						
19. Places specimen in biohazard bag for transport	4						
20. Takes or sends specimen to laboratory	4						
21. Replaces all equipment	3						
22. Washes hands	3						
23. Records/reports all required information	4						
Totals	100						

* Final Check: Instructor or authorized person evaluates.
** Points Earned: Points possible times each "yes" check.

UNIT 20:10D Evaluation Sheet

Name _____ Date _____

Evaluated by _____

DIRECTIONS: Practice collecting a stool specimen according to the criteria listed. When you are ready for your final check, give this sheet to your instructor.

PROFICIENT

Collecting a Stool Specimen	Points Possible	Peer Check Yes	No	Final Check* Yes	No	Points Earned**	Comments
1. Checks order or obtains authorization	4						
2. Assembles equipment and supplies	4						
3. Knocks on door, introduces self, identifies patient, and explains procedure	5						
4. Asks patient to use bedpan or specimen collector for next bowel movement	5						
5. Washes hands and puts on gloves to collect specimen	5						
6. Collects specimen in bedpan or specimen collector	5						
7. Allows patient to wash hands	5						
8. Takes specimen to bathroom	5						
9. Uses tongue blades to transfer specimen to container	6						
10. Discards tongue blades in plastic waste bag	6						
11. Removes gloves and washes hands	6						
12. Closes lid securely	6						
13. Labels container and lab requisition with:							
Type specimen	2						
Test ordered	2						
Patient's name	2						
Date/time	2						
Room number/address	2						
Physician's name	2						
14. Cleans and replaces all equipment used:							
Puts on gloves	2						
Cleans and disinfects bedpan	2						
Replaces all equipment used	2						
Removes gloves and washes hands	2						
15. Places specimen in biohazard bag for transport	5						
16. Keeps specimen warm and sends or takes to laboratory immediately	5						
17. Washes hands	4						
18. Records/reports all required information	4						
Totals	100						

* Final Check: Instructor or authorized person evaluates.
** Points Earned: Points possible times each "yes" check.

487

U N I T 20 : 10 E   E v a l u a t i o n   S h e e t

Name _____ Date _____

Evaluated by _____

DIRECTIONS: Practice preparing and testing a Hemoccult® slide according to the criteria listed. When you are ready for your final check, give this sheet to your instructor.

PROFICIENT

Preparing and Testing a Hemoccult® Slide	Points Possible	Peer Check Yes	No	Final Check* Yes	No	Points Earned**	Comments
1. Checks order or obtains authorization	3						
2. Assembles equipment and supplies	3						
3. Reads manufacturer's instructions	5						
4. Knocks on door, introduces self, identifies patient, and explains procedure	3						
5. Asks patient to use bedpan or specimen collector for next bowel movement	3						
6. Washes hands and puts on gloves to collect specimen	4						
7. Collects specimen in bedpan or specimen collector	3						
8. Allows patient to wash hands	3						
9. Takes specimen to bathroom	3						
10. Places Hemoccult slide packet on top of paper towel	5						
11. Opens front cover or flap of packet	5						
12. Uses tongue blade/ stick to smear small amount of stool specimen on correct area(s) of slide	5						
13. Discards tongue blade/stick in plastic waste bag	5						
14. Removes gloves and washes hands	4						
15. Closes cover or flap of packet	5						
16. Labels packet and lab requisition with:							
Patient's name	2						
Date and time	2						
Room number/address	2						
Physician's name	2						

20:10E (cont.)

Preparing and Testing a Hemoccult® Slide	Points Possible	Peer Check		Final Check*		Points Earned**	Comments
		Yes	No	Yes	No		
17. Develops test as follows:							
Opens back of packet	4						
Places correct amount of developer on guaiac paper	4						
Waits correct amount of time	4						
Reads test correctly	4						
18. Cleans and replaces all equipment used:							
Puts on gloves	2						
Discards remaining stool specimen	2						
Cleans and disinfects bedpan	2						
Replaces all equipment used	2						
19. Removes gloves and washes hands	4						
20. Records or reports all required information	5						
Totals	100						

* Final Check: Instructor or authorized person evaluates.
** Points Earned: Points possible times each "yes" check.

UNIT 20:11 GIVING ENEMAS AND RECTAL TREATMENTS

ASSIGNMENT SHEET

Grade _____ Name _____

INTRODUCTION: A variety of rectal treatments are administered to patients. This sheet will help you review the main facts.

INSTRUCTIONS: Read the text information about Giving Enemas and Rectal Treatments. In the space provided, print the word(s) that completes the statement or answers the question.

1. Define *enema*.

2. List two (2) purposes for enemas.

3. What is the difference between retention and nonretention enemas?

4. List the main purpose for each of the following types of enemas.
    a. Cleansing:
    b. Disposable:
    c. Oil retention:

5. What position is usually used for enemas? Why is this position used?

6. List three (3) points that should be noted after an enema has been given.

7. What is an impaction? How is it removed?

8. Why is a rectal tube inserted?

9. What is a suppository?

10. List three (3) purposes of suppositories.

Name _____ Date _____

Evaluated by _____

DIRECTIONS: Practice administering a soap-solution enema according to the criteria listed. When you are ready for your final check, give this sheet to your instructor.

PROFICIENT

Giving a Soap-Solution Enema	Points Possible	Peer Check Yes	No	Final Check* Yes	No	Points Earned**	Comments
1. Checks order or obtains authorization	2						
2. Assembles equipment and supplies	2						
3. Prepares container by connecting tubing and closing clamp	3						
4. Fills container with 1000 cc water at 105° F or 41° C	3						
5. Adds 20–30 cc soap gently to avoid suds	3						
6. Removes air from tubing	3						
7. Lubricates tip correctly	3						
8. Places all equipment on tray and takes to patient's room	2						
9. Knocks on door, introduces self, identifies patient, and explains procedure	2						
10. Closes door and screens unit	2						
11. Washes hands	2						
l2. Locks and elevates bed and lowers siderail if elevated	2						
13. Covers patient with bath blanket and fanfolds top linen	2						
14. Places underpad under patient's buttocks	2						
15. Positions patient in Sims' or in dorsal recumbent on bedpan	4						
16. Folds bath blanket at an angle to expose anal area	3						
17. Puts on gloves	3						
18. Raises buttock and exposes anus	3						
19. Inserts tip 2-4 inches into rectum	4						
20. Informs patient while inserting tube	3						
21. Opens clamp to allow solution to flow	3						

Giving a Soap-Solution Enema	Points Possible	Peer Check		Final Check*		Points Earned**	Comments
		Yes	No	Yes	No		
22. Raises container 12 inches to obtain slow flow	4						
23. Encourages patient to relax and breathe deeply	3						
24. Clamps tubing as soon as solution instilled to prevent air from entering rectum	3						
25. Informs patient while removing tip	3						
26. Encourages patient to retain enema as long as possible	3						
27. Positions patient on bedpan	2						
28. Places call signal and tissue in reach	2						
29. Answers call signal immediately	2						
30. Removes bedpan correctly	2						
31. Assists with perineal care and allows patient to wash hands	2						
32. Replaces sheets and removes bath blanket and underpad	2						
33. Observes following checks before leaving:							
Patient positioned in correct alignment	1						
Siderails elevated if indicated	1						
Bed at lowest level	1						
Call signal and supplies within reach	1						
Area neat and clean	1						
34. Observes contents of pan and notes following:							
Amount of stool	1						
Color of stool	1						
Type of stool	1						
35. Cleans and replaces all equipment used:							
Cleans and disinfects bedpan	1						
Places contaminated disposables in infectious waste bag	1						
Replaces all equipment	1						
36. Removes gloves and washes hands	2						
37. Records or reports all required information	3						
Totals	100						

* Final Check: Instructor or authorized person evaluates.
** Points Earned: Points possible times each "yes" check.

Name _____ Date _____

Evaluated by _____

DIRECTIONS: Practice administering a disposable enema according to the criteria listed. When you are ready for your final check, give this sheet to your instructor.

PROFICIENT

Giving a Disposable Enema	Points Possible	Peer Check Yes	No	Final Check* Yes	No	Points Earned**	Comments
1. Checks order or obtains authorization	2						
2. Assembles equipment and supplies	2						
3. Lubricates tip on enema unit	2						
4. Knocks on door, introduces self, identifies patient, and explains procedure	2						
5. Closes door and screens unit	2						
6. Washes hands	2						
7. Locks and elevates bed and lowers siderail if elevated	2						
8. Drapes with bath blanket	2						
9. Places underpad under patient's buttocks	2						
10. Positions patient in Sims'	3						
11. Folds bath blanket at angle to expose buttocks	2						
12. Puts on gloves	3						
13. Lifts buttock to expose anal area	3						
14. Squeezes container to get solution to top of tip	4						
15 Inserts tip 2-4 inches	4						
16. Informs patient while inserting tip	4						
17. Squeezes container in a spiral manner to expel solution	4						
18. Holds container at angle to avoid air bubbles	4						
19. Encourages patient to breathe deeply and retain solution	4						
20. Removes tip gently when all solution instilled	4						
21. Informs patient while removing tip	4						
22. Places container in infectious waste bag	3						

Giving a Disposable Enema	Points Possible	Peer Check		Final Check*		Points Earned**	Comments
		Yes	No	Yes	No		
23. Encourages patient to retain enema 5–10 minutes	4						
24. Positions patient on bedpan	2						
25. Places call signal and toilet tissue within reach	2						
26. Answers signal immediately	2						
27. Removes bedpan correctly	2						
28. Assists with perineal care and allows patient to wash hands	2						
29. Replaces top bed linens and removes underpad and bath blanket	2						
30. Observes following checks before leaving:							
Patient positioned in correct alignment	1						
Siderails elevated if indicated	1						
Bed at lowest level	1						
Call signal and supplies within reach	1						
Area neat and clean	1						
31. Observes contents of pan and notes following:							
Amount of stool	2						
Color of stool	2						
Type of stool	2						
32. Cleans and replaces all equipment:							
Cleans and disinfects bedpan	1						
Puts contaminated disposables in infectious waste bag	1						
Replaces all equipment	1						
33. Removes gloves and washes hands	2						
34. Records/reports all required information	4						
Totals	100						

* Final Check: Instructor or authorized person evaluates.
** Points Earned: Points possible times each "yes" check.

UNIT 20:11 C Evaluation Sheet

Name _____ Date _____

Evaluated by _____

DIRECTIONS: Practice administering an oil retention enema according to the criteria listed. When you are ready for your final check, give this sheet to your instructor.

PROFICIENT

Giving an Oil Retention Enema	Points Possible	Peer Check Yes	No	Final Check* Yes	No	Points Earned**	Comments
1. Checks order or obtains authorization	2						
2. Assembles equipment and supplies	2						
3. Lubricates tip of commercial enema	2						
4. Prepares oil enema if necessary:							
Warms oil	2						
Measures 4–6 ounces	2						
Fills irrigation container and closes clamp	2						
Lubricates tip	2						
5. Knocks on door, introduces self, identifies patient, and explains procedure	2						
6. Closes door and screens unit	2						
7. Washes hands	2						
8. Locks and elevates bed and lowers siderail if elevated	2						
9. Covers patient with bath blanket	2						
10. Places underpad under patient's buttocks	2						
11. Positions in Sims'	2						
12. Folds bath blanket at angle to expose buttocks	2						
13. Puts on gloves	2						
14. Lifts buttock to expose anal area	2						
15. Squeezes container to get oil to tip or fills tubing on irrigation container with oil by opening clamp	3						
16. Inserts tip 2–4 inches into rectum	3						
17. Informs patient while inserting tip	3						
18. Coils container to expel solution or raises level of irrigation container 12 inches	3						
19. Instills solution slowly	3						

495

Giving an Oil Retention Enema	Points Possible	Peer Check		Final Check*		Points Earned**	Comments
		Yes	No	Yes	No		
20. Encourages patient to breathe deeply and retain solution	3						
21. Removes tip gently when all oil is instilled	3						
22. Informs patient while removing tip	3						
23. Encourages patient to retain oil 30 minutes	3						
24. Places call signal within reach	2						
25. Removes gloves and washes hands	2						
26. Answers signal immediately	2						
27. Washes hands and puts on gloves	2						
28. Positions patient on bedpan	2						
29. Places call signal and toilet tissue within reach	2						
30. Answers signal immediately	2						
31. Removes bedpan correctly	2						
32. Assists with perineal care and allows patient to wash hands	2						
33. Replaces top linens and removes bath blanket and underpad	2						
34. Observes following checks before leaving:							
Patient in correct alignment	1						
Elevates siderails if indicated	1						
Bed at lowest position	1						
Call signal and supplies within reach of patient	1						
Area neat and clean	1						
35. Observes contents of pan and notes following:							
Amount of stool	2						
Color of stool	2						
Type of stool	2						
36. Cleans and replaces all equipment:							
Cleans and disinfects bedpan	1						
Places contaminated disposables in infectious waste bag	1						
Replaces all equipment	1						
37. Removes gloves and washes hands	2						
38. Records or reports all required information	3						
Totals	100						

* Final Check: Instructor or authorized person evaluates.
** Points Earned: Points possible times each "yes" check.

UNIT 20:11 D Evaluation Sheet

Name _____ Date _____

Evaluated by _____

DIRECTIONS: Practice inserting a rectal tube according to the criteria listed. When you are ready for your final check, give this sheet to your instructor.

Inserting a Rectal Tube	Points Possible	Peer Check Yes	No	Final Check* Yes	No	Points Earned**	Comments
1. Checks order or obtains authorization	2						
2. Assembles equipment and supplies	2						
3. Prepares rectal tube:							
Lubricates tip correctly	3						
Connects to flatus bag	3						
4. Knocks on door, introduces self, identifies patient, and explains procedure	3						
5. Closes door and screens unit	2						
6. Washes hands	2						
7. Locks and elevates bed and lowers siderail if elevated	2						
8. Positions patient in Sims'	3						
9. Positions underpad under patient's buttocks	3						
10. Folds top bedlinen at angle to expose buttocks	3						
11. Puts on gloves	3						
12. Raises buttock to expose anal area	3						
13. Inserts tube 2–4 inches into rectum	4						
14. Informs patient while inserting tube	4						
15. Tapes tube to patient's buttocks	4						
16. Places open end in basin or specimen bottle if flatus bag not used	4						
17. Positions patient as comfortably as possible with call signal in reach	3						
18. Removes gloves and washes hands	3						
19. Checks patient and tube at intervals during treatment	4						
20. Leaves in place as directed, usually 20–30 minutes	4						

PROFICIENT

Inserting a Rectal Tube	Points Possible	Peer Check Yes	No	Final Check* Yes	No	Points Earned**	Comments
21. At end of required time, washes hands and puts on gloves	3						
22. Removes tube gently	4						
23. Informs patient while removing tube	4						
24. Places disposable tube in infectious waste bag	3						
25. Asks patient how much flatus expelled or if patient feels better	3						
26. Observes following checks before leaving:							
Patient in correct alignment	1						
Siderails elevated if indicated	1						
Bed at lowest level	1						
Call signal and supplies within reach	1						
Area neat and clean	1						
27. Notes following points:							
Flatus in bag	2						
Drainage if any	2						
Comments of patient after treatment	2						
28. Cleans and replaces all equipment	2						
29. Removes gloves and washes hands	3						
30. Records/reports all required information and reports unusual observations immediately	3						
Totals	100						

* Final Check: Instructor or authorized person evaluates.
** Points Earned: Points possible times each "yes" check.

UNIT 20:12 APPLYING RESTRAINTS

ASSIGNMENT SHEET

Grade _____ Name _____

INTRODUCTION: Restraints are needed at times to protect patients. This sheet will help you review the main facts regarding their use.

INSTRUCTIONS: Read the information about Applying Restraints. In the space provided, print the word(s) that best completes the statement or answers the question.

1. What are physical restraints?

2. Identify four (4) principles based on OBRA legislation that must be followed before restraints can be applied.

3. List three (3) factors that must be included in a physician's order for a restraint.

4. List three (3) types of patients who may require restraints.

5. List three (3) types of restraints and briefly state the main use of each type.

6. How can you check to make sure limb restraints are not too tight?

7. List five (5) signs of poor circulation.

8. All restraints must be removed every _____ hours for at least _____ minutes. The patient should be _____, _____ exercises provided, and _____ care given.

9. List five (5) complications that can occur when restraints are applied.

10. Because complications can occur when restraints are applied, what must the staff decide before restraints are applied to the patient?

Name _____   Date _____

Evaluated by _____

DIRECTIONS: Practice applying limb restraints according to the criteria listed. When you are ready for your final check, give this sheet to your instructor.

Applying Limb Restraints	Points Possible	Peer Check Yes	No	Final Check* Yes	No	Points Earned**	Comments
1. Checks order or obtains authorization	2						
2. Assembles supplies	2						
3. Knocks on door, introduces self, identifies patient, and explains procedure	2						
4. Closes door and screens unit	2						
5. Washes hands	2						
6. Positions patient comfortably in correct alignment in bed/wheelchair	2						
7. Places soft edge against skin	5						
8. Wraps smoothly around limb	5						
9. Removes all wrinkles	5						
10. Pulls both straps through ring or tab	5						
11. Pulls restraint secure	5						
12. Tests fit by inserting two fingers between skin and restraint	5						
13. Positions limb in comfortable position	5						
14. Limits movement only as much as necessary	5						
15. Secures straps to frame with quick release tie	5						
16. Rechecks patient and restraint	5						
17. Observes following checks before leaving :							
Patient in alignment	1						
Siderails elevated if indicated	1						
Bed at lowest level	1						
Call signal and supplies within reach	1						
Area neat and clean	1						
18. Checks circulation below restraint every 15 to 30 minutes:							
Color	2						
Temperature	2						
Return of color after blanching nails	2						
Edema or swelling	2						
Complaints of pain /numbness /tingling	2						

20:12A (cont.)

Applying Limb Restraints	Points Possible	Peer Check		Final Check*		Points Earned**	Comments
		Yes	No	Yes	No		
19. Removes restraints every 2 hours for at least 10 minutes and:							
Repositions patient	3						
Provides range–of–motion exercises	3						
Gives skin care	3						
20. Removes restraint when authorized	5						
21. Replaces all equipment	2						
22. Washes hands	2						
23. Records or reports required information	5						
Totals	100						

* Final Check: Instructor or authorized person evaluates.
** Points Earned: Points possible times each "yes" check.

Name _____ Date _____

Evaluated by _____

DIRECTIONS: Practice applying a jacket restraint according to the criteria listed. When you are ready for your final check, give this sheet to your instructor.

		PROFICIENT					
Applying a Jacket Restraint	**Points Possible**	**Peer Check** Yes	No	**Final Check*** Yes	No	**Points Earned****	**Comments**
1. Checks order or obtains authorization	3						
2. Assembles supplies and follows manufacturer's instructions to obtain the correct size restraint for the patient	2						
3. Knocks on door, introduces self, identifies patient, and explains procedure	2						
4. Closes door and screens unit	2						
5. Washes hands	2						
6. Positions patient comfortably in correct alignment in bed/wheelchair	2						
7. Slips sleeves onto arms	5						
8. Positions open or V-neck on front for most security and follows manufacturer's instructions	5						
9. Brings strap through hole in jacket	5						
10. Crisscrosses straps in back	5						
11. Removes all wrinkles	5						
12. Checks tightness of jacket	5						
13. Positions patient comfortably	5						
14. Limits movement only as much as necessary	5						
15. Secures straps to frame with quick release tie	5						
16. Rechecks patient, restraint, and respirations	5						
17. Observes following checks before leaving:							
Patient in alignment	1						
Siderails elevated if indicated	1						
Bed at lowest level	1						
Call signal and supplies within reach of patient	1						
Area neat and clean	1						

20:12B (cont.)

Applying a Jacket Restraint	Points Possible	Peer Check		Final Check*		Points Earned**	Comments
		Yes	No	Yes	No		
18. Checks respirations, color, and temperature of skin every 15 to 30 minutes	6						
19. Removes restraints every 2 hours for at least 10 minutes and:							
Repositions patient	4						
Provides range–of–motion exercises	4						
Gives skin care	4						
20. Removes restraint when authorized	5						
21. Replaces all equipment	2						
22. Washes hands	2						
23. Records or reports required information	5						
Totals	100						

* Final Check: Instructor or authorized person evaluates.
** Points Earned: Points possible times each "yes" check.

UNIT 20:13 ADMINISTERING PRE- AND POSTOPERATIVE CARE

ASSIGNMENT SHEET

Grade _____ Name _____

INTRODUCTION: Since operative care involves many factors, this sheet will help you review some of the main facts.

INSTRUCTIONS: Read the information about Administering Pre- and Postoperative Care. In the space provided, print the word(s) that best completes the statement or answers the question.

1. List the three (3) phases of operative care.

2. List ten (10) points of care that may be ordered before surgery.

3. Why is a bath given the night before and the morning of surgery?

4. If a patient does not want to remove a wedding ring before surgery, what can you do?

5. Why is the skin shaved prior to surgery?

6. How can you determine the area that must be shaved for the skin preparation or surgical shave?

7. Briefly describe each of the following types of anesthesia.

    a. General:

    b. Local:

    c. Spinal:

8. A common postoperative problem with general anesthesia is _____.

9. List the main pieces of equipment that should be placed by the bed or on the bedside stand in a post-operative unit.

10. List five (5) types of care required for the postoperative patient.

11. What is the purpose of surgical or elastic hose?

12. What are Montgomery straps? Why are they used?

Name _____ Date _____

Evaluated by _____

DIRECTIONS: Practice shaving the operative area according to the criteria listed. When you are ready for your final check, give this sheet to your instructor.

PROFICIENT

Shaving the Operative Area	Points Possible	Peer Check Yes	No	Final Check* Yes	No	Points Earned**	Comments
1. Checks order or obtains authorization	3						
2. Assembles equipment and supplies	2						
3. Prepares tray or skin prep kit:							
Fills 2 bowls with water at 105°F or 41°C	4						
Mixes soap in one bowl	4						
Checks razor and blades	4						
Places all supplies on tray	4						
4. Knocks on door, introduces self, identifies patient, and explains procedure	3						
5. Closes door and screens unit	3						
6. Washes hands	3						
7. Locks and elevates bed and lowers siderail if elevated	3						
8. Drapes with bath blanket	3						
9. Places underpad at area to be shaved	3						
10. Positions light source to illuminate area	3						
11. Puts on gloves	3						
12. Shaves correct area:							
Starts at top of area to be shaved	4						
Applies soap to small area	4						
Holds skin taut	4						
Shaves in direction of hair growth	4						
Rinses razor	4						
Rubs razor on gauze to remove hairs	4						
13. Cleans umbilicus with applicators if abdomen is shaved	4						
14. Checks area with light and removes remaining hairs	4						
15. Washes, rinses, and dries entire area	4						

Shaving the Operative Area	Points Possible	Peer Check		Final Check*		Points Earned**	Comments
		Yes	No	Yes	No		
16. Replaces top linens and removes bath blanket and underpad	2						
17. Observes following checks before leaving:							
Patient in alignment	1						
Siderails elevated if indicated	1						
Bed at lowest level	1						
Call signal and supplies within reach	1						
Area neat and clean	1						
18. Puts disposable razor and blades in sharps container	3						
19. Cleans and replaces all equipment	2						
20. Removes gloves and washes hands	3						
21. Records or reports all required information	4						
Totals	100						

* Final Check: Instructor or authorized person evaluates.
** Points Earned: Points possible times each "yes" check.

Name _____ Date _____

Evaluated by _____

DIRECTIONS: Practice administering preoperative care according to the criteria listed. When you are ready for your final check, give this sheet to your instructor.

Administering Preoperative Care	Points Possible	Peer Check Yes	No	Final Check* Yes	No	Points Earned**	Comments
1. Checks order or obtains authorization	3						
2. Assembles equipment and supplies	2						
3. Knocks on door, introduces self, identifies patient, and explains procedure	2						
4. Reassures patient as needed	2						
5. Washes hands	2						
6. Closes door, screens unit, locks and elevates bed, and lowers siderail if elevated	2						
7. Checks ID band	5						
8. Completes oral hygiene and bath	5						
9. Removes clothes and places surgical gown on patient	5						
10. Removes hair pins, wigs, etc.	5						
11. Puts hair in cap	5						
12. Checks that nail polish and make-up removed	5						
13. Puts valuables in safe	5						
14. Tapes/ties wedding ring	5						
15. Removes dentures and places in labeled cup in safe area	5						
16. Removes glasses, prosthesis	5						
17. Encourages patient to void	5						
18. Takes/records vital signs	5						
19. Completes care one hour before scheduled surgery	5						
20. Elevates siderails immediately after preop medication administered	5						
21. Positions patient in comfortable position	3						
22. Encourages patient to relax	3						

PROFICIENT

20:13B (cont.)

Administering Preoperative Care	Points Possible	Peer Check		Final Check*		Points Earned**	Comments
		Yes	No	Yes	No		
23. Observes following checks before leaving:							
Makes sure drinking water removed from bedside	1						
Lowers bed to lowest level	1						
Places call signal in reach	1						
Leaves area neat and clean	1						
24. Cleans and replaces all equipment	2						
25. Washes hands	2						
26. Records or reports all required information	3						
Totals	100						

* Final Check: Instructor or authorized person evaluates.
** Points Earned: Points possible times each "yes" check.

UNIT 20:13 C Evaluation Sheet

Name _____ Date _____

Evaluated by _____

DIRECTIONS: Practice preparing a postoperative unit according to the criteria listed. When you are ready for your final check, give this sheet to your instructor.

PROFICIENT

Preparing a Postoperative Unit	Points Possible	Peer Check Yes	Peer Check No	Final Check* Yes	Final Check* No	Points Earned**	Comments
1. Assembles equipment and supplies	3						
2. Washes hands and puts on gloves if needed	3						
3. Makes a postoperative bed as follows:							
Removes soiled linen	5						
Makes foundation of bed	5						
Places extra drawsheet at head and tucks in place	5						
Makes cuffs on top linen at head and foot of bed	5						
Fanfolds top linen to side of bed correctly	5						
Places underpads at the operative site	5						
Ties pillow to head of bed	5						
Elevates bed to level of stretcher	5						
Elevates siderail on side opposite where stretcher will be positioned	5						
4. Tapes plastic cuffed bag to bed or table	5						
5. Removes all unnecessary articles from bedside table	5						
6. Places emesis basin and tissues on bedside table	5						
7. Places equipment for vital signs on bedside table	5						
8. Tapes padded tongue blade to head of bed	5						
9. Positions other furniture out of path of stretcher	5						
10. Positions IV standard in convenient location	5						
11. Checks area before leaving to be sure all supplies and equipment are in place	3						
12. Replaces all equipment	3						
13. Washes hands	3						
14. Records or reports required information	5						
Totals	100						

* Final Check: Instructor or authorized person evaluates.
** Points Earned: Points possible times each "yes" check.

UNIT 20:13D Evaluation Sheet

Name _____ Date _____

Evaluated by _____

DIRECTIONS: Practice applying surgical hose according to the criteria listed. When you are ready for your final check, give this sheet to your instructor.

Applying Surgical Hose	Points Possible	Peer Check Yes	No	Final Check* Yes	No	Points Earned**	Comments
1. Checks order or obtains authorization	3						
2. Assembles supplies	2						
3. Knocks on door, introduces self, identifies patient, and explains procedure	2						
4. Closes door and screens unit	3						
5. Washes hands	2						
6. Checks stockings for cleanliness	5						
7. Reads instructions on how to determine measurement for correct size	5						
8. Locks and elevates bed and lowers siderail if elevated	3						
9. Exposes legs correctly	3						
10. Turns hose smooth side out	5						
11. Tucks foot into heel of stocking	5						
12. Eases foot and heel into position	5						
13. Pulls stockings over foot to ankle with gentle motion	5						
14. Eases stocking up leg	5						
15. Avoids stretching stocking	5						
16. Removes wrinkles from stocking	6						
17. Checks position to be sure stocking below knee	6						
18. Smooths excess material with palms of hands as necessary	5						
19. Pulls toe forward slightly	5						
20. Observes following checks before leaving:							
Patient in alignment	1						
Siderails elevated if indicated	1						
Bed at lowest level	1						
Call signal and supplies within reach of patient	1						
Area neat and clean	1						
21. Checks stocking at intervals:							
Color of skin	2						
Temperature of skin	2						
Swelling	2						
22. Removes stocking at least once every eight hours and gives skin care	4						
23. Washes hands	2						
24. Records/reports all required information	3						
Totals	100						

* Final Check: Instructor or authorized person evaluates.
** Points Earned: Points possible times each "yes" check.

UNIT 20:14 APPLYING BINDERS

ASSIGNMENT SHEET

Grade _____ Name _____

INTRODUCTION: This assignment will help you review the main facts regarding binders.

INSTRUCTIONS: Read the information about Applying Binders. In the space provided, print the word(s) that best completes the statement or answers the question.

1. List five (5) functions of binders.

2. Binders must be applied _____ to prevent _____, which can lead to the formation of _____. No _____ or _____ should be present. They should fit _____ for support but not be so _____ they cause discomfort.

3. Straight binders are usually applied to what three (3) parts of the body?

4. If pins are used to hold a binder in place, they should be placed no further than _____ inches apart for maximum support.

5. If the waist on a binder is too large, what can you do?

6. Why are breast binders used?

7. What has replaced the use of T-binders?

8. Binders are usually put into position from the _____ (bottom or top) to the _____ (bottom or top) .

9. What two (2) things must always be checked after binders have been applied?

10. Why is it important to remove binders at frequent intervals?

UNIT 20:14 Evaluation Sheet

Name _____ Date _____

Evaluated by _____

DIRECTIONS: Practice applying a straight binder according to the criteria listed. When you are ready for your final check, give this sheet to your instructor.

Applying a Straight Binder	Points Possible	Peer Check Yes	Peer Check No	Final Check* Yes	Final Check* No	Points Earned**	Comments
		PROFICIENT					
1. Checks order or obtains authorization	3						
2. Assembles supplies	3						
3. Inserts pins in bar of soap	3						
4. Knocks on door, introduces self, identifies patient, and explains procedure	3						
5. Closes door and screens unit	3						
6. Washes hands	3						
7. Locks and elevates bed to working level and lowers siderail if elevated	3						
8. Fanfolds top linens to expose abdomen	4						
9. Folds binder in half with the inside facing out	6						
10. Instructs patient to raise hips correctly or turns patient on side	6						
11. Places binder under patient	6						
12. Centers on back by spine	6						
13. Opens binder	6						
14. Checks location so binder will not interfere with use of bedpan	6						
15. Fastens binder from bottom to top	6						
16. Checks waist	6						
17. Makes darts at waist and holds with vertical pins if necessary	6						
18. Checks binder for snug fit	6						
19. Observes following checks before leaving:							
Patient in alignment	1						
Siderails elevated if indicated	1						
Bed at lowest level	1						
Call signal and supplies within patient's reach	1						
Area neat and clean	1						
20. Replaces equipment	3						
21. Washes hands	3						
22. Records or reports all required information	4						
Totals	100						

* Final Check: Instructor or authorized person evaluates.
** Points Earned: Points possible times each "yes" check.

UNIT 20:15 ADMINISTERING OXYGEN

ASSIGNMENT SHEET

Grade _____ Name _____

INTRODUCTION: The following assignment will help you learn the main points of oxygen administration.

DIRECTIONS: Review the information on Administering Oxygen. Then print the word(s) that best completes the statement or answers the question.

1. Why is it important to check your legal responsibilities before administering oxygen?

2. Define *hypoxia.*

3. List three (3) signs of oxygen shortage.

4. List the four (4) main methods of administering oxygen. Then list the usual flow rate for each method.

   Method   *Flow Rate*

5. Why is oxygen usually passed through water before being administered to a patient?

6. Why is distilled water used in the oxygen humidifier?

7. List four (4) safety rules that must be observed when oxygen is in use.

8. What does a pulse oximeter measure?

9. A patient who is receiving oxygen must be checked frequently. List three (3) special checkpoints that must be observed.

10. Who is usually responsible for oxygen administration in health care facilities?

UNIT 20:15 Evaluation Sheet

Name _____ Date _____

Evaluated by _____

DIRECTIONS: Practice administering oxygen according to the criteria listed. When you are ready for your final check, give this sheet to your instructor.

Administering Oxygen	Points Possible	PROFICIENT Peer Check Yes	No	Final Check* Yes	No	Points Earned**	Comments
1. Checks doctor's order or obtains orders from immediate supervisor	4						
2. Assembles equipment and supplies	3						
3. Knocks on door, introduces self, and identifies patient	3						
4. Explains procedure to patient and reassures as needed	3						
5. Washes hands	3						
6. Connects tubing to mask/cannula	4						
7. Checks water supply if humidifier used and adds distilled water as needed	4						
8. Turns on oxygen supply	4						
9. Regulates gauge for ordered liter flow or sets as follows if no specific order:							
Mask: 6–8 liters	2						
Cannula: 2–6 liters	2						
Catheter: 2–6 liters	2						
Tent: 10–12 liters	2						
10. Checks for oxygen flow by placing hand at outlet	4						
11. Puts on gloves	4						
12. Applies mask:							
Positions over mouth and nose	3						
Adjusts strap until snug	3						
13. Applies cannula:							
Places tips in nostrils	3						
Adjusts straps so position of tips maintained	3						
Instructs patient to breathe through nose	3						
14. Applies tent:							
Fills with oxygen	3						
Tucks in all edges	3						

515

Administering Oxygen	Points Possible	Peer Check		Final Check*		Points Earned**	Comments
		Yes	No	Yes	No		
15. Checks area for all of the following safety precautions:							
Eliminates sources of sparks or flames	3						
Cautions everyone against smoking	3						
Posts sign in patient care area	3						
16. Checks patient and area frequently for following points:							
Respirations	2						
Color	2						
Restlessness/discomfort	2						
Provides skin care to face/nose/ears	2						
Checks water level if humidifier used	2						
Checks gauge for correct liter flow	2						
17. Reports any abnormal observations immediately	4						
18. Cleans and replaces all equipment after use	3						
19. Removes gloves and washes hands	3						
20. Records/reports all required information	4						
Totals	100						

* Final Check: Instructor or authorized person evaluates.
** Points Earned: Points possible times each "yes" check.

UNIT 20:16 GIVING POSTMORTEM CARE

ASSIGNMENT SHEET

Grade _____ Name _____

INTRODUCTION: Providing postmortem care is a difficult but essential part of patient care. This assignment will help you review the main facts about postmortem care.

INSTRUCTIONS: Read the information on Giving Postmortem Care. In the space provided, print the word(s) that best completes the statement or answers the question.

1. What is postmortem care?

2. If a health care assistant has cared for a patient for a period of time, when the patient dies it is natural to feel _____ and a sense of _____ . A natural expression of grief is _____ and you should not be _____ if you do. However, health care workers must also try to control their _____ because family members will need their _____ .

3. List four (4) things that may have to be done to prepare the body for viewing by the family.

4. Patient's _____ apply after death. The body should be treated with _____ and _____ . _____ should be provided at all times.

5. List six (6) items that might be present in a morgue kit.

6. If jewelry is present on the body, how is it cared for?

7. If the family wants a wedding ring left on the body, what should you do?

8. Who is usually responsible for the removal of tubes or intravenous (IV) needles?

UNIT 20:16 Evaluation Sheet

Name _____ Date _____

Evaluated by _____

DIRECTIONS: Practice giving postmortem care according to the criteria listed. When you are ready for your final check, give this sheet to your instructor.

Giving Postmortem Care	Points Possible	Peer Check Yes	No	Final Check* Yes	No	Points Earned**	Comments
1. Checks order or obtains authorization	2						
2. Assembles equipment and supplies	2						
3. Identifies patient by checking armband	2						
4. Closes door and screens unit	2						
5. Washes hands and puts on gloves	2						
6. Locks and elevates bed and lowers siderail if elevated	2						
7. Positions body lying flat with arms and legs straight	4						
8. Closes eyes gently and uses moist cotton ball if necessary	4						
9. Replaces dentures in mouth and applies chin strap	4						
10. Removes and replaces soiled dressings	4						
11. Follows agency policy for removal of tubes, IVs, catheters, and drainage bags	4						
12. Bathes and dries soiled body areas	4						
13. Combs hair if needed	4						
14. Places underpad/padding under buttocks at anal area	4						
15. Removes gloves and washes hands	3						
16. Places clean gown on body	4						
17. Follows agency policy to handle jewelry	4						
18. Fills out identification cards/tags and places on ankle/toe	4						
19. Provides privacy for family to view body	4						
20. Places body in shroud/body bag or sheet	4						
21. Attaches second identification card/tag to shroud/bag	4						

Name _____

20:16 (cont.)

Giving Postmortem Care	Points Possible	Peer Check Yes	No	Final Check* Yes	No	Points Earned**	Comments
22. Collects all belongings	3						
23. Checks belongings with admission clothing list	3						
24. Places belongings in bag/container	3						
25. Labels belongings with identification card/tag	3						
26. Transfers body to stretcher	3						
27. Transports body to morgue	3						
28. Returns to unit	2						
29. Strips and cleans unit according to agency policy	2						
30. Replaces all equipment and leaves area neat and clean	2						
31. Washes hands	2						
32. Records or reports all required information	3						
Totals	100						

* Final Check: Instructor or authorized person evaluates.
** Points Earned: Points possible times each "yes" check.

UNIT 21:1 PERFORMING RANGE-OF-MOTION (ROM) EXERCISES

ASSIGNMENT SHEET

Grade _____ Name _____

INTRODUCTION: Range-of-motion (ROM) exercises help keep muscles and joints functioning. This assignment will help you review the information on ROMs.

INSTRUCTIONS: Read the information on Performing Range-of-Motion (ROM) Exercises. In the space provided, print the word(s) that best completes the statement or answers the question.

PART A:

1. Why are range-of-motion (ROM) exercises done?

2. Who performs ROM exercises?

3. Identify six (6) problems caused by lack of movement and inactivity.

4. Briefly describe each of the following types of range of motion exercises, and state who does each type:
   a. active:
   b. passive:
   c. resistive:

5. In some states or health care facilities, only _____ or _____ may perform range-of-motion exercises to the _____ and _____. Some exercises may be restricted or limited after _____ or _____ replacement surgery.

6. Where should support be provided when ROMs are being performed?

7. How many times should each movement be performed?

8. What should you do if a patient complains of pain during ROMs?

9. Identify two (2) ways to provide privacy for the patient while providing ROMs.

PART B: In the space provided, place the letter from Column B that best describes the motion in Column A. Letters may be used once, more than once, or not at all.

Column A

_____ 1. Bending a body part

_____ 2. Turning a body part downward

_____ 3. Moving toward thumb side of hand

_____ 4. Turning a body part outward

_____ 5. Moving a part toward the midline

_____ 6. Swinging the arm in a circle

_____ 7. Excessive straightening of a body part

_____ 8. Moving the lower arm away from upper arm

_____ 9. Moving toward little finger side of hand

_____ 10. Turning palm up

_____ 11. Turning a body part inward

_____ 12. Straightening the foot away from the knee

_____ 13. Moving the arm out to the side

_____ 14. Turning the head from side to side

_____ 15. Moving a part away from the midline

_____ 16. Bending the fingers to make a fist

_____ 17. Straightening a body part

_____ 18. Bending top of hand back toward the forearm

_____ 19. Bending the foot toward the knee

_____ 20. Turning the foot inward

Column B

A. Abduction

B. Adduction

C. Circumduction

D. Dorsiflexion

E. Eversion

F. Extension

G. Flexion

H. Hyperextension

I. Inversion

J. Plantar flexion

K. Pronation

L. Radial deviation

M. Rotation

N. Supination

O. Ulnar deviation

UNIT 21:1 Evaluation Sheet

Name _____ Date _____

Evaluated by _____

DIRECTIONS: Practice performing range-of-motion (ROM) exercises according to the criteria listed. When you are ready for your final check, give this sheet to your instructor.

PROFICIENT

Performing Range-of-Motion (ROM) Exercises	Points Possible	Peer Check Yes	No	Final Check* Yes	No	Points Earned**	Comments
1. Checks order or obtains authorization	2						
2. Determines type of ROMs and limitations to movement	2						
3. Assembles supplies	1						
4. Knocks on door, introduces self, identifies patient, and explains procedure	2						
5. Closes door and screens unit	2						
6. Washes hands	2						
7. Locks bed, elevates bed, and lowers siderail if elevated	2						
8. Positions patient in supine position	2						
9. Drapes patient with bath blanket	2						
10. Performs all ROMs as follows:							
Proceeds in organized manner	2						
Performs each movement three to five times	2						
Provides support for body parts	2						
Uses correct body mechanics	2						
Stops exercise if patient complains of pain/discomfort	2						
11. Exercises neck, if authorized:							
Supports head properly	2						
Rotates by turning head side to side	1						
Flexes by moving head toward chest	1						
Extends by returning head to upright position	1						
Hyperextends by tilting head backward	1						
Flexes laterally by moving head toward shoulders	1						

523

Performing Range-of-Motion (ROM) Exercises	Points Possible	Peer Check		Final Check*		Points Earned**	Comments
		Yes	No	Yes	No		
12. Exercises nearest shoulder:							
Supports arm properly	2						
Abducts by bringing arm straight out	1						
Adducts by moving arm in to side	1						
Flexes by raising arm in front of body above head	1						
Extends by bringing arm to side from above head	1						
13. Exercises nearest elbow:							
Supports arm properly	2						
Flexes by bending forearm to shoulder	1						
Extends by straightening arm	1						
Pronates by turning forearm and palm of hand down	1						
Supinates by turning forearm and palm of hand up	1						
14. Exercises nearest wrist:							
Supports wrist properly	2						
Flexes by bending hand down toward forearm	1						
Extends by straightening hand	1						
Hyperextends by bending top of hand back toward forearm	1						
Deviates ulnarly by moving hand to little finger side	1						
Deviates radially by moving hand to thumb side	1						
15. Exercises nearest fingers and thumb:							
Supports hand properly	2						
Flexes by bending fingers in toward palm	1						
Extends by straightening fingers	1						
Abducts by spreading apart	1						
Adducts by moving together	1						
Performs opposition by touching thumb to each finger tip	1						
16. Exercises nearest hip:							
Supports leg properly	2						
Abducts by moving leg out to side	1						
Adducts by moving leg in toward body	1						
Flexes by bending knee and moving thigh toward abdomen	1						
Extends by straightening knee and leg away from abdomen	1						

Performing Range-of-Motion (ROM) Exercises	Points Possible	Peer Check		Final Check*		Points Earned**	Comments
		Yes	No	Yes	No		
Rotates medially by bending knee and turning leg in toward midline	1						
Rotates laterally by bending knee and turning leg out away from midline	1						
17. Exercises nearest knee:							
Supports leg properly	2						
Flexes by bending lower leg back toward thigh	1						
Extends by straightening leg	1						
18. Exercises nearest ankle:							
Supports foot properly	2						
Dorsiflexes by moving foot up toward knee	1						
Plantar flexes by moving foot down away from knee	1						
Inverts by turning inward	1						
Everts by turning outward	1						
19. Exercises nearest toes:							
Supports leg and foot on bed	2						
Abducts by separating	1						
Adducts by moving together	1						
Flexes by bending down to bottom of foot	1						
Extends by straightening	1						
20. Raises siderail, moves to opposite side, and lowers siderail	2						
21. Repeats steps 12 to 19 on remaining joints	3						
22. Positions patient in correct alignment	2						
23. Replaces bed covers and removes bath blanket	1						
24. Observes checkpoints before leaving:							
Elevates siderails if indicated	1						
Lowers bed to lowest level	1						
Places call signal and supplies within reach	1						
Leaves area neat and clean	1						
25. Washes hands	2						
26. Records or reports required information	2						
Totals	100						

* Final Check: Instructor or authorized person evaluates.
** Points Earned: Points possible times each "yes" check.

ASSIGNMENT SHEET

Grade _____ Name _____

INTRODUCTION: This assignment sheet will help you review the main facts on ambulation aids.

INSTRUCTIONS: Review the information about Ambulating Patients Who Use Transfer (Gait) Belts, Crutches, Canes, or Walkers. In the space provided, print the word(s) that best completes the statement or answers the question.

1. When a patient is being fitted for crutches, the following measurement points should be noted:

   Height of heels on shoes:_____

   Position crutches:_____ inches to the side and front of the patient's foot.

   Distance between axilla and axillary bar: _____

   Degree angle for elbows: _____

2. If a patient can bear weight on both legs, the _____ gait is usually taught first. When the patient has mastered this gait, the _____ gait is taught next. After the patient gains strength in the arms and shoulders, faster gaits such as the _____ or_____ are taught last.

3. If a patient can bear weight on only one leg, the first crutch gait taught is the _____. When the patient gains strength in the arms and shoulders, faster gaits such as the _____ or _____ are taught.

4. Why is it important to avoid pressure on the axillary area when fitting a patient for crutches?

5. Canes should generally be used on the _____ side.

6. The cane handle should be level with _____. The elbow should be flexed at a/an _____ degree angle while using the cane.

7. Handles on a walker should be level with the _____. The elbows should be flexed at a/an _____ degree angle.

8. Why are the legs of the walker fitted with rubber tips?

9. Why is it important to caution a patient against sliding a walker?

10. What type of grasp should be used with a transfer belt? Why?

Name _____ Date _____

Evaluated by _____

DIRECTIONS: Practice ambulating a patient with a transfer (gait) belt according to the criteria listed. When you are ready for your final check, give this sheet to your instructor.

PROFICIENT

Ambulating a Patient with a Transfer (Gait) Belt	Points Possible	Peer Check		Final Check*		Points Earned**	Comments
		Yes	No	Yes	No		
1. Checks order or obtains authorization	2						
2. Assembles equipment and supplies	2						
3. Introduces self, identifies patient, and explains procedure	2						
4. Closes door and screens unit	2						
5. Washes hands	3						
6. Locks bed to prevent movement and lowers siderail if elevated	2						
7. Assists patient to sitting position	2						
8. Puts on robe	2						
9. Applies transfer (gait) belt:							
Checks for correct size	2						
Places on top of clothing	2						
Positions around waist	2						
Positions buckle/clasp slightly off center	2						
Makes sure belt is smooth and wrinkle free	2						
10. Tightens and closes belt correctly:							
Pulls belt snugly against patient	2						
Secures clasp or buckle	2						
Inserts two fingers under belt	2						
11. Checks belt:							
Checks that belt is comfortable	2						
Checks respirations	2						
Makes sure breasts not under belt	2						
12. Puts on patient's shoes/slippers	2						
13. Assists patient to standing position:							
Faces patient and gets broad base of support	2						
Grasps loops or places hands under sides of belt	2						
Bends at knees	2						
Gives signal for patient to stand	2						
Keeps back straight and straightens knees as patient stands	2						

Ambulating a Patient with a Transfer (Gait) Belt	Points Possible	Peer Check		Final Check*		Points Earned**	Comments
		Yes	No	Yes	No		
14. Moves to position behind patient:							
Supports patient in standing position	2						
Keeps one hand firmly on side of belt	2						
Moves other hand to grasp back of belt	2						
Moves second hand from side to back	2						
Moves behind patient	2						
15. Ambulates patient with belt:							
Keeps firm underhand grasps on belt	3						
Walks slightly behind patient	3						
Encourages patient to walk slowly	2						
Encourages patient to use handrails	2						
16. Assists patient if patient starts to fall:							
Keeps firm grip on belt	2						
Braces patient with body	2						
Eases patient slowly to floor	2						
Protects patient's head	2						
Calls for help but remains with patient	2						
Makes no attempt to get patient up until help arrives	2						
17. Returns patient to bed after ambulation	2						
18. Removes the belt	2						
19. Observes following checks before leaving:							
Patient in correct alignment	1						
Siderails elevated if indicated	1						
Bed at lowest level	1						
Call signal and supplies within reach	1						
Area neat and clean	1						
20. Replaces all equipment used	2						
21. Washes hands	3						
22. Records or reports all required information	3						
Totals	100						

* Final Check: Instructor or authorized person evaluates.
** Points Earned: Points possible times each "yes" check.

UNIT 21:2B Evaluation Sheet

Name _____   Date _____

Evaluated by _____

DIRECTIONS: Practice ambulating a patient with crutches according to the criteria listed. When you are ready for your final check, give this sheet to your instructor.

PROFICIENT

Ambulating a Patient Who Uses Crutches	Points Possible	Peer Check Yes	No	Final Check* Yes	No	Points Earned**	Comments
1. Checks order or obtains authorization	3						
2. Assembles equipment and supplies	2						
3. Checks rubber tips on ends	3						
4. Checks padding on axillary bar and handrest	3						
5. Introduces self, identifies patient, and explains procedure	3						
6. Washes hands	2						
7. Assists patient to put on shoes:							
Low broad heel	2						
Heel 1 to 1 ½ inches high	2						
Nonskid soles	2						
8. Puts transfer (gait) belt on patient, assists patient to standing position, and positions crutches	3						
9. Checks measurement of crutches for following:							
Crutches 4 to 6 inches in front of feet	2						
Crutches 4 to 6 inches to side of feet	2						
2 inch gap between axilla and bar	2						
Elbow flexed at 25–30° angle	2						
10. Assists with 4 point gait:							
Moves right crutch forward	3						
Moves left foot forward	3						
Moves left crutch forward	3						
Moves right foot forward	3						
11. Assists with 3 point gait:							
Advances both crutches and affected foot	3						
Transfers body weight forward to crutches	3						
Advances unaffected foot	3						

Ambulating a Patient Who Uses Crutches	Points Possible	Peer Check		Final Check*		Points Earned**	Comments
		Yes	No	Yes	No		
12. Assists with 2 point gait:							
Moves right foot and left crutch forward together	4						
Moves left foot and right crutch forward together	4						
13. Assists with swing to gait:							
Balances weight on foot/feet	3						
Moves both crutches forward	3						
Transfers weight forward	3						
Swings feet up to crutches	3						
14. Assists with swing-through gait:							
Balances weight on foot/feet	2						
Advances both crutches	2						
Transfers weight forward	2						
Swings feet up to and through crutches	2						
Stops slightly in front of crutches	2						
15. Checks that patient does not rest weight on axillary rest or bar	3						
16. Limits distances so patient not moving too far at one time	3						
17. Removes transfer belt, positions patient comfortably, and observes safety checks when ambulation complete	3						
18. Replaces equipment	2						
19. Washes hands	2						
20. Records or reports required information	3						
Totals	100						

* Final Check: Instructor or authorized person evaluates.
** Points Earned: Points possible times each "yes" check.

UNIT 21:2C Evaluation Sheet

Name _____ Date _____

Evaluated by _____

DIRECTIONS: Practice ambulating a patient using a cane according to the criteria listed. When you are ready for your final check, give this sheet to your instructor.

PROFICIENT

Ambulating a Patient Who Uses a Cane	Points Possible	Peer Check Yes	No	Final Check* Yes	No	Points Earned**	Comments
1. Checks order or obtains authorization	4						
2. Assembles equipment and supplies	3						
3. Checks rubber suction tip	4						
4. Introduces self, identifies patient, and explains procedure	3						
5. Washes hands	3						
6. Assists patient to put on shoes:							
Low broad heel	2						
Heel 1 to 1½ inches high	2						
Nonskid soles	2						
7. Puts transfer (gait) belt on patient, assists patient to standing position, and positions cane	4						
8. Checks measurement of cane for following points:							
Positions cane 6–10 inches from side of unaffected foot	4						
Top of cane at top of femur at the hip joint	4						
Elbow flexed at 25–30° angle	4						
9. Tells patient to use cane on unaffected side	4						
10. Assists patient with 3 point gait: Balances weight on unaffected foot	3						
Moves cane forward	3						
Moves affected foot forward	3						
Transfers weight forward to cane	3						
Moves unaffected foot forward	3						
11. Assists patient with 2 point gait: Balances weight on unaffected foot	3						
Moves cane and affected foot forward	3						
Keeps cane close to body	3						
Transfers weight forward to cane	3						
Moves unaffected foot forward	3						
12. Remains alert at all times and watches patient closely to ensure that patient maintains balance	4						
13. Assists patient on steps:							
Steps first with unaffected foot	3						
Follows with cane and affected foot	3						

Ambulating a Patient Who Uses a Cane	Points Possible	Peer Check		Final Check*		Points Earned**	Comments
		Yes	No	Yes	No		
14. Gives verbal clues to assist patient in performing proper gait pattern	4						
15. Removes transfer belt, positions patient comfortably, and observes safety checks when ambulation complete	3						
16. Replaces equipment	3						
17. Washes hands	3						
18. Records or reports patient's progress and any problems noted	4						
Totals	100						

* Final Check: Instructor or authorized person evaluates.
** Points Earned: Points possible times each "yes" check.

UNIT 21:2D Evaluation Sheet

Name _____ Date _____

Evaluated by _____

DIRECTIONS: Practice ambulating a patient using a walker according to the criteria listed. When you are ready for your final check, give this sheet to your instructor.

PROFICIENT

Ambulating a Patient Who Uses a Walker	Points Possible	Peer Check Yes	No	Final Check* Yes	No	Points Earned**	Comments
1. Checks order or obtains authorization	4						
2. Assembles equipment and supplies	2						
3. Checks walker for following points:							
Rubber suction tips secure	4						
No rough or damaged edges on hand rests	4						
4. Introduces self, identifies patient, and explains procedure	3						
5. Washes hands	2						
6. Assists patient to put on shoes:							
Low broad heel	2						
Heel 1 to 1$\frac{1}{2}$ inches high	2						
Nonskid soles	2						
7. Puts transfer (gait) belt on patient, assists patient to standing position, positions walker, and asks patient to grasp hand rests securely	5						
8. Checks height of walker for following points:							
Hand rests at level of top of femur at the hip joint	4						
Elbows flexed at 25–30° angle	4						
9. Starts with patient standing inside walker	6						
10. Tells patient to lift walker forward so back legs are even with patient's toes	6						
11. Cautions patient against sliding walker	6						
12. Tells patient to transfer weight slightly forward to walker	6						
13. Tells patient to use walker for support while walking into walker	6						
14. Walks to side and slightly behind patient	5						
15. Remains alert and watches patient closely to ensure that patient maintains balance	5						

Ambulating a Patient Who Uses a Walker	Points Possible	Peer Check		Final Check*		Points Earned**	Comments
		Yes	No	Yes	No		
16. Checks that patient is lifting walker	5						
17. Checks that patient is placing walker just to toes	5						
18. Positions patient comfortably, removes transfer belt, and observes safety checks when ambulation complete	3						
19. Replaces all equipment	2						
20. Washes hands	2						
21. Records or reports patient's progress and any problems noted	5						
Totals	100						

* Final Check: Instructor or authorized person evaluates.
** Points Earned: Points possible times each "yes" check.

UNIT 21:3 ADMINISTERING HEAT/COLD APPLICATIONS

ASSIGNMENT SHEET

Grade _____ Name _____

INTRODUCTION: This sheet will help you review the main facts regarding heat and cold applications.

INSTRUCTIONS: Review the information about Administering Heat/Cold Applications. In the space provided, print the word(s) that best completes the statement or answers the question.

1. How do blood vessels react when heat applications are applied?

   How does this affect the blood supply to the area?

2. How do blood vessels react when cold applications are applied?

   How does this affect the blood supply to the area?

3. List three (3) reasons why cold applications are done.

4. List three (3) reasons why heat applications are done.

5. Define the following words, and list two (2) examples for each type of application.
   a. moist cold:
   b. dry cold:
   c. moist heat:
   d. dry heat:

6. What is the purpose of a sitz bath?

7. What are hydrocollator packs?

8. Paraffin wax treatments are often used for _____ or prior to _____.

9. A/An _____ order is needed before heat or cold applications can be applied to a patient.

10. Name three (3) things that should be checked frequently while a heat or cold application is in place.

535

Name _____ Date _____

Evaluated by _____

DIRECTIONS: Practice applying an ice bag/collar according to the criteria listed. When you are ready for your final check, give this sheet to your instructor.

PROFICIENT

Applying an Ice Bag or Ice Collar	Points Possible	Peer Check Yes	No	Final Check* Yes	No	Points Earned**	Comments
1. Checks order or obtains authorization	2						
2. Assembles equipment and supplies	2						
3. Washes hands	2						
4. Fills bag with water to check leaks	4						
5. Rinses ice cubes to remove sharp edges	4						
6. Uses scoop or cup without bottom to fill bag	4						
7. Fills one-half full	4						
8. Expels air from bag	4						
9. Secures cap in place	4						
10. Dries outside of bag	4						
11. Covers bag correctly	4						
12. Knocks on door, introduces self, identifies patient, and explains procedure	4						
13. Washes hands and puts on gloves if needed	3						
14. Positions ice bag gently with metal cap away from patient's skin	4						
15. Checks patient and position of application before leaving	4						
16. Places call signal within reach	3						
17. Removes gloves and washes hands before leaving room	2						
18. Checks following points at frequent intervals:							
Checks bag for coldness	2						
Refills as necessary	2						
Checks condition of skin	3						
Removes immediately if skin mottled or discolored	3						
19. Leaves application in place for ordered length of time	4						

21:3A (cont.)

Applying an Ice Bag or Ice Collar	Points Possible	Peer Check Yes	No	Final Check* Yes	No	Points Earned**	Comments
20. Removes ice bag/collar at correct time	3						
21. Checks condition of skin	4						
22. Notes patient's comments	4						
23. Observes following checks before leaving:							
Patient in correct alignment	1						
Siderails elevated if indicated	1						
Bed at lowest level	1						
Call signal and supplies in reach	1						
Area neat and clean	1						
24. Empties ice bag or collar and wipes with a disinfectant	2						
25. Inflates with air for storage	2						
26. Replaces all equipment	2						
27. Washes hands	2						
28. Records or reports all required information	4						
Totals	100						

* Final Check: Instructor or authorized person evaluates.
** Points Earned: Points possible times each "yes" check.

UNIT 21:3B Evaluation Sheet

Name _____ Date _____

Evaluated by _____

DIRECTIONS: Practice applying a warm water bag according to the criteria listed. When you are ready for your final check, give this sheet to your instructor.

Applying a Warm Water Bag	Points Possible	Peer Check Yes	No	Final Check* Yes	No	Points Earned**	Comments
1. Checks order or obtains authorization	2						
2. Assembles equipment and supplies	2						
3. Washes hands	2						
4. Fills with water or air to check for leaks	4						
5. Fills pitcher with water at 115–120° F or 46–49° C	4						
6. Fills bag 1/3–1/2 full	4						
7. Expels air from bag	4						
8. Closes bag correctly	4						
9. Dries outside with towels	4						
10. Checks for signs of leaks	4						
11. Covers bag properly	4						
12. Knocks on door, introduces self, identifies patient, and explains procedure	4						
13. Washes hands and puts on gloves if needed	2						
14. Applies bag gently to affected area	4						
15. Positions bag on top of affected area	4						
16. Checks patient comfort and position of bag before leaving	4						
17. Places call signal within reach	3						
18. Removs gloves and washes hands before leaving room	2						
19. Rechecks at frequent intervals for following points:							
Notes pain, extreme redness	3						
Removes immediately if signs of burn present	3						
Refills as necessary	3						
20. Removes application at end of ordered time period	4						

PROFICIENT

21:3B (cont.)

Applying a Warm Water Bag	Points Possible	Peer Check Yes	No	Final Check* Yes	No	Points Earned**	Comments
21. Checks skin carefully	4						
22. Notes patient's comments	4						
23. Observes following checks before leaving:							
Patient in correct alignment	1						
Siderails elevated if indicated	1						
Bed at lowest level	1						
Call signal and supplies within reach	1						
Area neat and clean	1						
24. Empties water from bag and wipes with a disinfectant	3						
25. Fills bag with air before storing it	3						
26. Replaces all equipment	2						
27. Washes hands	2						
28. Records or reports all required information	3						
Totals	100						

* Final Check: Instructor or authorized person evaluates.
** Points Earned: Points possible times each "yes" check.

UNIT 21:3C Evaluation Sheet

Name _____ Date _____

Evaluated by _____

DIRECTIONS: Practice applying an aquamatic pad according to the criteria listed. When you are ready for your final check, give this sheet to your instructor.

Applying an Aquamatic Pad	Points Possible	Peer Check Yes	No	Final Check* Yes	No	Points Earned**	Comments
PROFICIENT							
1. Checks orders or obtains authorization	3						
2. Assembles equipment and supplies	2						
3. Knocks on door, introduces self, identifies patient, and explains procedure	3						
4. Washes hands and puts on gloves if needed	2						
5. Places unit on solid table	4						
6. Checks cord carefully	4						
7. Attaches tubing to main unit and aquamatic pad if necessary	4						
8. Fills unit to fill line with distilled water	4						
9. Screws cap in place and loosens 1/4 turn	4						
10. Plugs in cord	4						
11. Sets temperature at 95–105° F or 35–41° C, or as ordered	4						
12. Turns unit on	4						
13. Checks for leaks and warmth	4						
14. Coils tubing to facilitate water flow, checks tubing for kinks or obstructions, and rechecks level of water in reservoir	4						
15. Covers pad properly	4						
16. Places pad on correct area	4						
17. Places call signal within reach	3						
18. Removes gloves if worn and washes hands before leaving room	2						
19. Rechecks patient and pad at intervals for following:							
Checks condition of skin	3						
Removes if skin burned or patient complains of pain	3						
Refills unit as necessary	3						
20. Removes pad at end of ordered time period	4						

21:3C (cont.)

Applying an Aquamatic Pad	Points Possible	Peer Check		Final Check*		Points Earned**	Comments
		Yes	No	Yes	No		
21. Checks condition of skin	4						
22. Notes patient's comments on effectiveness	4						
23. Observes following checks before leaving:							
Patient in correct alignment	1						
Siderails elevated if indicated	1						
Bed at lowest level	1						
Call signal and supplies within reach	1						
Area neat and clean	1						
24. Empties pad and control unit	2						
25. Disinfects unit and pad correctly or discards pad if disposable	2						
26. Replaces all equipment	2						
27. Removes gloves if worn and washes hands	2						
28. Records or reports all required information	3						
Totals	100						

* Final Check: Instructor or authorized person evaluates.
** Points Earned: Points possible times each "yes" check.

Name _____ Date _____

Evaluated by _____

DIRECTIONS: Practice applying a moist compress according to the criteria listed. When you are ready for your final check, give this sheet to your instructor.

PROFICIENT

Applying a Moist Compress	Points Possible	Peer Check Yes	No	Final Check* Yes	No	Points Earned**	Comments
1. Checks order or obtains authorization	4						
2. Assembles equipment and supplies	2						
3. Knocks on door, introduces self, identifies patient, and explains procedure	2						
4. Closes door and screens unit	2						
5. Washes hands and puts on gloves if necessary	2						
6. Elevates bed and lowers siderail if elevated	2						
7. Positions underpad or bed protector by area to be treated	4						
8. Fills basin with correct temperature water:							
Checks temperature with bath thermometer	4						
Uses cold water and at times ice cubes for cold compress	4						
Uses 100–105° F or 37.8–41° C for hot compress	4						
9. Puts compress in water	5						
10. Wrings out compress to remove excess water	5						
11. Applies compress to correct area	5						
12. Covers compress with plastic sheet and towel or underpad	5						
13. Covers with ice bag/aquamatic pad if indicated	4						
14. Places call signal in reach	4						
15. Removes gloves if worn and washes hands before leaving room	2						

Name _____

21:3D (cont.)

Applying a Moist Compress	Points Possible	Peer Check Yes	No	Final Check* Yes	No	Points Earned**	Comments
16. Checks compress at frequent intervals:							
Changes compress and remoistens as necessary	3						
Checks condition of skin	3						
Notes pain, extreme redness	3						
Removes immediately if signs of burn present	3						
17. Removes application at end of ordered time period	5						
18. Checks skin carefully	5						
19. Notes patient's comments	5						
20. Observes following checks before leaving:							
Patient in correct alignment	1						
Siderails elevated if indicated	1						
Bed at lowest level	1						
Call signal and supplies within reach	1						
Area neat and clean	1						
21. Replaces all equipment	2						
22. Removes gloves if worn and washes hands	2						
23. Records or reports all required information	4						
Totals	100						

* Final Check: Instructor or authorized person evaluates.
** Points Earned: Points possible times each "yes" check.

UNIT 21:3E Evaluation Sheet

Name _____ Date _____

Evaluated by _____

DIRECTIONS: Practice administering a sitz bath according to the criteria listed. When you are ready for your final check, give this sheet to your instructor.

PROFICIENT

Administering a Sitz Bath	Points Possible	Peer Check Yes	No	Final Check* Yes	No	Points Earned**	Comments
1. Checks order or obtains authorization	3						
2. Assembles equipment and supplies	3						
3. Knocks on door, introduces self, identifies patient, and explains procedure	3						
4. Washes hands	3						
5. Prepares sitz chair:							
Sets temperature at 105° F or 41° C	3						
Fills with water	3						
Plugs in cord	3						
Drapes bottom with towel or bath blanket	3						
6. Prepares tub or sitz tub:							
Regulates temperature of water at 105° F or 41° C	3						
Fills with water to correct level	3						
Places towel or bath blanket in bottom of tub	3						
7. Prepares portable unit:							
Fills container with water at 105° F or 41° C	3						
Positions container on commode or toilet seat	3						
Connects tubing correctly	3						
Clamps tubing	3						
Positions holes on tubing to face side	3						
Fills bag with water at 110–115° F or 43–46° C	3						
8. Positions patient in bath with perineal area in water	5						
9. Covers legs/shoulders with bath blanket	5						
10. Observes patient for signs of weakness or fainting	5						

544   Copyright © 2001 Delmar Thomson Learning. All rights reserved.

21:3E (cont.)

Administering a Sitz Bath	Points Possible	Peer Check		Final Check*		Points Earned**	Comments
		Yes	No	Yes	No		
11. Maintains temperature by adding water to tub or allowing water to flow from bag on portable unit	5						
12. Continues treatment 20 minutes or as ordered	5						
13. Dries patient and replaces clothes at end of bath	5						
14. Returns patient to bed	3						
15. Observes following checks before leaving:							
Patient in alignment	1						
Siderails elevated if indicated	1						
Bed at lowest level	1						
Call signal and supplies within reach	1						
Area neat and clean	1						
16. Wears gloves to empty and disinfect tub or chair	2						
17. Cleans and replaces all equipment	2						
18. Removes gloves and washes hands	3						
19. Records or reports all required information	4						
Totals	100						

* Final Check: Instructor or authorized person evaluates.
** Points Earned: Points possible times each "yes" check.

UNIT 22:1 FILING RECORDS

ASSIGNMENT SHEET

Grade _____ Name _____

INTRODUCTION: This assignment will help you review the main facts on filing systems and methods of filing.

INSTRUCTIONS: Read the information about Filing Records. In the space provided, print the word(s) that best completes the statement or answers the question.

1. What is filing?

2. List two (2) reasons why filing methods are necessary.

3. Briefly describe how records are filed in each of the following systems.

   a. Alphabetical:

   b. Numerical:

   c. Geographic:

   d. Subject:

4. Why are cross indexes or references essential in a filing system?

5. List two (2) ways cross indexes or references can be kept.

6. The filing folders should be _____ and of good _____. Files should be _____ located. Filing cabinets should be _____ and equipped with _____. Sufficient file space must be provided so that records are not _____.

7. Where is the data for computerized "paperless" files stored?

8. How does color coded indexing help prevent errors?

9. Why is it easier to locate a file that is out of place when the files are color coded?

UNIT 22:1A FILING RECORDS USING THE ALPHABETICAL OR NUMERICAL SYSTEM

ASSIGNMENT SHEET #1

Grade _____ Name _____

INTRODUCTION: The following assignment will allow you to practice the basic principles of filing.

INSTRUCTIONS: Read the information section on Filing Using the Alphabetical or Numerical System. In the space provided, list the correct filing order.

1. Alphabetical Filing: For each group of names below, index each name correctly in the space provided. Then, in the last column, place the indexed names (from each group) in the correct filing order. See first example.

Group 1	Indexing Order	Filing Order
Mary K. Brown	Brown, Mary K.	Bell, Arlet Ann
June J. Smith		
Betty M. Stanton		
Jesse Tom Thomas		
Arlet Ann Bell		
C. M. James		
Mary S. Jones		

Group 2	Indexing Order	Filing Order
A. Barr		
Bruce Arnold Barr		
B. D. Barr		
Bruce A. Barr		
Arnold Barr		
David B. Barr		
Bruce Barr		

Group 3	Indexing Order	Filing Order
Cynthia Macerow		
Michael M. O'Rouge		
Camelia MacDanner		
Carol McDavis		
Carl M. O'Brian		
Mary DuBarry		
Charles M. Macer		
Clair C. McDowell		
Christopher C. Mack		
Mary D. Ducan		
Mack M. Mt. John		
Jean Mount-Smith		

Group 4	*Indexing Order*	*Filing Order*
Carl Kirk (Clinton, Iowa)		
Carol Kirk		
Carl Kirk (Ashland, Ohio)		
C. Kirk		
Harry Kirk, RN (Ash, Ohio)		
Genevieve Krirk		
Roger Krickey		
Michael Mounts		
Lanna McKirk		
Mike Mt. Kirk		
Harry Kirk, MD (Bath, Ohio)		
Harry Kirk, DDS (Sandusky, Ohio)		

2. Numerical Order: Place the following numbers in numerical order. Remember to ignore zeros that come before the number while filing but do not eliminate them.

249

588

456

0987

00034

5678

0086

00289

0039

288

00250

9870

3. Terminal number system: Below are numbers for two systems. Divide the numbers into two systems, and then place each system in correct numerical order.

		System 1	*System 2*
08–99–90	70–67–90		
07–77–90	45–34–88		
06–76–88	02–34–88		
05–65–90	52–45–88		
04–66–88	03–94–90		
55–34–88	22–43–88		
43–42–90	24–32–88		
45–33–90	06–82–90		
34–33–90	62–62–88		
62–66–88	00–94–90		

ASSIGNMENT SHEET #2

Grade _____ Name _____

INTRODUCTION: This assignment will allow you additional practice in correct methods of filing.

INSTRUCTIONS: Review information. Learn from the corrected errors of assignment # 1. Then complete the following information.

1. Alphabetical Filing: For each group of names below, index each name in the space provided. Then place the indexed names in correct filing order.

Group 1	Indexing Order	Filing Order
Judy Sainer		
Stacy St. John		
John S. Stacy		
Jill Stadler		
Joseph St. Clair		
Michael Scott		
Lois Scanlon		
Bob Scodova		
Frederick C. Set		
Mike M. Sanborn		
John Stanton		
Mike Sanborn		

Group 2	Indexing Order	Filing Order
Henry Russ		
Rupert C. Rush		
Herbert Rusk		
Henry C. Russ		
Orville D. Rush		
Tom D. Rush, Sr		
Robert A. Rusell		
Barbara D. Russell		
Tom Dean Rush, Jr		
Michael Rurals		
Brent T. Rusiska		
Bonnie F. Russell		
Kenneth K. Russel		
Lennie L. Ruster		
Mable M. Rustert		
Florence C. Rusher		
Connie S. O'Rush		
Mary Russell-Brown		

Group 3   *Indexing Order*   *Filing Order*

Third Street Ambulance Supplies

EMS Supply Corporation

4th Street Medical Supplies

Mike Smith, DDS, Miami, Florida

American Medical Association

American Nurses Association

A. M. Albian Company

Dr. John's Foot Pads

Mike Smith, MD, Lakeland, Florida

Mike A. Smith, ATR, Arcadia, Florida

The Company for Medical Supplies

M. A. Smith Pharmacy

Smith Medical Equipment of Miami Florida

2nd Avenue Pharmacy

2. Numerical Order: Place the following numbers in numerical order. Start with the left hand answer column from top to bottom and then use the right hand column.

05820	50
0582	0062
5822	555
0058	005821
0005	00555
0085	082
008	080
0850	00088
0567	85200

3. Terminal Number System: Below are two systems of numbers. Divide the numbers into two separate systems (using terminal digits) and then place each system in correct numerical order.

		System 1	*System 2*
5862–77	5682–77		
4657–77	4004–77		
4328–65	4328–77		
3333–65	0333–65		
0324–65	3245–65		
2435–65	3425–65		
3891–77	0020–77		
0002–77	0002–65		
0200–77	0033–65		
0020–65	5865–77		

551

Name _____ Date _____

Evaluated by _____

DIRECTIONS: Practice filing records according to the criteria listed. When you are ready for your final check, give this sheet to your instructor.

PROFICIENT

Filing Records Using Alphabetical or Numerical Systems	Points Possible	Peer Check Yes	No	Final Check* Yes	No	Points Earned**	Comments
Files series of 50 names alphabetically meeting all of the following points:							
Indexes personal names							
Indexes names of businesses and organizations							
Indexes words such as "of," and," etc.							
Files names in strict alphabetical order							
Files "nothing" before "something" (Boon, W. before Boon, Will)							
Treats prefixes as part of the name							
Uses hyphenated names as one unit							
Spells out known abbreviations such as "Mt"							
Ignores titles, degrees, or seniority as indexing unit							
Uses geographic location as final indexing unit							
Spells out numbers as letters (3rd as "third")							
2 points for each name in correct filing order	100						
Totals	100						
Files series of 50 numbers meeting the following criteria:							
Puts numbers in order from small to large							
Disregards zeros placed in front of numbers							
2 points for each number in correct filing order	100						
Totals	100						
Files 50 numbers in a terminal number system (5 terminal digits with 10 numbers in each digit system) meeting the following criteria:							
Separates numbers into five terminal digit systems							
Arranges each system in correct numerical order							
Places five terminal digit systems in correct numerical order							
2 points for each number in correct filing order	100						
Totals	100						

* Final Check: Instructor or authorized person evaluates.
** Points Earned: Points possible times each "yes" check.

UNIT 22:2 USING THE TELEPHONE

ASSIGNMENT SHEET

Grade _____ Name _____

INTRODUCTION: This assignment will help you review the main facts about correct telephone techniques.

INSTRUCTIONS: In the space provided, print the word(s) that answers the question or completes the statement. Refer to the information on Using the Telephone, as needed.

1. List two (2) qualities that should be present in your voice when answering a telephone.

2. Always answer the telephone _____ and answer with a/an _____.

3. List five (5) points that should be noted on a memorandum or message sheet.

4. Reword the following phrases so they follow the correct rules for telephone techniques.

   a. "Hi"

   b. "Who is this?"

   c. "What do you want?"

   d. "What's your name again?"

   e. "The physician is playing golf."

   f. "Huh?"

   g. "Give me your name, or I won't connect you."

   h. "He don't talk to salespersons."

   i. "Bye"

   j. "He's busy, call back."

5. Why do you screen calls instead of just putting all calls through right away?

6. Identify two (2) types of information you must obtain from the caller to screen telephone calls.

7. What is telephone triage?

8. Why should you allow the caller to hang up first?

9. What is the purpose of an automated routing unit in a telephone system?

10. List two (2) reasons why a cellular telephone is more efficient than a paging system.

11. Why is it important to *never* discuss confidential patient information on a cellular telephone?

12. Can confidential patient information be sent by electronic mail (e-mail)? Why or why not?

13. Identify three (3) ways to meet legal and confidentiality requirements while faxing medical records.

14. You are employed by Dr. Myra Jones. Read the following facts and record each on the sample telephone message pads. Print all information clearly.

   a. Mrs. Smith calls Dr. Jones at 8:30 AM. Her daughter Melinda has a fever of 102. She wants the physician to either see the child or call in a prescription. No other signs or symptoms are present. She can't bring the child in until 4:00 PM. Her phone number is 522-5409.

   b. Dr. Peterson calls at 9:15 AM. He has seen Mrs. Complaint, a patient Dr. Jones referred to him for consultation. He would like to tell Dr. Jones his findings. He will be in his office from 1-4 PM. His office number is 528-0991. From 4-6 PM he will be at extension 34 at the hospital. The hospital number is 524-2118. After 7 PM, he will be at home. His home number is 756-6677.

   c. Ace Medical supply salesman, John Cauffwell, calls at 9:30 AM. He is calling in regard to the EKG paper the physician ordered. Paper number 524 is no longer available. He can send the new substitute, model 529, but it is more expensive. He could also try to locate some old stock of model 524. He feels that both are of equal quality. His number is (442) 560-4560, ext. 110.

   d. The hospital calls at 9:45 AM in regard to Johnny Pothman. Johnny started vomiting bright red blood at 9:40 AM after his T and A surgery. The nurse calling is Mrs. Efficient. She is on ward 5B, extension 5566. The hospital number is 524-2118. They want the physician to call stat.

   e. Review the messages you recorded on the four situations above. Are they concise but thorough? Are all words spelled correctly? Are all telephone numbers and extensions accurate? Are they printed clearly? Did you record the date and time of the message?

   f. The physician is due at the office at 10:00 AM. Look at the messages and determine which one should be seen immediately. Mark this message with a number 1. Now determine which message is second in importance, and label it with a number 2. Mark the remaining messages 3 and 4 in their order of importance. This is how you would arrange them in the physician's office. In this way, the physician would respond to the most important message immediately and not waste time reading many other messages.

Telephone Message

To _____

From _____

Phone _____ Ext. _____

_____ Please call _____ Will call back

Message _____

_____

_____

_____

_____

_____

_____

Date _____ Time _____ In. _____

Telephone Message

To _____

From _____

Phone _____ Ext. _____

_____ Please call _____ Will call back

Message _____

_____

_____

_____

_____

_____

_____

Date _____ Time _____ In. _____

Telephone Message

To _____

From _____

Phone _____ Ext. _____

_____ Please call _____ Will call back

Message _____

_____

_____

_____

_____

_____

_____

Date _____ Time _____ In. _____

Telephone Message

To _____

From _____

Phone _____ Ext. _____

_____ Please call _____ Will call back

Message _____

_____

_____

_____

_____

_____

_____

Date _____ Time _____ In. _____

UNIT 22:2 Evaluation Sheet

Name _____ Date _____

Evaluated by _____

DIRECTIONS: Practice using the telephone according to the criteria listed. When you are ready for your final check, give this sheet to your instructor.

PROFICIENT

Using the Telephone	Points Possible	Peer Check Yes	No	Final Check* Yes	No	Points Earned**	Comments
1. Assembles equipment	3						
2. Answers telephone correctly:							
Answers with a smile	3						
Answers promptly	3						
Identifies agency	3						
Identifies self	3						
3. Determines who is calling	5						
4. Asks caller to spell name or checks name correctly	5						
5. Determines purpose of call	5						
6. Obtains all pertinent information	5						
7. Screens calls correctly	5						
8. Uses the following voice qualities while talking:							
Low pitched	2						
Clear and distinct	2						
Interested	2						
9. Uses correct grammar	5						
10. Holds telephone correctly	5						
11. Ends conversation correctly:							
Thanks caller	3						
Says Good-bye	3						
Allows caller to hang up first	3						
Replaces receiver gently	3						
12. Records all information accurately on message	5						
13. Responds correctly to the following situations:							
Caller refuses to give name	6						
Caller refuses to state purpose of call	6						
Caller wants person who is not available	6						
Caller has emergency and no one else is available	6						
14. Replaces equipment	3						
Totals	100						

* Final Check: Instructor or authorized person evaluates.
** Points Earned: Points possible times each "yes" check.

UNIT 22:3 SCHEDULING APPOINTMENTS

ASSIGNMENT SHEET #1

Grade _____ Name _____

INTRODUCTION: This assignment will provide practice in scheduling appointments. Try to do it as neatly and efficiently as possible.

INSTRUCTIONS: Use the appointment book worksheet or computer software to schedule all of the following appointments. Print all information neatly.

1. In the date columns on your appointment sheet, print Monday and a date on the top of one column. Print Tuesday and the next day's date at the top of the second column.

2. The physician is not in the office until 9:00 AM because he makes hospital rounds early in the morning. Lunch is scheduled from 12 Noon to 1:00 PM.

3. On Tuesday, the physician has a medical board meeting at the hospital from 12:30 until 2:30 PM. He should return to the office by 3:00 PM.

4. Mrs. Nellie Smith (John) calls and wants an appointment for a physical examination on Tuesday afternoon. The physical will take one hour. Telephone number is 589–2008.

5. Mrs. Maddie East (Mike) calls and needs an appointment for an allergy shot early Monday morning. The nurse gives the injection and the patient does *not* have to see the physician. The time required is 15 minutes because the patient is watched for reactions.Telephone number is 756–1824.

6. Mrs. Frieda Shade (Randy) calls and needs an appointment for her triplets. They also need immunization shots. Each child will take about 10 minutes. She prefers an early appointment on Monday afternoon. The names are Ron, Bob, and Bozo. Telephone number is 522–8680.

7. Mrs. Carol Bjore (Chuck) calls and needs an early appointment Monday morning to have a wart removed from her foot. This will take approximately one-half hour. Telephone number is 589–2897.

8. Mrs. Kim Staup (Dave) calls and wants an appointment for 9:45 Tuesday morning. She has a cold. The appointment should require 15 minutes. Telephone number is 522–2321.

9. Mrs. Beth Wilfong (Randy) calls and wants an appointment Tuesday morning for a Pap test. This requires 15 minutes. Telephone number is 522–0689.

10. Ms. Ann Henegar calls and wants an appointment for a physical examination. She prefers early Tuesday morning. This requires one hour. Telephone number is 756–1184.

11. Ms. Melody Jett calls and wants an early morning appointment for Monday. She has laryngitis. This should require about 15 minutes. Telephone number is 524–9293.

12. Mrs. Tami Conery (Scott) calls and wants an appointment Monday morning for surgery on her ingrown toenail. This should require 45 minutes. Telephone number is 797–6116.

13. Ms. Lisa Haumesser calls and wants an appointment for Monday morning. She has an ear infection. This should require 15 minutes. Telephone number is 522–7723.

14. Ms. Sandy Riggenbach calls and wants an 11:00 appointment Tuesday morning for a physical examination. This will take one hour. Telephone number is 797–2418.

15. Ms. Debbie Hillborn (Terry) calls. She needs an appointment for her four children. She prefers Monday at 2:00. They all have colds, and they should require about 10 minutes apiece. Telephone number is 589–0302.

16. Chris Frey calls. She needs to have a growth removed from her right arm. She prefers Monday morning. The surgery will require one hour. Telephone number is 524–8713.

17. Ms. Sue Hockensmith (Ray) calls. She has a skin rash and will require one-half hour for allergy tests. She prefers Tuesday morning. Telephone number is 524–9964.

18. Mr. Duane Yoder calls. He needs a 4:00 appointment for Tuesday. His cough must be checked and a chest X ray must be done. Time required is one-half hour. Telephone number is 589–0020.

19. Diana Fletcher calls. She needs a physical examination. She can come anytime after 3:00 Monday. Time required is one hour. Telephone number is 797–5433.

20. Debbie Koppert calls. She has stomach cramps. Her exam will take one-half hour. She can come anytime after 3:00 Monday. Telephone number is 522–5564.

21. Mr. Jim Johnson needs an appointment for a repeat X ray on his fractured arm. This should take 15 minutes. He can come anytime Monday afternoon. Telephone number is 589–3156.

22. Mr. Robert Hephner calls. He needs an appointment on Monday afternoon for allergy shots. He must be checked by the physician. This should require 15 minutes. Telephone number is 589–8152.

Grade _____ Name _____

APPOINTMENT BOOK WORKSHEET

Day _____ Date _____   Day _____ Date _____

8:00 _____	8:00 _____
8:15 _____	8:15 _____
8:30 _____	8:30 _____
8:45 _____	8:45 _____
9:00 _____	9:00 _____
9:15 _____	9:15 _____
9:30 _____	9:30 _____
9:45 _____	9:45 _____
10:00 _____	10:00 _____
10:15 _____	10:15 _____
10:30 _____	10:30 _____
10:45 _____	10:45 _____
11:00 _____	11:00 _____
11:15 _____	11:15 _____
11:30 _____	11:30 _____
11:45 _____	11:45 _____
12:00 _____	12:00 _____
12:15 _____	12:15 _____
12:30 _____	12:30 _____
12:45 _____	12:45 _____
1:00 _____	1:00 _____
1:15 _____	1:15 _____
1:30 _____	1:30 _____
1:45 _____	1:45 _____
2:00 _____	2:00 _____
2:15 _____	2:15 _____
2:30 _____	2:30 _____
2:45 _____	2:45 _____
3:00 _____	3:00 _____
3:15 _____	3:15 _____
3:30 _____	3:30 _____
3:45 _____	3:45 _____
4:00 _____	4:00 _____
4:15 _____	4:15 _____
4:30 _____	4:30 _____

UNIT 22:3 SCHEDULING APPOINTMENTS

ASSIGNMENT SHEET #2

Grade _____ Name _____

INTRODUCTION: This sheet will provide you with a second chance to practice scheduling appointments. Note the changes or corrections from Scheduling Appointments assignment #1.

INSTRUCTIONS: Use the appointment book worksheet or computer software to schedule all of the following appointments. Make sure all notations are printed clearly and spelled correctly.

1. In the date columns, place Wednesday and a date at the top of the left-hand column. Place Thursday and the next day's date at the top of the right-hand column.

2. The physician is not in the office until 9:00 each morning. Lunch is scheduled from 12 Noon until 1:00 PM.

3. The physician will not be in the office from 1–3 on Wednesday. He has an appointment with his dentist for endodontic care.

4. Sandy Kirk calls and wants an appointment for a physical examination right after lunch on Thursday. This will require one hour. Telephone number is 522–1190.

5. Mrs. Jill Johnson (Mike) calls and wants surgery on the warts on her foot Wednesday morning. This will take about one and one-half hours. Telephone number is 589–7191.

6. Rose Neptune calls and needs a tetanus shot. She prefers an early appointment Thursday morning. This will take 15 minutes. Telephone number is 526–3678.

7. Mrs. Lisa Goldsmith calls. She wants an appointment for her infant. The infant has diarrhea. She prefers Tuesday or Wednesday afternoon. This will require 15 minutes. Telephone number is 524–8750.

8. Mrs. Linda Clow (Mike) needs an appointment for check-ups on her triplets. Each infant should take 10 minutes. She prefers Thursday morning right before lunch. Telephone number is 589–4746.

9. Chris Bell calls because of a burn on her arm. She can come in early Wednesday morning. She requires 15 minutes. Telephone number is 522–1948.

10. Mrs. Jody Albanese (Mike) calls. She has laryngitis. She prefers a Wednesday afternoon appointment. This will require 15 minutes. Telephone number is 589–6151.

11. Mrs. Tara Stimson (Roger) calls and needs an appointment for a Pap test. This should take 15 minutes. She prefers early Thursday morning. Telephone number is 524–3107.

12. Mrs. Cindy Gross (Mike) calls. She needs a physical exam. She prefers Wednesday morning. Time required is one hour. Telephone number is 525–1149.

13. Ms. Kim Cantrell needs an allergy shot. She prefers Thursday afternoon. This requires 15 minutes. Telephone number is 886–2108.

14. Bonnie Secrist calls for an appointment for minor surgery on her nose. She prefers Wednesday afternoon. This will take one-half hour. Telephone number is 589–4265.

15. Ms. Tina Shepher needs an appointment for her injured knee. She prefers Wednesday morning. This requires 15 minutes. Telephone number 886–7022.

16. Miss Cheryl Crupper needs a physical exam. She prefers 10:00 Thursday morning. Time required is one hour. Telephone number is 524–6505.

17. Mr. Ron Dillon needs an appointment due to frequent headaches. He will require 15 minutes and prefers 4:00 Thursday afternoon. Telephone number is 747–4858.

18. Shelley Jones has stomach pain. She needs a late appointment Wednesday afternoon. It requires 15 minutes. Telephone number is 756–6632.

19. Mrs. Janet Pifer (Frederick) wants a physical exam Thursday afternoon. Time required is one hour. Telephone number is 529–5209.

20. Ms. Belinda Nelson needs her monthly blood test. She can come either morning. This takes 15 minutes. Telephone number is 756–8032.

21. Mrs. Erin McKevitt (Ron) needs a VDRL for marriage license. She prefers early Thursday morning and requires 15 minutes. Telephone number is 589–3626.

22. Mrs. Brenda Kelser (Ron) calls for an appointment to check her blood pressure. She prefers late Thursday afternoon. This requires 15 minutes. Telephone number is 589–5289.

23. Cindy Hagedorn needs a physical exam. She just had one so this exam should only take about one-half hour. She prefers Thursday morning. Telephone number is 756–7487.

24. Mari Martin needs a Pap test. She can come Wednesday afternoon or Thursday morning. This requires 15 minutes. Telephone number is 522–5048.

25. Polly Troupe needs an examination for gastritis and blood pressure. She prefers Thursday afternoon. It will require 15 minutes. Telephone number is 886–4885.

26. Cindy Taylor needs surgery on her ingrown toenail. This requires one-half hour. She prefers the afternoon. Telephone number is 747–7501.

27. Mary Wadley calls for an appointment because she has pain in her elbow. She prefers Wednesday afternoon. This should require 15 minutes. Telephone number is 756–6346.

28. Mr. Roger Daugherty calls to get his blood pressure checked. He prefers an afternoon appointment. It will take about 15 minutes. Telephone number is 524–1652.

Grade _____   Name _____

APPOINTMENT BOOK WORKSHEET

Day _____ Date _____   Day _____ Date _____

8:00 _____	8:00 _____
8:15 _____	8:15 _____
8:30 _____	8:30 _____
8:45 _____	8:45 _____
9:00 _____	9:00 _____
9:15 _____	9:15 _____
9:30 _____	9:30 _____
9:45 _____	9:45 _____
10:00 _____	10:00 _____
10:15 _____	10:15 _____
10:30 _____	10:30 _____
10:45 _____	10:45 _____
11:00 _____	11:00 _____
11:15 _____	11:15 _____
11:30 _____	11:30 _____
11:45 _____	11:45 _____
12:00 _____	12:00 _____
12:15 _____	12:15 _____
12:30 _____	12:30 _____
12:45 _____	12:45 _____
1:00 _____	1:00 _____
1:15 _____	1:15 _____
1:30 _____	1:30 _____
1:45 _____	1:45 _____
2:00 _____	2:00 _____
2:15 _____	2:15 _____
2:30 _____	2:30 _____
2:45 _____	2:45 _____
3:00 _____	3:00 _____
3:15 _____	3:15 _____
3:30 _____	3:30 _____
3:45 _____	3:45 _____
4:00 _____	4:00 _____
4:15 _____	4:15 _____
4:30 _____	4:30 _____

563

Name _____ Date _____

Evaluated by _____

DIRECTIONS: Practice scheduling appointments according to the criteria listed. When you are ready for the final check, give this sheet to your instructor.

Scheduling Appointments	Points Possible	Peer Check Yes	No	Final Check* Yes	No	Points Earned**	Comments
1. Uses pencil or computer software and printer to complete all information	10						
2. Lists day and date in correct area	10						
3. Marks times unavailable for appointments with an X through time area	10						
4. Prints all notations for appointments:							
Schedules correct time and preferred day	10						
Prints name correctly	10						
Notes husband's name if patient married	10						
Records purpose for the appointment	10						
Prints telephone number clearly	10						
5. With arrows, marks out correct amount of time for each appointment	10						
6. Prints all information clearly so it is easy to read	10						
Totals	100						

* Final Check: Instructor or authorized person evaluates.
** Points Earned: Points possible times each "yes" check.

ASSIGNMENT SHEET

Grade _____ Name _____

INTRODUCTION: This assignment sheet will help you review basic facts about medical records.

INSTRUCTIONS: Read the information on Completing Medical Records and Forms. In the space provided, print the word(s) that best completes the statement or answers the question.

1. List two (2) standard names for two types of medical records.

2. List five (5) kinds of information that are usually found on any statistical data sheet.

3. Information on medical records is _____

   and should not be released without the _____

   of the patient. The records should be _____ when not in use.

4. Briefly describe facts included under each of the following sections of the medical history.

   a. General Statistical Data:

   b. Family History:

   c. Past History:

   d. Personal History:

   e. Present illness or ailment:

5. Print the meaning of the following symbols or abbreviations commonly found or used on medical records.

   a. S –   e. O –

   b. M –   f. 1 & w –

   c. W –   g. NA –

   d. D –   h. d –

Grade _____   Name _____

PATIENT INFORMATION   DATE:

PATIENT'S NAME	MARITAL STATUS					DATE OF BIRTH	SOCIAL SECURITY NO.	
	S	M	W	DIV	SEP			

STREET ADDRESS ☐ PERMANENT ☐ TEMPORARY	CITY AND STATE	ZIP CODE	HOME PHONE NO.

PATIENT'S EMPLOYER	OCCUPATION (INDICATE IF STUDENT)	HOW LONG EMPLOYED?	BUSINESS PHONE NO.

EMPLOYER'S STREET ADDRESS	CITY AND STATE	ZIP CODE

IN CASE OF EMERGENCY CONTACT:	DRIVERS LIC. NO.

SPOUSE'S NAME

SPOUSE'S EMPLOYER	OCCUPATION (INDICATE IF STUDENT)	HOW LONG EMPLOYED?	BUSINESS PHONE NO.

EMPLOYER'S STREET ADDRESS	CITY AND STATE	ZIP CODE

WHO REFERRED YOU TO THIS PRACTICE?

IF THE PATIENT IS A MINOR OR STUDENT

MOTHER'S NAME	STREET ADDRESS, CITY, STATE AND ZIP CODE	HOME PHONE NO.

MOTHER'S EMPLOYER	OCCUPATION	HOW LONG EMPLOYED?	BUSINESS PHONE NO.

EMPLOYER'S STREET ADDRESS	CITY AND STATE	ZIP CODE

FATHER'S NAME	STREET ADDRESS, CITY, STATE AND ZIP CODE	HOME PHONE NO.

FATHER'S EMPLOYER	OCCUPATION	HOW LONG EMPLOYED?	BUSINESS PHONE NO.

EMPLOYER'S STREET ADDRESS	CITY AND STATE	ZIP CODE

INSURANCE INFORMATION

PERSON RESPONSIBLE FOR PAYMENT, IF NOT ABOVE	STREET ADDRESS, CITY, STATE AND ZIP CODE	HOME PHONE NO.	

☐ COMPANY NAME & ADDRESS	NAME OF POLICYHOLDER	CERTIFICATE NO.	GROUP NO.
☐ COMPANY NAME & ADDRESS	NAME OF POLICYHOLDER	POLICY NO.	
☐ COMPANY NAME & ADDRESS	NAME OF POLICYHOLDER	POLICY NO.	

☐ MEDICARE	MEDICARE NO.	☐ MEDICAID	PROGRAM NO.	COUNTY NO.	ACCOUNT NO.

In order to control our cost of billing, we request that office visits be paid at the time service is rendered. We would rather control our billing costs than be forced to raise our fees.

AUTHORIZATION: I hereby authorize the physician indicated above to furnish information to insurance carriers concerning this illness/accident, and I hereby irrevocably assign to the doctor all payments for medical services rendered. I understand that I am financially responsible for all charges whether or not covered by insurance.

Responsible Party Signature

Grade _____ Name _____

MEDICAL HISTORY FORM

Date _____

Patient's name _____

| Age | Date of birth | Sex |
| Address | City | State | Zip code |

Phone ( )

Insurance company	Policy number
Place of employment	Address
Phone ( )	Job responsibilities

Parent/Guardian if minor

| Address | City | State | Zip code |

Phone ( )

Family History:

List family members: (mother, father, brothers, sisters, grandparents, etc.)—ages and health status (if deceased write their age at the time of their death and the cause). List allergies and/or any conditions or diseases they may have or have had, such as asthma, arthritis, tuberculosis, diabetes, cancer, heart disease, hypertension, kidney disease, mental illness, depression, or any other health problems that you know of in your family.

_____

_____

_____

Patient's Past History: Mark the boxes to the right either "yes" or "no" for the following questions:*

Do you ever have or have you ever had any of the following: **(yes) (no)**

SKIN

| Rashes, hives, itching or other skin irritations | ( ) ( ) |

EYES, EARS, NOSE, THROAT

Headaches, dizziness, fainting	( ) ( )
Blurred or impaired vision	( ) ( )
Hearing loss or ringing in the ears	( ) ( )
Discharge from eyes or ears	( ) ( )
Sinus trouble/colds/allergies	( ) ( )
Asthma or hay fever	( ) ( )
Sore throats/hoarseness	( ) ( )

CARDIOPULMONARY

Shortness of breath	( ) ( )
Persistent cough or coughing up blood or other secretions	( ) ( )
Chills and/or fever	( ) ( )
Night sweats	( ) ( )
Tuberculosis or exposed to TB	( ) ( )

Scarlet fever or rheumatic fever	( ) ( )
Chest pain	( ) ( )
Heart palpitations or rapid heart-beat or pulse	( ) ( )
High blood pressure	( ) ( )
Swelling of hands and/or feet	( ) ( )

GASTROINTESTINAL

Heartburn or indigestion	( ) ( )
Nausea and/or vomiting	( ) ( )
Loss of appetite	( ) ( )
Belching or gas	( ) ( )
Peptic ulcer, gallbladder or liver disease	( ) ( )
Yellow jaundice or hepatitis	( ) ( )
Diarrhea or constipation	( ) ( )
Dysentery	( ) ( )
Rectal bleeding, hemorrhoids (piles)	( ) ( )
Tarry or clay-colored stools	( ) ( )

GLANDS

| Weight gain or loss | ( ) ( ) |

Diabetes	( ) ( )
Thyroid or goiter	( ) ( )
Swollen glands	( ) ( )

GENITOURINARY

Kidney disease or stones, or Bright's disease	( ) ( )
Painful, frequent or urgent urination	( ) ( )
Blood or pus in urine	( ) ( )
Sexually transmitted disease (venereal disease)	( ) ( )
Been sexually active with anyone who has AIDS or HIV or hepatitis	( ) ( )

NEUROMUSCULAR

Problems with becoming tired and/or upset easily	( ) ( )
Nervous breakdown/depression	( ) ( )
Poliomyelitis (infantile paralysis)	( ) ( )
Convulsions	( ) ( )
Joint and/or muscular pain	( ) ( )
Back pain or injury/osteomyelitis/ rheumatism	( ) ( )

| Are you currently taking any medications? | Yes ( ) No ( ) |

If yes, please list them _____

Have you ever had or been treated for cancer or any tumors?	( ) ( )
Are you anemic or have you ever had to take iron medication?	( ) ( )
Do you use tobacco?	( ) ( )

What type? _____

| Do you use IV drugs or alcohol? | ( ) ( ) |

WOMEN ONLY

Painful menstrual periods	( ) ( )
Pregnancy/abortion/miscarriage	( ) ( )
Vaginal infection or discharge/ abnormal bleeding	( ) ( )

Last menstrual period _____

Birth control _____

List dates of all operations/surgeries, injuries, and illnesses that required hospitalization:

_____

_____

Did you ever receive benefits from a medical insurance claim due to illness or injury?	Yes ( ) No ( )
Were you ever rejected from the military or for employment?	( ) ( )
Were you ever absent from school/work in the past 10 years because of illness or injury?	( ) ( )
Did you ever file a Workers' Compensation claim?	( ) ( )
Did you ever seek psychological or psychiatric treatment?	( ) ( )

*Please use the back of this form to explain any "yes" answers. Thank you.

UNIT 22:4 Evaluation Sheet

Name _____ Date _____

Evaluated by _____

DIRECTIONS: Practice completing medical records and forms according to the criteria listed. When you are ready for your final check, give this sheet to your instructor.

Completing Medical Records and Forms	Points Possible	Peer Check Yes	No	Final Check* Yes	No	Points Earned**	Comments
1. Assembles equipment	3						
2. Questions patient in a private area	5						
3. Completes statistical data sheet as follows:							
Asks questions politely	4						
Speaks clearly and distinctly	4						
Rechecks and repeats numbers for accuracy	4						
Types, keys, or prints all information neatly and legibly	4						
Completes all parts of the sheet with accurate information	6						
Uses correct abbreviations	4						
Avoids blanks—uses "none" or "NA"	4						
Draws red line through error, initials, and inserts correct information	4						
4. Completes medical history record:							
Asks questions clearly	4						
Obtains all pertinent information	4						
Allows patient time to think about answers	4						
Repeats questions or explains points to be sure patient understands questions	4						
Asks the correct questions to complete each of the following sections accurately:							
Statistical data	3						
Family history	3						
Past history	3						
Personal history	3						
Present ailment	3						
Types, keys, or prints all information neatly and legibly	4						
Uses correct abbreviations	4						
Avoids blanks—prints a zero, none, or "NA"	4						
Draws red line through error, initials, and inserts correct information	4						
Rechecks form at end to be sure all information is complete and accurate	4						
Notes any additional pertinent information the patient relates	4						
5. Replaces all equipment	3						
Totals	100						

* Final Check: Instructor or authorized person evaluates.
** Points Earned: Points possible times each "yes" check.

UNIT 22:5 COMPOSING BUSINESS LETTERS

ASSIGNMENT SHEET

Grade _____ Name _____

INTRODUCTION: A professional business letter will create a positive impression. This sheet will help you review the main facts about business letters.

INSTRUCTIONS: Read the information on Composing Business Letters. In the space provided, print the word(s) that best completes the statement or answers the question.

1. Briefly list the main reason why each of the following types of letters are written.

   a. collection:

   b. appointment:

   c. recall:

   d. consultation:

   e. inquiry:

2. Identify the following parts of a letter.

   a. section that includes the address of the person sending the letter and the date:

   b. section with name and address of the person to whom the letter is being sent:

   c. phrase such as "Dear Mr. Brown:":

   d. phrase such as "Sincerely,":

   e. section containing message:

   f. initials of person preparing the letter:

3. Most letters should include at least three paragraphs. Briefly list what should be included in each of the sections.

   a. paragraph 1:

   b. paragraph 2:

   c. paragraph 3:

4. How does a modified block style letter differ from a block style letter?

5. At the end of a letter reference initials can be given for one or two persons. Who are they?

6. List the correct abbreviations for each of the following states:

   a. Ohio: c. Alaska: e. Washington: g. Missouri:

   b. Utah: d. Idaho: f. Indiana: h. Virginia:

UNIT 22:5 Evaluation Sheet

Name _____ Date _____

Evaluated by _____

DIRECTIONS: Practice composing business letters according to the criteria listed. When you are ready for your final check, give this sheet to your instructor.

PROFICIENT

Composing Business Letters	Points Possible	Peer Check Yes	No	Final Check* Yes	No	Points Earned**	Comments
Note: Use either modified block (noted as MB) or block style (noted as B)							
1. Inserts heading as follows:							
Spaces down approximatelty 15 lines from top of paper	2						
Starts at center line (MB) or left margin line (B)	2						
Keys number and name of street in full	2						
Keys city, state, zip code	2						
Keys month, day, year	2						
Note: If letterhead paper is used, keys full date two lines under letterhead, starting at center (MB) or left margin line (B) (10 points if correct)							
2. Inserts inside address:							
Spaces 4 lines under heading or letterhead date	2						
Starts at left margin line	2						
Keys name and/or title	2						
Keys number and street name in full	2						
Keys city, state, zip code	2						
3. Inserts salutation:							
Spaces 1 line under end of inside address	2						
Starts at left margin line	2						
Keys name correctly	2						
Keys colon after name	2						
4. Composes body:							
Keys each paragraph with single spacing	2						
Leaves double space between paragraphs	2						
Starts all information on left margin line	2						
States reason for writing in first paragraph	3						
States main facts in second paragraph	3						
Signs off in third paragraph	3						
5. Inserts complimentary close:							
Spaces 1 line under last line in body	2						
Uses capital letter for first word only	2						
Punctuates with comma at end of closing	2						
Starts at center line (MB) or left margin line (B)	2						

Name _____

Composing Business Letters	Points Possible	Peer Check		Final Check*		Points Earned**	Comments
		Yes	No	Yes	No		
6. Inserts signature:							
Spaces 3 lines for written signature	2						
Keys name correctly	2						
Keys title correctly	2						
Starts on center line (MB) or left margin line (B)	2						
7. Inserts reference initials:							
Spaces 1 line under printed name/title	2						
Keys initials correctly	2						
Uses slash for small letters or colon for capital letters to separate 2 sets of initials	2						
Starts on left margin line	2						
8. Sets margins evenly maintaining correct width	4						
9. Includes all required information in letter	8						
10. Uses complete sentences and correct punctuation	8						
11. Spells all words correctly	8						
12. Prepares neat, clear, legible letter	5						
Totals	100						

* Final Check: Instructor or authorized person evaluates.
** Points Earned: Points possible times each "yes" check.

UNIT 22:6 COMPLETING INSURANCE FORMS

ASSIGNMENT SHEET

Grade _____ Name _____

INTRODUCTION: This assignment will help you review the main facts regarding insurance forms.

INSTRUCTIONS: Read the information on Completing Insurance Forms. In the space provided, print the word(s) that best completes the statement or answers the question.

1. Where is information regarding a patient's insurance coverage usually recorded?

2. Why is it wise to check with a patient periodically regarding his/her insurance coverage?

3. Before you accept insurance forms from a patient, there are some points you should check. List two (2) of these points.

4. What is an *Authorization to Release Benefits* form? Why is it used?

5. What term is used to describe the person to whom the insurance contract has been issued?

6. What is a HCFA-1500 form?

7. What is the name of the book containing ICD-9-CM codes?

8. Define *diagnosis.*

9. If a patient has three (3) different diagnoses, how should they be listed on the insurance form?

10. Explain what each of the following digits of an ICD-9-CM code represents:

    a. first three digits:

    b. fourth digit:

    c. fifth digit:

11. What word would you look up in the *International Classification of Diseases and Operations* for a diagnosis of "inflammation of the right bronchus?"

12. What is the name of the book containing CPT codes?

13. How many digits are present in a CPT code?

14. Why are modifiers used for a CPT code?

    How are modifiers separated from a CPT code?

15. Policy numbers or contract numbers frequently include a/an _____ or series of _____, which must be included on the form in the correct area. If a question does not apply to a particular patient, put _____ or a/an _____ in the space. Answer _____ questions on the form.

16. What is a NPI? Where is it inserted on an insurance form?

U N I T 2 2 : 6 E v a l u a t i o n S h e e t

Name _____ Date _____

Evaluated by _____

DIRECTIONS: Practice completing insurance forms according to the criteria listed. When you are ready for your final check, give this sheet to your instructor.

Completing Insurance Forms	Points Possible	Peer Check Yes	Peer Check No	Final Check* Yes	Final Check* No	Points Earned**	Comments
1. Inserts all of the following patient information accurately on the form:							
Full name and address	5						
Company name and address	5						
Contract numbers	5						
Dates requested	5						
2. Inserts all of the following supplier information accurately on the form:							
Full name and address	5						
Dates requested	5						
Diagnosis and services	5						
Charges for services	5						
3. Checks to be sure all of the following signatures are complete on the form:							
Patient	5						
Insured	5						
Physician/supplier	5						
4. Uses correct codes on the form for place of service, diagnosis, and treatment	15						
5. Answers all questions on the form or marks blank areas with a dash or *NA*	10						
6. Prepares form so it is aligned, neat, accurate, and properly corrected if necessary	10						
7. Uses correct spelling and punctuation on all parts of the form	10						
Totals	100						

(Column group header above table: **PROFICIENT**)

* Final Check: Instructor or authorized person evaluates.
** Points Earned: Points possible times each "yes" check.

ASSIGNMENT SHEET #1

Grade _____ Name _____

INTRODUCTION: This assignment will help you review the main facts about the pegboard bookkeeping system.

INSTRUCTIONS: Read the information on Maintaining a Bookkeeping System. In the space provided, print the word(s) that best completes the statement or answers the question.

1. Briefly list the main purpose of each of the following records in the bookkeeping system:

   a. day sheet or daily journal:

   b. statement-receipt record:

   c. charge slip:

   d. ledger card:

2. What advantage is there to using the three layer version of the statement-receipt record in regard to insurance claims?

3. How can the ledger card serve as a monthly statement or bill for the patient?

4. A current balance is determined by adding the previous _____ and _____ and then subtracting the _____ made.

5. Why is it important to use a ballpoint pen and pressure while recording information on the pegboard system?

6. What should you do if you make an error while recording information in a pegboard bookkeeping system?

7. What is meant by the letters *ROA?*

8. Identify four (4) types of information in the database of a computerized bookkeeping system.

9. Why is it important to make daily tape or disk backups of a computerized bookkeeping system?

10. A patient has a previous balance owed of $50.00. The office visit today has a charge of $25.00. The patient pays $30.00 by check. What is the current balance?

UNIT 22:7 MAINTAINING A BOOKKEEPING SYSTEM

ASSIGNMENT SHEET #2

Grade _____ Name _____

INTRODUCTION: Keeping accurate records in an office is essential. This assignment will help you practice the pegboard system.

INSTRUCTIONS: Read the information and procedure sheets on Maintaining a Bookkeeping System. Then complete a series of records using the following information provided.

1. Take out two ledger cards. On the first card write *Smith, John, 1 South Main Street, America, U.S.A.* On the second card write *Mendez, Mike, 2 South Fifth Street, America, U.S.A.* Place *00. 00* in the top current balance space of each.

2. Place a day sheet on the pegboard. Place a series of statement receipt blanks over the daysheet. Make sure they are lined up correctly.

3. Record the following visits. Use correct ledger cards for each patient. Follow the instructions on the procedure sheet for the correct methods of recording. Check all addition and subtraction for accuracy. Complete a deposit slip at the same time by making sure your paper is folded under on the daysheet or positioned correctly.

   A. On 5/1/— Joan Smith, wife of John Smith, visits the office. She has an examination and a prophylaxis treatment. The exam charge is $25, and the prophy charge is $15. She pays $30 in cash. Her next appointment is 5/30/—.

   B. Mike Mendez visits the office on 5/1/—. He has a root canal treatment. The charge is $60.00. He pays $40 by check. His next appointment is 5/23/—.

   C. Mary Smith, the daughter of John Smith, visits the office on 5/1/—. She has an amalgam restoration for a charge of $25.00. She does not pay. Her next appointment is 6/15/—.

   D. Jane Mendez visits the office on 5/1/—. She is Mike's wife. She has a composite restoration for a charge of $20.00. She pays $15 by check. Her next appointment is 6/3/—.

   E. Joe Smith, John's son, visits the office on 5/1/—. He has an extraction, and the charge is $45. He pays $20 in cash. His next appointment is 5/16/—.

   F. John Smith visits the office on 5/1/—. He receives his partial denture. The charge is $200.00. He pays $10 by check. His next appointment is 9/15/—.

   G. Quick-Pay Insurance Company sends in a payment of $200 by check for John Smith. Record this payment.

4. Total all amounts columns and check these by using the "proof of posting" box on the daysheet. Also total the bank deposit slip.

UNIT 22:7 MAINTAINING A BOOKKEEPING SYSTEM

ASSIGNMENT SHEET #3

Grade _____ Name _____

INTRODUCTION: This assignment will give you a second chance to record on a pegboard system. Note errors or corrections from assignment #2.

INSTRUCTIONS: Use the same day sheet and ledger cards you used on the previous assignment. Follow the procedure sheet to record the information.

1. Line up all sheets correctly on the pegboard. Make sure that the current balance on both ledger cards is correct.

2. The Mendez family visits the office on 5/2/—. The following family members are seen by the physician:

   Jane Mendez: Examination and prophylactic treatment. Cost is $52. She does not pay. Next appointment 5/15/—.

   Mike Mendez: Amalgam restoration and anesthetic. Charge for the anesthetic is $25 and for the amalgam is $30. He pays $31 in cash. Next appointment 6/28/—.

   Nellie Mendez: Composite restoration for $20. She pays $10 by check. Next appointment 10/4/—.

3. The Smith family also visits the office on 5/2/—. The following family members are treated.

   Joe Smith: Complete denture fitted for a cost of $650. He pays $100 by check. No appointment scheduled.

   Mary Smith: Endodontic treatment for a cost of $68. She pays $20 in cash. Next appointment is 7/8/—.

   Brad Smith: Examination and prophylactic treatment. Exam costs $25 and prophy treatment costs $20. He pays $32 in cash.

4. Square Deal Dental Insurance sends a check to the office for Joe Smith. The check is for $440.00.

5. Total all amount columns on the day sheet. Check your totals by using the proof of posting area. Correct any errors noted. Also, total the bank deposit slip.

UNIT 22:7 Evaluation Sheet

Name _____ Date _____

Evaluated by _____

DIRECTIONS: Practice maintaining a bookkeeping system according to the criteria listed. When you are ready for your final check, give this sheet to your instructor.

Maintaining a Bookkeeping System	Points Possible	Peer Check Yes	Peer Check No	Final Check* Yes	Final Check* No	Points Earned**	Comments
1. Records all of the following information on ledger cards correctly:							
Patients' names/addresses	4						
Descriptions of services	4						
Payments, charges, and current balances	10						
2. Records all of the following information on the statement-receipt forms:							
Patients' names and dates	4						
Descriptions of services	4						
Charges, payments made, and current balances	10						
Next appointment date/time	5						
3. Records all of the following information on the day sheet:							
Date and names of patients	4						
Descriptions of services	4						
Correct previous balances from current balances on ledger cards	10						
Charges, payments made or received, current balances	10						
Receipt numbers from statement-receipt forms	5						
Figures in cash column	5						
Figures in check column	5						
Final totals for deposit slip	6						
Final figures in proof of posting boxes	10						
Totals	100						

PROFICIENT

* Final Check: Instructor or authorized person evaluates.
** Points Earned: Points possible times each "yes" check.

UNIT 22:8 WRITING CHECKS, DEPOSIT SLIPS, AND RECEIPTS

ASSIGNMENT SHEET #1

Grade _____ Name _____

INTRODUCTION: The assignment below will help you review the main facts about checks, deposit slips, and receipts.

INSTRUCTIONS: Read the information about Writing Checks, Deposit Slips, and Receipts. In the space provided, print the word(s) that best completes the statement or answers the question.

1. Checks and receipts help provide a record of _____ that occur.

2. A written order for the payment of money through a bank is a/an _____.

   A record of money or goods received is a/an _____.

3. Define the following words.

   a. payee:

   b. originator or maker:

   c. endorsement:

4. Why must all checks and receipts be written in ink or printed on a computer printer?

5. List four (4) things you should observe on a check you receive from a patient.

6. Why are most checks received in an agency stamped "For deposit only to the account of . . ."?

7. When should a check be endorsed by a person who wants to cash the check?

8. If a patient makes a payment, a/an _____ can be given to the patient as _____ of payment. All information must be _____ and _____ and written in _____ to prevent alteration.

9. Why should cash or checks be deposited in the bank as soon as possible?

10. Two patients make payments in cash with the exact amount of money. One pays $48.32 and one pays $35.80. The amount of currency recorded for deposit is _____, and the amount of coin deposited is _____.

UNIT 22:8 WRITING CHECKS, DEPOSIT SLIPS, AND RECEIPTS

ASSIGNMENT SHEET #2

Grade _____ Name _____

INTRODUCTION: The following assignment will let you practice the correct way of writing checks, deposit slips, and receipts.

INSTRUCTIONS: Follow the directions in each step to complete the financial records. Use the sample checks, deposit slips, and receipts provided.

1. The checking account has a current balance of $19,102.39. Record this balance on the first "balance" line of the first check stub.

2. The physician buys pharmaceutical supplies from Ace Drug Co. on May 1, —. The total cost of the drugs is $802.36. Write check stub and check #1 for this amount.

3. On May 2, — the physician buys stationery for the office from Physician's Stationery Supply Company. The total amount is $506.28. Write check stub and check #2 for this amount.

4. On May 3, —, the following payments are received. Write receipts for the following.

   a. Mrs. James Johnson pays $1,500.90 by check for her surgery.

   b. Mr. Jerry Casper pays $1,250.70 in cash for an x-ray machine he purchases from the physician.

   c. Mrs. Kenneth Meyers pays $450.10 for the medical bill from her hospitalization. She pays by check.

5. Make out a deposit slip for the payments received in #4. Deposit this amount in the checking account. Note the deposit on the next check stub.

6. On May 3, — the office rent is due. Make out check #3 to Business Rentals, Incorporated for $1,225.00.

7. On May 4, —, the electric bill is due. Write check #4 to the Tri-County Electric Company for $278.85.

8. Write the following receipt for May 5, —.

   Mrs. Kathy Wrenner pays $150.00 by check for a physical examination.

9. Make out a deposit slip for the amount in #8. Deposit this amount in the checking account. Complete the check stub.

10. On May 6, —, write a check to Bowman Medical Supplies for medical supplies purchased. The amount for check # 5 is $908.10.

11. On May 7, —, write check #6 to Cardio-Supply Company for ECG paper and electro pads. The amount due is $604.86.

SAMPLE CHECKS

No. ____ $ _____
Date _____ 20__
To _____
For _____

Balance		
Am't Dep.		
Total		
Am't Ck.		
Balance		

Happy Doctor, MD
1 Healthy Lane
Fitness, OH 11133

Pay to the
Order of: _____ $____

_____ Dollars

First Money Bank
1 Rich Lane
Wealthy, OH 11133
00098-5567
Memo _____

No. _____

_____ 20 __

By _____

No. ____ $ _____
Date _____ 20__
To _____
For _____

Balance		
Am't Dep.		
Total		
Am't Ck.		
Balance		

Happy Doctor, MD
1 Healthy Lane
Fitness, OH 11133

Pay to the
Order of: _____ $____

_____ Dollars

First Money Bank
1 Rich Lane
Wealthy, OH 11133
00098-5567
Memo _____

No. _____

_____ 20 __

By _____

No. ____ $ _____
Date _____ 20__
To _____
For _____

Balance		
Am't Dep.		
Total		
Am't Ck.		
Balance		

Happy Doctor, MD
1 Healthy Lane
Fitness, OH 11133

Pay to the
Order of: _____ $____

_____ Dollars

First Money Bank
1 Rich Lane
Wealthy, OH 11133
00098-5567
Memo _____

No. _____

_____ 20 __

By _____

SAMPLE CHECKS

No. _____ $ _____
Date _____ 20__
To _____
For _____

Balance		
Am't Dep.		
Total		
Am't Ck.		
Balance		

Happy Doctor, MD
1 Healthy Lane
Fitness, OH 11133

Pay to the
Order of: _____

_____ Dollars

First Money Bank
1 Rich Lane
Wealthy, OH 11133
00098-5567
Memo _____

No. _____

_____ 20 ___

_____ $____

By _____

No. _____ $ _____
Date _____ 20__
To _____
For _____

Balance		
Am't Dep.		
Total		
Am't Ck.		
Balance		

Happy Doctor, MD
1 Healthy Lane
Fitness, OH 11133

Pay to the
Order of: _____

_____ Dollars

First Money Bank
1 Rich Lane
Wealthy, OH 11133
00098-5567
Memo _____

No. _____

_____ 20____

_____ $____

By _____

No. _____ $ _____
Date _____ 20__
To _____
For _____

Balance		
Am't Dep.		
Total		
Am't Ck.		
Balance		

Happy Doctor, MD
1 Healthy Lane
Fitness, OH 11133

Pay to the
Order of: _____

_____ Dollars

First Money Bank
1 Rich Lane
Wealthy, OH 11133
00098-5567
Memo _____

No. _____

_____ 20 ___

_____ $____

By _____

SAMPLE DEPOSIT SLIPS

Happy Doctor, MD
1 Healthy Lane
Fitness, OH 11133

Date _____ 20 _____
Signature _____
(If cash received)

	Currency		
	Coin		
	Checks _____		
	_____		
	_____		
	TOTAL		
	Less Cash		
	TOTAL DEPOSIT		

First Money Bank
1 Rich Lane
Wealthy, OH 11133
0098-5567

Happy Doctor, MD
1 Healthy Lane
Fitness, OH 11133

Date _____ 20 _____
Signature _____
(If cash received)

	Currency		
	Coin		
	Checks _____		
	_____		
	_____		
	TOTAL		
	Less Cash		
	TOTAL DEPOSIT		

First Money Bank
1 Rich Lane
Wealthy, OH 11133
0098-5567

SAMPLE RECEIPTS

No. _____   No. _____   Date _____ 20 ___
Date _____   Received From _____
To _____   _____ Dollars
For _____   For _____
Amount· _____ $ _____   _____

No. _____   No. _____   Date _____ 20 ___
Date _____   Received From _____
To _____   _____ Dollars
For _____   For _____
Amount _____ $ _____   _____

No. _____   No. _____   Date _____ 20 ___
Date _____   Received From _____
To _____   _____ Dollars
For _____   For _____
Amount _____ $ _____   _____

No. _____   No. _____   Date _____ 20 ___
Date _____   Received From _____
To _____   _____ Dollars
For _____   For _____
Amount _____ $ _____   _____

UNIT 22:8 WRITING CHECKS, DEPOSIT SLIPS, AND RECEIPTS

ASSIGNMENT SHEET #3

Grade _____ Name _____

INTRODUCTION: Note any changes on assignment #2. Then use this assignment sheet to provide additional practice in writing checks, deposit slips, and receipts.

INSTRUCTIONS: Follow these directions to complete the sample checks, deposit slips, and receipts.

1. The checking account has a current balance of $10,089.78. Note this on the next check stub to be used.

2. On May 1, —, the physician buys an x-ray machine from Dr. Jones. Make out check #1 for $6,220.00 to Jeremy Jones, MD.

3. On May 1, —, make out check #2 to United Telephone Company for $223.92. This is for the telephone bill.

4. On May 3, —, the physician buys drugs from Medico Drug Company for $1,102.30. Write check #3 for this amount.

5. On May 3, —, the following payments are received. Write receipts to the following people:

   a. Mrs. Estelle McCall pays $1,206.55 by check for her surgery.

   b. Mrs. Floyd Stark pays $120.00 cash for a physical examination.

   c. Mr. Duane Yoder pays $225.00 by check for suturing the lacerations on his hand.

   d. Mr. Jim Johnson pays $820.50 by check for treatment of a fractured jaw.

6. Make out a bank deposit slip for the above payments in #5. Deposit this amount in the checking account. Note the new amount on the next check stub.

7. On May 5, —, the office rent is due. Make out check #4 to Business Rentals for $1,200.75.

8. Write check #5 to Maria Sardina for $52.91. This is a refund for overpayment on her account. It is May 6, —.

9. On May 7, —, write check #6 to Global Insurance Company for liability insurance for the month. Amount due is $929.70.

No. _____ $ _____
Date _____ 20__
To _____
For _____

Balance		
Am't Dep.		
Total		
Am't Ck.		
Balance		

Happy Doctor, MD
1 Healthy Lane
Fitness, OH 11133

Pay to the
Order of: _____ $____

_____ Dollars

First Money Bank
1 Rich Lane
Wealthy, OH 11133
00098-5567
Memo _____

No. _____

_____ 20 __

By _____

No. _____ $ _____
Date _____ 20__
To _____
For _____

Balance		
Am't Dep.		
Total		
Am't Ck.		
Balance		

Happy Doctor, MD
1 Healthy Lane
Fitness, OH 11133

Pay to the
Order of: _____ $____

_____ Dollars

First Money Bank
1 Rich Lane
Wealthy, OH 11133
00098-5567
Memo _____

No. _____

_____ 20 __

By _____

No. _____ $ _____
Date _____ 20__
To _____
For _____

Balance		
Am't Dep.		
Total		
Am't Ck.		
Balance		

Happy Doctor, MD
1 Healthy Lane
Fitness, OH 11133

Pay to the
Order of: _____ $____

_____ Dollars

First Money Bank
1 Rich Lane
Wealthy, OH 11133
00098-5567
Memo _____

No. _____

_____ 20 __

By _____

SAMPLE CHECKS

No. _____ $ _____
Date _____ 20__
To _____
For _____

Balance		
Am't Dep.		
Total		
Am't Ck.		
Balance		

Happy Doctor, MD
1 Healthy Lane
Fitness, OH 11133

No. _____

_____ 20 __

Pay to the
Order of: _____ $____

_____ Dollars

First Money Bank
1 Rich Lane
Wealthy, OH 11133
00098-5567   By _____
Memo _____

No. _____ $ _____
Date _____ 20__
To _____
For _____

Balance		
Am't Dep.		
Total		
Am't Ck.		
Balance		

Happy Doctor, MD
1 Healthy Lane
Fitness, OH 11133

No. _____

_____ 20 __

Pay to the
Order of: _____ $____

_____ Dollars

First Money Bank
1 Rich Lane
Wealthy, OH 11133
00098-5567   By _____
Memo _____

No. _____ $ _____
Date _____ 20__
To _____
For _____

Balance		
Am't Dep.		
Total		
Am't Ck.		
Balance		

Happy Doctor, MD
1 Healthy Lane
Fitness, OH 11133

No. _____

_____ 20 __

Pay to the
Order of: _____ $____

_____ Dollars

First Money Bank
1 Rich Lane
Wealthy, OH 11133
00098-5567   By _____
Memo _____

SAMPLE DEPOSIT SLIPS

Happy Doctor, MD
1 Healthy Lane
Fitness, OH 11133

Date _____ 20 _____
Signature _____
            (If cash received)

First Money Bank
1 Rich Lane
Wealthy, OH 11133
0098-5567

Currency		
Coin		
Checks _____		
_____		
TOTAL		
Less Cash		
TOTAL DEPOSIT		

Happy Doctor, MD
1 Healthy Lane
Fitness, OH 11133

Date _____ 20 _____
Signature _____
            (If cash received)

First Money Bank
1 Rich Lane
Wealthy, OH 11133
0098-5567

Currency		
Coin		
Checks _____		
_____		
TOTAL		
Less Cash		
TOTAL DEPOSIT		

SAMPLE RECEIPTS

No. _____	No. _____	Date _____ 20 ___
Date _____	Received From _____	
To _____	_____ Dollars	
For _____	For _____	
Amount· _____	$ _____ _____	

No. _____	No. _____	Date _____ 20 ___
Date _____	Received From _____	
To _____	_____ Dollars	
For _____	For _____	
Amount _____	$ _____ _____	

No. _____	No. _____	Date _____ 20 ___
Date _____	Received From _____	
To _____	_____ Dollars	
For _____	For _____	
Amount _____	$ _____ _____	

No. _____	No. _____	Date _____ 20 ___
Date _____	Received From _____	
To _____	_____ Dollars	
For _____	For _____	
Amount _____	$ _____ _____	

UNIT 22:8A Evaluation Sheet

Name _____   Date _____

Evaluated by _____

DIRECTIONS: Practice writing checks according to the criteria listed. When you are ready for your final check, give this sheet to your instructor.

PROFICIENT

Writing Checks	Points Possible	Peer Check		Final Check*		Points Earned**	Comments
		Yes	No	Yes	No		
1. Uses ink at all times	6						
2. Completes the stubs first with the following points:							
Inserts correct number	4						
Fills in amount in numbers by $ sign close to sign and writes cents as fractions	5						
Writes month, day, year in "Date" area	4						
Writes full name in "To" area	4						
Writes brief purpose for writing check in "For" area	4						
Inserts current balance	5						
Inserts any deposits made	5						
Totals current balance and any deposit noted	5						
Inserts correct amount of check written	5						
Subtracts correctly to obtain final balance	6						
3. Writes checks correctly as follows:							
Inserts correct number	4						
Writes month, day, year in "Date" area	4						
Writes full name of payee at left of line	6						
Prints amount in numbers at $ sign close to sign with cents as fractions	6						
Writes words for amount on dollar line, starting at left of line with cents as fractions and no blanks	6						
Writes purpose on "Memo" line	4						
Leaves "By" line blank to obtain authorized signature	5						
4. Completes all checks and obtains a correct final balance in the account	6						
5. Writes neatly and legibly and forms numbers clearly	6						
Totals	100						

* Final Check: Instructor or authorized person evaluates.
** Points Earned: Points possible times each "yes" check.

Name _____ Date _____

Evaluated by _____

DIRECTIONS: Practice writing deposit slips according to the criteria listed. When you are ready for your final check, give this sheet to your instructor.

PROFICIENT

Writing Deposit Slips	Points Possible	Peer Check Yes	No	Final Check* Yes	No	Points Earned**	Comments
1. Uses ink at all times	8						
2. Writes month, day, year in "Date" area	8						
3. Inserts correct amount of currency with "00" in cents column	10						
4. Inserts correct total for coins with dollar amounts to left and cents amount to right of line	10						
5. Lists all checks separately in spaces provided	10						
6. Adds all numbers together to obtain correct total	10						
7. Leaves "Less Cash" blank unless receiving cash	8						
8. Subtracts "Less Cash" amount if any present to obtain correct final total deposit, or moves above total down if no cash retained	10						
9. Leaves "Signature" area blank unless cash received and then obtains authorized signature	8						
10. Adds total of deposit to stub on next check in checking account correctly	10						
11. Writes neatly and legibly and forms numbers clearly	8						
Totals	100						

* Final Check: Instructor or authorized person evaluates.
** Points Earned: Points possible times each "yes" check.

UNIT 22:8C Evaluation Sheet

Name _____ Date _____

Evaluated by _____

DIRECTIONS: Practice writing receipts according to the criteria listed. When you are ready for your final check, give this sheet to your instructor.

Writing Receipts	Points Possible	Peer Check Yes	No	Final Check* Yes	No	Points Earned**	Comments
		PROFICIENT					
1. Uses ink at all times	8						
2. Completes stubs first with the following points:							
Inserts correct number	6						
Writes month, day, year in "Date" area	6						
Writes full name of person to whom receipt issued in "To" area	6						
Writes brief reason why receipt issued in "For" area	6						
Prints amount in numbers with cents as fractions	6						
Notes if receipt for cash or check	6						
3. Writes receipts correctly observing following:							
Fills in correct number	6						
Writes month, day, year in "Date" area	6						
Writes full name of person or company receipt for on "Received From" line starting at left of line	6						
Writes amount in words on dollars line starting at left with cents as fractions and no blanks	8						
Writes brief reason for receipt on "For" space	6						
Inserts amount in numbers on "$" area with numbers close to sign and cents as fractions	8						
Signs own name as signature	8						
4. Writes neatly and legibly and forms numbers clearly	8						
Totals	100						

* Final Check: Instructor or authorized person evaluates.
** Points Earned: Points possible times each "yes" check.

INDEX

593

Trendelenberg position, 372, 376
Trimming models, 302
Tub bath, 448
Turning patients, 408, 412-413
Tympanic temperature, 165
Typing blood, 349-350

Ultrasonic, 138-140
Universal Numbering System, 262-265, 266-267
Universal precautions. *See* Standard precautions
Urinal, 468, 471-472
Urinary
   catheter care, 473-475
   drainage unit, 473, 476-477
   sediments, 363-364
   system, 67-68
Urine
   specimens, 481-486
   tests, 356-364
Urinometer, 361-362

Varnish, dental, 309, 310
Vision screening, 377-378
Vital signs, 155-187

Walker, 526, 533-534
Wallet card, 242
Warm water bag, 538-539
Washing hands, 124-125
Weight and height, 365-371
Wheelchair, 416-417
White blood cells, counting, 338-341, 344-345
Word parts, 27-32
Wounds, 201-204
Wrapping autoclave, 132-133
Wright's stain, 346, 348

X rays, dental, 317-319

Zinc oxide eugenol, 309, 313